HUMAN NUTRITION

	DATE DUE	
25 ... 2001		
2 1 FEB 2002		
0 9 APR 2002		
0 3 JUL 2002		
1 0 APR 2003		

Executive Editor: Richard A. Weimer
Production Editor and Designer: Michael Rogers
Art Director: Don Sellers, AMI
Illustrator: Joe Vitek

HUMAN NUTRITION:
A Self-Instructional Text
Sandy J. Wickham, MA, RD

Robert J. Brady Co. • Bowie, Maryland 20715
A PRENTICE-HALL PUBLISHING AND COMMUNICATIONS COMPANY

Library of Congress Cataloging in Publication Data

Wickham, Sandy J., 1944-
  Human nutrition.

  Bibliography: p.
  Includes index.
  1. Nutrition—Programmed instruction.   2. Diet in disease—Programmed instruction.   I. Title.
QP141.W463   641.1'07'7   81-10248
ISBN 0-87619-857-4   AACR2

Prentice-Hall International, Inc., London
Prentice-Hall of Australia, Pty., Ltd., Sydney
Prentice-Hall of India Private Limited, New Delhi
Prentice-Hall of Japan, Inc., Tokyo
Prentice-Hall of Southeast Asia Pte. Ltd., Singapore
Whitehall Books, Limited, Petone, New Zealand

Printed in the United States of America

82 83 84 85 86 87 88 89 90 91 92   10 9 8 7 6 5 4 3 2 1

CONTENTS

To all my teachers who made a difference:
some extraordinary persons,
some revered books,
in the hopes that this text will be a
useful teaching tool

TO THE READER

One of the major objectives of this text is to get the reader *involved* with nutrition. The rudiments of nutrition must be learned in order to understand the why's and how's of body mechanisms which make use of food to accomplish the various chemical and physical activities of the body. The results of various nutrition studies have demonstrated repeatedly that greater familiarity with different foods, varied food experiences, and *use* of sound nutrition principles promote behavioral change and favor development of beneficial food habits. *Understanding* specific nutrition terminology and nutritional processes within the body improves the ability to differentiate between accurate and inaccurate nutrition information. The sheer wealth of nutrition and diet information presented in popular communication media underlines the importance of sound nutrition education and the need for each person to become an able discriminator between nutritional fallacy and fact.

Nutrition is perhaps best described as a multi-faceted science developed from an accumulation of interrelated scientific data of chemical, physical, biological, cultural, and anthropological origin. The nutrition information presented in this text is representative of data obtained from legitimate research conducted by researchers professionally recognized within their respective fields of study. The sources cited within the text, tables, and charts, are those to whom credit should be given for original research, original statements or ideas, or specific location of presented information. As an introductory level text this book does not purport to present information obtained from original research of the author but rather previously established nutrition fact. The originality of this text lies in its self-instructional method of material presentation. The teaching aids and self-instructional techniques used in this text are intended to facilitate the learning of basic nutrition facts and principles as well as to personalize the learning experience.

A Key Points outline is given at the end of each topic section which presents definitions of nomenclature important and appropriate to each section, an outline of text material, and/or selective major points of emphasis. The Key Points provide a condensation of content in each section and perform as a tool for learning through summary and repetition.

Following the Key Points outline is a series of questions designed to reinforce and clarify text content. Answers to the questions are provided. Emphasis is placed upon defining terminology important to the study of nutrition. Some questions strive to facilitate learning through repetition or to emphasize an important point. Other questions are intended to stimulate deductive reasoning. Various situation episodes are presented in order to develop the reader's ability to appropriately apply sound nutrition principles in the selection of foods and composition of diets which meet individual nutritional needs. No question is intended to "trick"; all the questions are intended to "teach."

In some cases, additional nutrition information is given within the questions. Some questions are organized in such a way as to lead the reader to a correct conclusion in a discovery approach. In most cases, a variety of question formats is used in each section in order to avoid repetition of style and boredom of exercise.

Processes involved in the digestion, absorption, and metabolism of protein, carbo-hydrate, and fat are described in the chapters appropriate to each of those macronutrients. The chapter on digestion, absorption and metabolism (Chapter Six) is designed specifically as a reference section and outline, especially by visual representation, of organs involved, interrelated functions, and location of major events. Definitions of important terms are stressed and these terms are alphabetized in appropriate sections for ease of reference.

Diet-related health conditions of current popular interest and significant incidence such as atherosclerosis, hypertension, and tooth decay are addressed. Even data obtained from studies concerning these subject areas which is yet inconclusive and often contradictory is presented and examined.

Questions are given which require the reader to refer to supplemental information contained within footnotes, tables, charts, figures, and food labels in order to develop the reader's appreciation and use of such valuable information resources. Extra care was taken to choose footnote references specifically appropriate in content and reading level for beginning nutrition students. For the more advanced or inquisitive student, primary and more technical references can be found within the references cited.

For the student not yet familiar with the metric system, an appendix section on metrics, including a practice unit, is provided for reference. Nutrients and food portions given in the food composition tables and other reference sources are usually stated in metric terms which have little meaning for the student who cannot "visualize" metric units. A somewhat detailed presentation of kidney anatomy and function is given in an appendix section to facilitate understanding of that organ's functions, especially control of water and acid-base balance. The 1980 RDAs express vitamin A recommendations only in retinol equivalents. Vitamin A recommendations formerly were stated in terms of International Units. The vitamin A content of food is still expressed in International Units in most food composition tables. In view of the rather complicated nature of computing retinol equivalents, the conversion information for determining retinol equivalents from various standards is given in detail in another appendix section. Dietary goals for Americans, though controversial in content and priorities, exemplify attempts by politicians and nutritionists to formulate a national nutritional policy and are discussed often enough in popular literature to warrant presentation in yet another appendix section.

Classroom instruction and other nutrition reference texts are expected to supplement the information within this text. Conduction of a personal diet study is highly recommended for practicum in analyzing and improving individual diet selection and consumption.

Above all, the recurrent theme expressed in this text is the need to eat a variety of foods selected from as well as within all food groups. For the healthy individual, appropriate food selections can be made even though choices are limited by individual food preferences, socio-cultural-religious diet restrictions and energy requirements. Developing an ability to make wise personal food choices in light of current scientific knowledge from the wide selection of foods available is a goal of nutrition education. Though the scope of this text is limited to presentation of the fundamentals of nutrition, it is hoped that the information and learning techniques employed in this text will aid attainment of sound nutrition knowledge which in turn will increase the reader's awareness of his or her place as a consumer of food from a limited world-wide market place. Additionally, it is hoped that such awareness will inspire in the reader a desire to obtain maximum benefit from available food resources.

SJW

ACKNOWLEDGMENTS

I would like to express my gratitude to Dr. Elveda Smith and Dr. Rose Tseng for their original suggestions instrumental to the development of a "different" teaching technique for certain aspects of nutrition as my Master's Thesis Project. The research I conducted for that first project included a review of programmed instructional materials. I became convinced of the value of self-instructional programmed materials but felt that they had greater merit when combined with techniques that required the physical involvement of the learner. The expansion of those thoughts and that first project has finally resulted in this self-instructional workbook-text.

I am also grateful to my friend and teacher, Betty Clamp, for her cheerful acceptance to review this manuscript when her own time is filled with nutrition education as well as personal activities.

To my daughters, Paige and Nikki, I wish to express my loving thanks for allowing me the time to devote to this favorite project. And, lastly, I wish to express my appreciation to my husband, Roger, for not only overlooking the many hours I spent on this project but for his support and assistance that made it all possible.

HUMAN NUTRITION

1
FUNDAMENTALS OF NUTRITION

Every specialized field of study has a language of its own. Comprehending a study's "language" enables the novice to learn facts and form generalizations—the bones in the skeletal framework upon which larger concepts are built. How could there be lively debates or fruitful discussions leading to the understanding and sharing of ideas without the use of a language composed of terms with commonly accepted meanings? Therefore, a primary objective of this introductory level workbook is presentation and explanation of appropriate, correct, and professionally accepted nutrition-related terminology. The learning of nutrition terms is stressed in each chapter, and exercises are given to reinforce learning.

Let us begin with a frankly basic concept: What is food? Food is that material of plant or animal origin which nourishes and sustains the human body and enables the body to grow. Food is influenced by various cultural factors and fulfills individual psychological and social needs as well as physiological needs. Specific materials which are accepted as food by one society may not be accepted as food by another. *for optimal health*

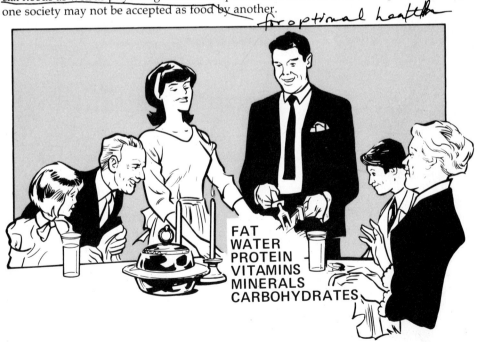

Figure 1-1. *Food is potentially nourishing. A simple but important concept is that food must be consumed to fulfill its potential.*

Food is composed of nutrients. The various functions of these nutrients are to supply energy, to promote growth and repair, and to regulate body processes. Individual nutrients may perform all or only some of these functions. In addition, food may contain other substances which cannot be classified as nutrients.

Nutrients in food. The six classes of nutrients in food are carbohydrate, fat, protein, vitamins, minerals, and water. First, nutrients are ingested in the form of food. Nutrients are then broken down during the process of digestion. Then they are absorbed, metabolized, and reassembled into the same or frequently different compounds. Often they are even excreted.

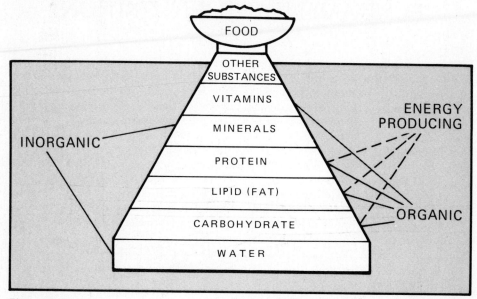

Figure 1-2.

Three of the nutrients are termed energy nutrients: carbohydrate, protein, and fat. These nutrients are oxidized in the body to produce heat and energy.[1] This energy is used to make new body compounds and to produce movement.

Four of the nutrients are organic nutrients: carbohydrate, fat, protein, and vitamins. *Organic compounds contain the element carbon.* Organic nutrients can be altered or destroyed by chemical and physical agents, such as acid and heat. When organic materials are oxidized heat and/or other forms of energy and the by-products carbon dioxide and water are produced.

Vitamins are relatively small molecular organic compounds which are needed in very small quantities in the diet. They perform specific metabolic functions vital to life. Vitamins assist in the biochemical[2] reactions necessary in the digestion, absorption, and metabolism[3] of the energy nutrients. Though vitamins are not direct sources of energy, they are necessary for the production of energy from carbohydrates, fats, and proteins.

Although carbohydrate, protein, fat, and vitamins are complex compounds, minerals are not. Minerals are simple inorganic chemical elements. The ash that remains when a food is completely burned (oxidized) in the presence of air is composed of minerals.

When an individual first approaches the study of nutrition he or she may overlook water as a nutrient needed in the human diet. However, death will occur sooner from a lack of this nutrient than from the lack of any other nutrient. Water, another inorganic compound, is the medium in which body chemical reactions occur and is the transporter of necessary materials to the cells and metabolic wastes from the cells.[4] Water is a participant in some body chemical reactions, a component of various body secretions such as hormones and saliva, and a requisite in the maintenance of constant body temperature. There are several body mechanisms for regulating water intake and excretion so maintenance of a controlled body water balance is possible.

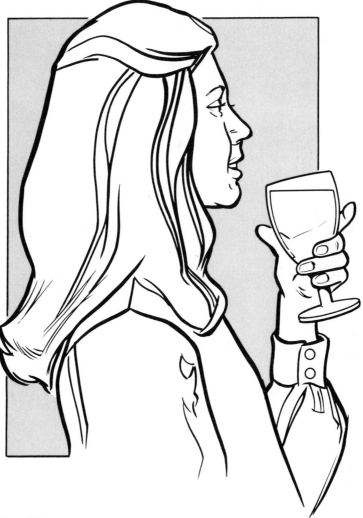

Figure 1-3.

Definitions of terms. Because food habits are influenced by non-nutritional factors, such as a person's culture as well as social and psychological needs, a discussion of food and/or nutrition will elicit emotional responses from most people. Nutritional terms with a chemical or clinical background have clearly defined scientific meanings. However, many terms used by nutritionists or lay persons referring to nutrition have more nebulous meanings which are often individually interpreted on an emotional level. A meaningful discussion of nutrition must contain words and terms which convey the same meaning to all readers and listeners; they should be clear, specific, and with an accepted definition.

Todhunter has set forth the following definitions in an effort to clarify nutritional terms[5]:

Nutrition is the process by which the human body (or other living organism) utilizes food for the maintenance of life, for growth, for the normal functioning of every organ and tissue, and for the production of energy . . . Nutrition is a subject matter field; it is the science in which one studies the chemical reactions involved in the nutritional processes within the body in response to foods of varying kinds and amounts and under different conditions of age, health, and disease.

Malnutrition is . . . a state in which a prolonged lack of one or more nutrients retards physical development or causes the appearance of specific clinical conditions such as anemia, goiter, and rickets.

Undernutrition is . . . the state of the body arising from an inadequate intake of food and thus a caloric deficiency resulting in reduced body weight.

Overnutrition is a poorly conceived term that is misleading and confusing to the public and which should be replaced by a term more correctly describing the condition. There are several terms from which to choose: "overconsumption," "overeating," "excessive caloric intake," or by naming the nutrient in excess which could be harmful such as "excessive fat intake" (or sugar, or vitamin A, or vitamin D).

Some other terms requiring clarification are:

Nutritious which refers to those foods which nourish or contribute to body requirements for sustaining life and providing for growth and energy, i.e. contain nutrients. A more specific definition would require the density of nutrients in a particular food to be significant when compared to the energy or caloric value of the food.[6]

Organic is frequently defined by food faddists as foods grown without the addition of chemical fertilizers or insecticide sprays. *However, the only scientifically accepted definition of organic is a compound containing carbon.*

Empty calories is a term representative of foods which contain a high amount of calories but a small or even negligible amount of nutrients.

Dietary fiber refers to the combined, undigested carbohydrates in food and encompasses the cellulose and lignin found in crude fiber as well as hemicellulose, pectic substances, gums, and other carbohydrates which are not normally digested by man.[7]

Junk food is a term with no specific, accepted meaning and is generally used according to the bias of the speaker or writer.

Health food is another term for which there is no scientifically accepted definition. *There is no single food or food group which has the ability to impart special health benefits to the consumer.*

Essential nutrient is one that is necessary for proper functioning of the body but cannot be made within the body or cannot be manufactured in amounts necessary. Consequently, essential refers specifically to those nutrients which must be supplied from the diet.

Key Points: Fundamentals of Nutrition

I. Food nourishes and sustains the human body and enables the body to grow.
   A. Food is influenced by cultural factors.
   B. Food fulfills psychological/social/physiological needs.
II. Nutrients supply energy, promote growth and repair, and regulate the various body processes.
   A. The six classes of nutrients are: carbohydrate, fat, protein, vitamins, minerals, and water.
   B. The energy nutrients are carbohydrate, protein, and fat.
   C. The organic nutrients contain the element carbon in their chemical structure: carbohydrate, fat, protein, and vitamins.
   D. Vitamins are organic compounds needed in small amounts to assist the biochemical reactions necessary to life.

E. Minerals are simple, inorganic chemical elements.

III. Many nutritional terms do not have scientifically established meanings.

Questions: Fundamentals of Nutrition

1. In order for the human body to be nourished and sustained as well as to grow, _____ is needed with regularity and in adequate amounts.

2. The components in food which supply energy, promote growth and repair, and regulate body processes are termed _____ .

3. How many classes of nutrients are there?
    a. 3
    b. 4
    c. 6

4. There are substances in food other than nutrients which are ingested and even retained in the body when food is eaten.
    a. True
    b. False

5. Oxidation of food in the body produces _____and/or _____ with the by-product formation of _____ and _____ .

6. Match the appropriate lettered descriptive term (or terms) to the six nutrients.
    _____ 1. carbohydrate   a. inorganic
    _____ 2. water   b. organic
    _____ 3. protein   c. energy nutrient
    _____ 4. minerals
    _____ 5. vitamins
    _____ 6. fat

7. Match the phrase on the right to the term on the left which most correctly identifies the term.
    _____ 1. organic   a. organic compounds assisting chemical
    _____ 2. vitamins   reactions
    _____ 3. minerals   b. nourishes, sustains, and enables the
    _____ 4. energy nutrients   body to grow
    _____ 5. water   c. any compound containing carbon
    _____ 6. food   d. transporter of necessary nutrients to
                                       and from cells
                                   e. simple chemical elements
                                   f. carbohydrate, protein, and fat

8. This term refers to all the changes that occur to nutrients from the time they are ingested and utilized until they are excreted: _____ .

9. The prefix "bio" means:
    a. metabolism
    b. complex
    c. life

10. Approximately what percentage of the human body by weight is composed of minerals?
    a. 2
    b. 4
    c. 10

11. Identify the following parts of a cell:

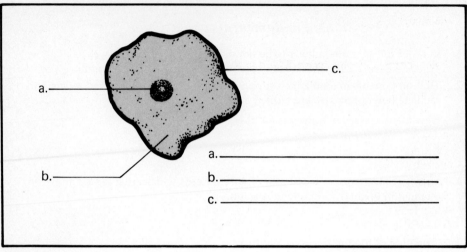

a.

c.

b.

a. _____

b. _____

c. _____

Figure 1-4.

12. Members of the African Masai tribe consume the blood of cattle and goats as part of their diet. The Eskimos eat the visible animal fat (blubber) of animals. Though influenced by different cultural factors and consisting of different items, the diet of these two peoples include blood and blubber respectively as _____.

13. There is no individual food which imparts special health properties to the consumer.
    a. True
    b. False

14. Why is the term "health food" misleading?

15. Why is "overnutrition" an unfavorable term?

16. Why may an overweight person still be malnourished?

17. Match the phrases on the right to the terms on the left which each phrase best describes:

    _____ 1. fiber
    _____ 2. overnutrition
    _____ 3. nutrition
    _____ 4. nutritious
    _____ 5. junk food
    _____ 6. empty calories
    _____ 7. undernutrition
    _____ 8. malnutrition
    _____ 9. organic

    a. the process of food utilization
    b. a more specific phrase for this word would be "excessive caloric intake"
    c. a descriptive term for a food with a high nutrient density
    d. descriptive term for a food high in calories but negligible in nutrients
    e. compounds containing carbon
    f. a state of retarded development due to a lack of one or more nutrients
    g. undesirable reduced body weight due to inadequate caloric intake
    h. undigestible carbohydrates in food
    i. a term which simply expresses a food bias of the user

Answers: Fundamentals of Nutrition

1. food
2. nutrients
3. c
4. a
5. heat; energy; carbon dioxide (CO_2); water (H_2O)
6. 1. b, c
   2. a
   3. b, c
   4. a
   5. b
   6. b, c
7. 1. c
   2. a
   3. e
   4. f
   5. d
   6. b
8. metabolism
9. c
10. b
11. a. nucleus
    b. cytoplasm
    c. cell membrane
12. food
13. a
14. Because it implies that a certain food imparts special health benefits.
15. It is too vague. The best terms are those which are specific.
16. Excessive caloric intake does not insure adequate intake of all nutrients.
17. 1. h
    2. b
    3. a
    4. c
    5. i
    6. d
    7. g
    8. f
    9. e

REFERENCES

[1] Oxidation is the chemical reaction in which a substance combines with oxygen, a removal of hydrogen occurs, or there is an increase in the positive valence. In the body, the energy nutrients are oxidized in the various body tissues by the oxygen transported there by the blood.

[2] Biochemical refers to the chemistry of living processes (bio=life).

[3] Metabolism is the sum of all the chemical processes within a living cell. It includes those changes that occur to the nutrients from their absorption, utilization for energy or body structures, to their excretion.

[4] A cell is a small structural unit of living substance consisting of three basic components: cell membrane, cytoplasm, and a nucleus. Some of the many other important parts of a cell are:

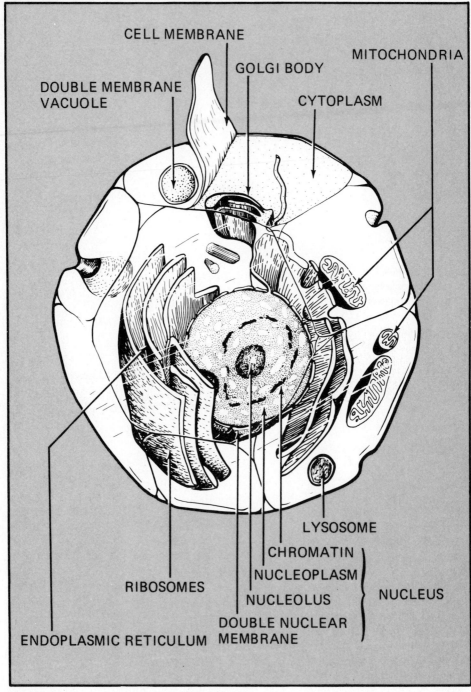

Figure 1-5. *Some major components of a human cell.*

mitochondria—round or rod-shaped structures where the chemical reactions of energy-producing oxidation take place.

lysosomes—small bodies containing digestive enzymes.

endoplasmic reticulum—a tubular system of channels.

Golgi complex—a body where concentrated enzymes are stored and secreted.

ribosomes—an area associated with the endoplasmic reticulum where protein synthesis takes place.

[5] Todhunter EN: The words we use and misuse in nutrition. Food and Nutrition News, 48, March-April 1977, pages 1 and 4. Reprinted with permission.

[6] A good review of the various attempts toward defining a nutritious food is by Guthrie HA: Concept of a nutritious food. Journal of the American Dietetic Association, 71, July 1977

[7] Leveille GA: Dietary fiber. Food and Nutrition News, 47, February 1976, p. 1. Reprinted with permission.

2

FOOD GUIDES USEFUL FOR MAKING APPROPRIATE FOOD SELECTIONS

This text stresses in each chapter the importance of eating a variety of foods chosen from many different types of food. The Recommended Dietary Allowances and the U.S. Recommended Dietary Allowances are guides for daily nutrient allowances associated with the maintenance of healthy individuals. These RDAs are useful tools for evaluating the adequacy of diets. However, their use requires working numerical computations and researching sources for the detailed nutrient composition of foods. The RDAs and U.S. RDAs also emphasize consumption of nutrients, rather than the consumption of food. It is unlikely that the average consumer would be motivated to use the RDAs and U.S. RDAs to evaluate diets planned except as a spot checking device.

The consumer is more likely to think in terms of foods, not nutrients, when planning menus. Several food plans which guide the consumer in making appropriate food selections for daily diets are the Basic Four Food Groups, the Modified Basic Four, the INQ system, and the Food Exchange System. Use of any of these food guides is helpful in meal planning if the one of your choice is used to plan diets which supply adequate nutrients, and a variety of foods which suit your personal food preferences.

The RDAs—What Are They?

The RDAs are the Recommended Dietary Allowances established by the Food and Nutrition Board of the National Academy of Sciences-National Research Council (NAS-NRC) for many nutrients *consumed* by the American population.[1] These nutrients are protein, three fat-soluble vitamins, seven water-soluble vitamins, and six minerals. A recommendation is also made for calories according to mean heights and weights for children, adults doing light work, and older adults with reduced basal metabolic rates and activity energy requirements. The calorie recommendations as well as accepted deviation ranges are based upon professionally recognized height/weight tables, median energy intakes of children, and established methods of computing decreased energy needs of older persons. It is necessary to read the explanatory text included with the Mean Heights and Weights and Recommended Energy Intake for clarification of methods of establishing caloric recommendations.

The revised 1980 RDA publication consists of the RDA table, Mean Heights and Weights and Recommended Energy Intake table, Estimated Safe and Adequate Daily Dietary Intakes of Additional Selected Vitamins and Minerals table, and an explanatory text. The RDA table is divided into groups for infants, children, males, females, and pregnant and lactating females. The male and female sections are subdivided into five age groups as well.

The following statement is taken directly from the text of the 1980 publication:[2]

Recommended Dietary Allowances are the levels of intake of essential nutrients considered, in the judgment of the committee on Dietary Allowances of the Food and Nutrition Board on the basis of available scientific knowledge, to be adequate to meet the known nutritional needs of practically all healthy persons.

Since the body of scientific knowledge is constantly being enlarged and refined, the RDAs are periodically revised. The last revision was published in 1980 and is given in this chapter. The Board recognizes that not all nutrients necessary for humans have a requirement established, and that some necessary nutrients may as yet be undiscovered. *Consequently, the Board urges food choices to be selected from many different common foods.*

The allowances recommended for the various nutrients take into consideration the variation that occurs in physiological need between individual healthy persons. Except for calories all the allowances are set higher than average need. In the case of protein, the average amount of protein intake by healthy persons was determined. In accordance with a bell-shaped curve on a graph showing normal distribution this average represented the point at which half of the American population would consume enough protein and half would not. Therefore, in order to prevent a deficit intake recommendation the allowance was set statistically at a point where over 95 percent of the population would have at least an adequate intake.

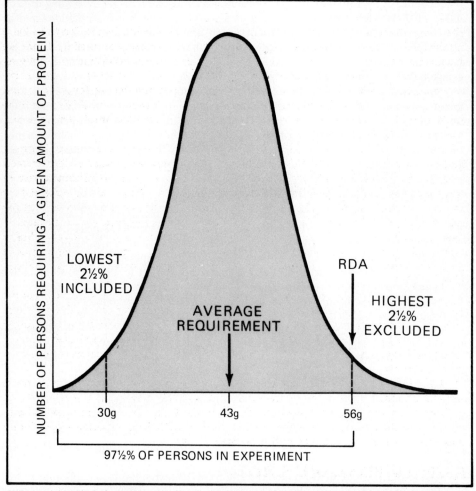

Figure 2-1.   Protein requirements of a large population. From McNutt KW and McNutt DR: Nutrition and Food Choices. Science Research Associates,   1978. Reproduced by permission.

The protein allowance also took into account the fact that different food sources of protein have significantly different protein quality values. Those of the highest value are generally from animal protein sources such as meat, poultry, fish, and milk. Those of lesser quality are generally of plant sources such as grains and legumes (peas, beans, and lentils). The RDA for protein is based upon a mixed diet which contains about 75 percent high quality protein. Protein need is computed on a gram protein per kilogram of body weight basis with a .8g/kg factor used for adult men and women.

Because of the relatively generous allowances made for individual variations it is generally accepted that consumption of ⅔ or more of the RDA is adequate for most healthy persons. A diet that supplies less than ⅔ of the allowances for one or more nutrients would seem probable to become nutritionally inadequate over an extended period of time.[3] In other words, the further below the RDA the individual intake is for any nutrient over an extended period of time, the greater the likelihood of developing a deficiency for that nutrient.

In order to better understand the RDAs, and attempt to avoid their misuse and misinterpretation, it is useful to divide descriptive statements about them into two categories: *What they are* and *what they are not* (See Table 2-1.)

The U.S. RDAs

The U.S. RDA's are different from the RDA's and are established by the Food and Drug Administration (FDA). They are used as a standard for nutritional labeling. There are actually four different sets of U.S. RDAs in order to meet nutrition labeling needs: one set for infants 12 months of age and under used with baby foods; one set for youngsters between the ages of one and four years used for "junior" foods; another set for pregnant and lactating women who have special nutrient needs; and one for adults and children over the age of four.[4] It is the latter set, based on the 1968 tables of the Food and Nutrition Board, which is used the majority of the time.

Although the 1974 Revised and 1980 Revised RDA tables had some changes in values for certain nutrients from the 1968 table, the U.S. RDA reference standards were retained based on the 1968 RDA. This decision was made in order to speed up implementation of nutrition labeling. The U.S. RDA nutrient values were generally chosen from the highest amounts recommended for each in the 1968 RDA table. Consequently, almost all of the values represent those set for adult men who seem to have the greatest nutrient requirements of the general population.[5] The one notable exception to this rule is the value chosen for iron. Women have a greater need for iron intake than men, especially those women in the child-bearing years. Therefore, the adult female requirement was chosen as the U.S. RDA.

The U.S. RDA for protein has two values given for each set. You will notice that the protein quality is measured according to the reference standard of casein, the protein of milk. If a protein source has a protein efficiency ratio (PER)[6] equal to or better than casein the smaller figure is used. If a protein source has a protein efficiency ratio less than that of casein the larger figure is used. This method of dividing protein allowances better serves nutrition labeling needs.

The FDA elected to set recommended amounts for biotin, pantothenic acid, copper, and zinc although these nutrients were not included in the 1968 RDA. The FDA felt that setting amounts for the nutrients would allow manufacturers to list them in nutrition labeling if they wished to do so.[7] As with the RDAs, the U.S. RDAs were expected to have future revisions utilizing new scientific nutrition data.

Key Points: RDAs and U.S. RDAs

I.   The RDAs and U.S. RDAs emphasize nutrient consumption rather than food consumption, and are useful in a variety of situations, including the setting up of intake guidelines and evaluating nutrient intake for *populations* of healthy individuals.

II.   The RDAs are set high enough to cover individual variations in nutrient needs between most healthy individuals.

III. The energy allowances of the RDAs represent *average* energy requirements.

IV.   The U.S. RDAs were established by the FDA and based on the 1968 RDAs in order to best meet nutrition labeling needs.

V.   The U.S. RDAs are broader in scope in nutrient intake recommendations for various population groups than are the RDAs.

Table 2-1.   What the RDAs are and are not.

RDAs are:	RDAs are *not*:
1. Intake guidelines for a population group.	1. Intended for application to specific individuals.
2. Set high enough to allow for individual differences. (However, the energy allotments represent average energy requirements.)	2. *Minimum* requirements.
3. Estimates of nutrients *consumed*.	3. Estimates of the nutrient content of foods.
4. Intended for healthy persons.	4. Intended for persons with illness, disease, or conditions requiring special nutritional considerations.
5. The nutrients for which there is a currently known human requirement.	5. Necessarily the only nutrients required in the diet of healthy persons.
6. Recommended to be obtained from a variety of common foods.	6. Recommended to be obtained largely or solely from synthetic foods.

Table 2-2. Recommended Dietary Allowances, Revised 1980.* Designed for the maintenance of good nutrition of practically all healthy people in the U.S.A. Food and Nutrition Board, National Academy of Sciences, National Research Council.

age and sex group	weight		height		protein	fat-soluble vitamins			water-soluble vitamins							minerals					
	kg.	lb.	cm.	in.	gm	vitamin A μg. R.E.†	vitamin D μg.‡	vitamin E mg.α T.E.#	vitamin C	thiamin mg	riboflavin	niacin mg N.E.¶	vitamin B₆ mg	folacin μg	vitamin B₁₂	calcium	phosphorus	magnesium mg	iron	zinc	iodine μg
infants																					
0.0-0.5 yr	6	13	60	24	kg×2.2	420	10	3	35	0.3	0.4	6	0.3	30	0.5**	360	240	50	10	3	40
0.5-1.0 yr	9	20	71	28	kg×2.0	400	10	4	35	0.5	0.6	8	0.6	45	1.5	540	360	70	15	5	50
children																					
1-3 yr	13	29	90	35	23	400	10	5	45	0.7	0.8	9	0.9	100	2.0	800	800	150	15	10	70
4-6 yr	20	44	112	44	30	500	10	6	45	0.9	1.0	11	1.3	200	2.5	800	800	200	10	10	90
7-10 yr	28	62	132	52	34	700	10	7	45	1.2	1.4	16	1.6	300	3.0	800	800	250	10	10	120
males																					
11-14 yr	45	99	157	62	45	1,000	10	8	50	1.4	1.6	18	1.8	400	3.0	1,200	1,200	350	18	15	150
15-18 yr.	66	145	176	69	56	1,000	10	10	60	1.4	1.7	18	2.0	400	3.0	1,200	1,200	400	18	15	150
19-22 yr	70	154	177	70	56	1,000	7.5	10	60	1.5	1.7	19	2.2	400	3.0	800	800	350	10	15	150
23-50 yr	70	154	178	70	56	1,000	5	10	60	1.4	1.6	18	2.2	400	3.0	800	800	350	10	15	150
51+ yr	70	154	178	70	56	1,000	5	10	60	1.2	1.4	16	2.2	400	3.0	800	800	350	10	15	150
females																					
11-14 yr	46	101	157	62	46	800	10	8	50	1.1	1.3	15	1.8	400	3.0	1,200	1,200	300	18	15	150
15-18 yr.	55	120	163	64	46	800	10	8	60	1.1	1.3	14	2.0	400	3.0	1,200	1,200	300	18	15	150
19-22 yr	55	120	163	64	44	800	7.5	8	60	1.1	1.3	14	2.0	400	3.0	800	800	300	18	15	150
23-50 yr.	55	120	163	64	44	800	5	8	60	1.0	1.2	13	2.0	400	3.0	800	800	300	18	15	150
51+ yr	55	120	163	64	44	800	5	8	60	1.0	1.2	13	2.0	400	3.0	800	800	300	10	15	150
pregnancy					+30	+200	+5	+2	+20	+0.4	+0.3	+2	+0.6	+400	+1.0	+400	+400	+150	††	+5	+25
lactation					+20	+400	+5	+3	+40	+0.5	+0.5	+5	+0.5	+100	+1.0	+400	+400	+150	††	+10	+50

*The allowances are intended to provide for individual variations among most normal persons as they live in the United States under usual environmental stresses. Diets should be based on a variety of common foods in order to provide other nutrients for which human requirements have been less well defined. See text for detailed discussion of allowances and of nutrients not tabulated. See preceding table for weights and heights by individual year of age and for suggested average energy intakes.

†Retinol equivalents; 1 retinol equivalent = 1μg. retinol or 6μg. β-carotene. See text for calculation of vitamin activity of diets as retinol equivalents.

‡As cholecalciferol: 10 μg. cholecalciferol = 400 I.U. vitamin D.

\#∝ocopherol equivalents: 1 mg d∝ tocopherol = 1∝T.E. See text for variation in allowances and calculation of vitamin E activity of the diet as ∝ tocopherol equivalents.

¶1 N.E. (niacin equivalent) = 1 mg niacin or 60 mg dietary tryptophan.

||The folacin allowances refer to dietary sources as determined by *Lactobacillus casei* assay after treatment with enzymes ("conjugases") to make polyglutamyl forms of the vitamin available to the test organism.

**The RDA for vitamin B$_{12}$ in infants is based on average concentration of the vitamin in human milk. The allowances after weaning are based on energy intake (as recommended by the American Academy of Pediatrics) and consideration of other factors, such as intestinal absorption; see text.

††The increased requirement during pregnancy cannot be met by the iron content of habitual American diets or by the existing iron stores of many women; therefore, the use of 30 to 60 mg supplemental iron is recommended. Iron needs during lactation are not substantially different from those of non-pregnant women, but coninued supplementation of the mother for two to three months after parturition is advisable in order to replenish stores depleted by pregnancy.

(*From:* Recommended Dietary Allowances, Ninth Revised Edition, 1980. With permission of the National Academy of Sciences, Washington, DC)

Table 2-3. Estimated safe and adequate daily dietary intakes of additional selected vitamins and minerals.*

age group	vitamins				trace elements†						electrolytes		
	vitamin K	biotin	pantothenic acid	copper	manganese	fluoride	chromium	selenium	molybdenum		sodium	potassium	chloride
	µg →							mg →					
infants													
0.0–0.5 yr	12	35	2	0.5–0.7	0.5–0.7	0.1–0.5	0.01–0.04	0.01–0.04	0.03–0.06		115–350	350–925	275–700
0.5–1.0 yr	10–20	50	3	0.7–1.0	0.7–1.0	0.2–1.0	0.02–0.06	0.02–0.06	0.04–0.08		250–750	425–1,275	400–1,200
children and adolescents													
1–3 yr	15–30	65	3	1.0–1.5	1.0–1.5	0.5–1.5	0.02–0.08	0.02–0.08	0.05–0.1		325–975	550–1,650	500–1,500
4–6 yr	20–40	85	3–4	1.5–2.0	1.5–2.0	1.0–2.5	0.03–0.12	0.03–0.12	0.06–0.15		450–1,350	775–2,325	700–2,100
7–10 yr	30–60	120	4–5	2.0–2.5	2.0–3.0	1.5–2.5	0.05–0.2	0.05–0.2	0.1–0.3		600–1,800	1,000–3,000	925–2,775
11 + yr	50–100	100–200	4–7	2.0–3.0	2.5–5.0	1.5–2.5	0.05–0.2	0.05–0.2	0.15–0.5		900–2,700	1,525–4,575	1,400–4,200
adults	70–140	100–200	4–7	2.0–3.0	2.5–5.0	1.5–4.0	0.05–0.2	0.05–0.2	0.15–0.5		1,100–3,300	1,875–5,625	1,700–5,100

*From Recommended Dietary Allowances, Revised 1980. Food and Nutrition Board, National Academy of Sciences—National Research Council. Because there is less information on which to base allowances, these figures are not given in the main table of the RDAs and are provided here in the form of ranges of recommended intakes.

†Since the toxic levels for many trace elements may be only several times usual intakes, the upper levels for the trace elements given in this table should not be habitually exceeded.

(*From:* Recommended Dietary Allowances, Ninth Revised Edition, 1980. With the permission of the National Academy of Sciences, Washington, DC)

Table 2-4.   Mean heights and weights and recommended energy intake.*

age and sex group	weight		height		energy		
	kg	lb	cm	in	needs		range in kcal
					MJ	kcal	
infants							
0.0-0.5 yr	6	13	60	24	kg × 0.48	kg × 115	95-145
0.5-1.0 yr	9	20	71	28	kg × 0.44	kg × 105	80-135
children							
1-3 yr	13	29	90	35	5.5	1,300	900-1,800
4-6 yr	20	44	112	44	7.1	1,700	1,300-2,300
7-10 yr	28	62	132	52	10.1	2,400	1,650-3,300
males							
11-14 yr	45	99	157	62	11.3	2,700	2,000-3,700
15-18 yr	66	145	176	69	11.8	2,800	2,100-3,900
19-22 yr	70	154	177	70	12.2	2,900	2,500-3,300
23-50 yr	70	154	178	70	11.3	2,700	2,300-3,100
51-75 yr	70	154	178	70	10.1	2,400	2,000-2,800
76+ yr	70	154	178	70	8.6	2,050	1,650-2,450
females							
11-14 yr	46	101	157	62	9.2	2,200	1,500-3,000
15-18 yr	55	120	163	64	8.8	2,100	1,200-3,000
19-22 yr	55	120	163	64	8.8	2,100	1,700-2,500
23-50 yr	55	120	163	64	8.4	2,000	1,600-2,400
51-75 yr	55	120	163	64	7.6	1,800	1,400-2,200
76+ yr	55	120	163	64	6.7	1,600	1,200-2,000
pregnancy						+300	
lactation						+500	

*From Recommended Dietary Allowances, Revised 1980, Food and Nutrition Board, National Academy of Sciences—National Research Council, Washington, D.C. The data in this table have been assembled from the observed median heights and weights of children, together with desirable weights for adults for mean heights of men (70 in.) and women (64 in.) between the ages of eighteen and thirty-four as surveyed in the U.S. population (DHEW/NCHS data).

Energy allowances for the young adults are for men and women doing light work. The allowances for the two older age groups represent mean energy needs over these age spans, allowing for a 2 percent decrease in basal (resting) metabolic rate per decade and a reduction in activity of 200 kcal per day for men and women between fifty-one and seventy-five years; 500 kcal for men over seventy-five years; and 400 kcal for women over seventy-five (see text). The customary range of daily energy output is shown for adults in the range column and is based on a variation in energy needs of ± 400 kcal at any one age (see text and Garrow, 1978), emphasizing the wide range of energy intakes appropriate for any group of people.

Energy allowances for children through age eighteen are based on median energy intakes of children of these ages followed in longitudinal growth studies. Ranges are the 10th and 90th percentiles of energy intake, to indicate range of energy consumption among children of these ages (see text).

(*From* Recommended Dietary Allowances, Ninth Revised Edition, 1980. With the permission of the National Academy of Sciences, Washington, DC)

Table 2-5.   U.S. Recommended Daily Allowance (U.S. RDA).
(for use in nutrition labeling of foods, including foods that also are vitamin and mineral supplements)

	Adults and Children Over 4 years		Children Under 4 years		Infants Under 13 months		Pregnant or Lactating Women	
Protein	65	g*	28	g*	25	g*	65	g*
Vitamin A	5,000	IU	2,500	IU	2,500	IU	8,000	IU
Vitamin C	60	mg	40	mg	40	mg	60	mg
Thiamin	1.5	mg	0.7	mg	0.7	mg	1.7	mg
Riboflavin	1.7	mg	0.8	mg	0.8	mg	2.0	mg
Niacin	20	mg	9.0	mg	9.0	mg	20	mg
Calcium	1.0	g	0.8	g	0.8	g	1.3	g
Iron	18	mg	10	mg	10	mg	18	mg
Vitamin D	400	IU	400	IU	400	IU	400	IU
Vitamin E	30	IU	10	IU	10	IU	30	IU
Vitamin B_6	2.0	mg	0.7	mg	0.7	mg	2.5	mg
Folacin	0.4	mg	0.2	mg	0.2	mg	0.8	mg
Vitamin B_{12}	6	mcg	3	mcg	3	mcg	8	mcg
Phosphorus	1.0	g	0.8	g	0.8	g	1.3	g
Iodine	150	mcg	70	mcg	70	mcg	150	mcg
Magnesium	400	mg	200	mg	200	mg	450	mg
Zinc	15	mg	8	mg	8	mg	15	mg
Copper	2	mg	1	mg	1	mg	2	mg
Biotin	0.3	mg	0.15	mg	0.15	mg	0.3	mg
Pantothenic acid	10	mg	5	mg	5	mg	10	mg

* If protein efficiency ratio of protein is equal to or better than that of casein, U.S. RDA is 45g for adults and pregnant or lactating women, 20g for children under 4 years of age and 18g for infants.
(From: Nutrition Labeling-How It Can Work for You. Bethesda, MD, National Nutrition Consortium Inc. with Ronald M. Deutsch, 1975, pp. 122-123. Used by permission.)

Questions: The RDAs—What Are They? and The U.S. RDAs

1. Match the items on the right to the phrases on the left which best *describe* each item.

    _____ 1. recommended allow-   a. RDA
    ances set by the Food   b. U.S. RDA
    and Nutrition Board of
    the NAS-NRC

    _____ 2. recommended allow-
    ances set by FDA

    _____ 3. has allowances recom-
    mended for different
    age groups within the
    two sex divisions

    _____ 4. has a protein allow-
    ance based on .8 g pro-
    tein/kg body weight
    for adults

_____ 5. has a protein allowance based on com-
parison to PER of ca-
sein

_____ 6. has its most used
allowances generally
stated for adults and
children over four
years old with no sub-
division by sex

_____ 7. recommended allowances devised to meet
the needs of nutrition
labeling

a. RDA
b. U.S. RDA

2. Have all essential nutrients been identified?
   a. Yes
   b. Probably not

3. Why is it recommended _not_ to obtain 100 percent of the RDAs from synthetic or processed foods?

4. RDAs are minimum nutrient requirements for individuals.
   a. True
   b. False

5. Consider the following situations and choose those for which application of the RDAs is valid:
   a. as guidelines for planning elementary school cafeteria lunch menus.
   b. for establishing guidelines for nutritional labeling of food stuffs.
   c. for assessing nutritional needs of persons with various illnesses.
   d. as a useful guide in planning nutrition education programs.

6. Individuals vary a great deal in the amount of calcium they absorb from their diet due to several different factors. Check the recommended intake for all age/sex categories in the RDA. Now, can you briefly explain why the U.S. RDA for calcium was set at 1000 mg (1 g)?

7. Explain the difference between the RDA and the U.S. RDA values for vitamin B_{12}.

8. Would the following amounts be nutritionally adequate _estimates_ of allowances for individual daily intake according to the RDA table (Yes or No)?
   _____ a. 45 g protein for a 160 pound 25-year-old man?
   _____ b. 27 g protein for a 130 pound 20-year-old woman?
   _____ c. 10 mg iron for a 16-year-old 120 pound young woman?
   _____ d. 45 mg ascorbic acid (vitamin C) for a 40-year-old 125 pound woman?

9. Energy intakes for children through age 18 are based on what criteria?

10. Why is there a separate table for Estimated Safe and Adequate Daily Dietary Intakes of Additional Selected Vitamins and Minerals included in the RDAs?

Answers: The RDAs—What Are They? and The U.S. RDAs

1. 1. a
   2. b
   3. a
   4. a
   5. b

6. b
7. b

2. b

3. Because synthetic foods, though they may be fortified with 100 percent RDA, will probably not supply other nutrients not yet determined as necessary in human nutrition, or nutrients for which requirements have not yet been defined which may be incidentally supplied in common foods.

4. b

5. a, b, d

6. 1 g of calcium lies in the mid-range of extremes of calcium recommendations for all age/sex groups other than infants. This relatively high amount helps to increase the margin of safety against deficiency due to individual differences in absorption and utilization.

7. The U.S. RDA was based upon the 1968 Revised RDA which had different recommendations for this nutrient.

8. a. Yes, 45 g is greater than two-thirds of the RDA for protein in this case. (Remember .8 g protein/kg body weight)
    b. No, 27 g is less than two-thirds of the RDA for protein in this case. (Remember .8 g protein/kg body weight)
    c. No, 10 mg iron is less than two-thirds of the RDA for iron in this case.
    d. Yes, 45 mg is greater than two-thirds of the RDA for ascorbic acid in this case.

9. The energy intakes for children through age 18 were based upon the median energy intakes of children these ages followed in longitudinal growth studies. The values for deviations given in parentheses within Table 2-4 for these children are 10th and 90th percentiles of energy intake.

10. Because there is less information on which to base allowances for nutrients listed in this table. Consequently, these nutrients and figures are not given in the main table of the RDA and ranges are given for recommended intake values versus more specific values.

THE BASIC FOUR FOOD GROUPS

The Basic Four Food Groups system was developed by the Institute of Home Economics of the Agricultural Research Service of the U.S. Department of Agriculture. The food groups and their recommended serving sizes are intended to provide the skeleton for a daily meal plan adequate in both calories and nutrients for most healthy individuals. As shown by the Recommended Daily Pattern, adjustments in numbers of servings for various population groups are necessary. In addition, it is assumed that smaller portions will comprise the servings for small children.

The adult pattern (2-2-4-4) supplies approximately 1200 calories. Additional calories to fill the caloric needs of persons requiring daily diets of more than 1200 kcal are expected to be obtained from Group Five, the "Other" foods: concentrated sweets and fats, as well as by additional servings or increased serving portions of foods from the Basic Four Food Groups.

The greatest deviation between the population categories occurs with the milk group. Teenagers, along with lactating and pregnant women, require the largest number of servings. The milk servings for small children may need to be decreased appropriate to the child's smaller size.

Servings of foods from each group are counted whether eaten alone or in a food product. In other words, a cup of milk counts as one serving whether it is consumed alone or in a one cup serving of custard or pudding. A casserole containing two ounces (56 to 60g) of chicken, one-half cup (120-125 mL) of broccoli, and one-half cup (120-125 mL) of milk per serving would actually provide one serving from the meat group, one serving from the vegetable group, and one-half serving from the milk group.

Table 2-6.   The Basic Four Food Plan.

1. Milk Group: These foods supply significant amounts of calcium, riboflavin, and protein.
   1 cup milk, plain yogurt, or calcium equivalent:
   > 1½ oz cheddar cheese
   > 1 cup pudding
   > 1¾ cups ice cream
   > 2 cups cottage cheese

2. Meat Group: These foods supply significant amounts of protein, niacin, iron, and thiamin.
   2 oz cooked lean meat, fish, poultry, or protein equivalent:
   > 2 eggs
   > 2 oz cheddar cheese
   > ½ cup cottage cheese
   > 1 cup cooked, dried beans or peas
   > 4 tbsp peanut butter

3. Fruit-Vegetable Group: Orange or dark green leafy vegetables and fruit are recommended 3 or 4 times weekly for vitamin A. Citrus fruit is recommended daily for vitamin C.
   Example of serving sizes:
   > ½ cup cooked vegetable or fruit, or juice
   > 1 cup raw
   > Portion commonly served, such as a medium-size apple or banana

Some good sources of vitamin A:	Some good sources of vitamin C:
Dark green leafy and deep yellow vegetables and a few fruits:	Citrus fruits
apricots	grapefruit, an orange, or orange juice
broccoli	cantaloupe
cantaloupe	strawberries
carrots	broccoli
chard, collards, cress, kale, turnip greens	brussels sprouts
pumpkin	potatoes, baked in the jacket
spinach	apples
sweet potatoes	
tomatoes	
winter squash	

4. Grain Group (whole grain, fortified or enriched): These foods supply significant amounts of carbohydrate, thiamin, iron, and niacin.
   Example of serving sizes:
   > 1 slice bread
   > 1 cup ready-to-eat cereal
   > ½ cup cooked cereal, pasta, or grits

5. Others: Foods and condiments such as oils and sugars complement, but do not replace, foods from the four groups. Amounts consumed should be determined by individual caloric needs.

(*From* A Guide to Good Eating—A Recommended Daily Pattern. Courtesy of National Dairy Council.)

Table 2-7.   **Recommended Daily Pattern to be used with the Basic Four Food Groups.**

Recommended Number of Servings

Food Group	Child	Teenager	Adult	Pregnant Woman	Lactating Woman
Milk	3	4	2	4	4
Meat	2	2	2	3	2
Fruit-Vegetable	4	4	4	4	4
Grain	4	4	4	4	4
Other	Amounts should be determined by individual caloric needs				

Key Points: The Four Food Groups

I.   The four food groups and their recommended serving sizes are intended to provide a good foundation for a daily meal plan for most *healthy* individuals.

II. Modification of food portion sizes and selections must be made in order to meet individual needs for calories and nutrients.

III. Portion sizes need to be reasonably decreased for small children.

IV. In addition to a recommendation for a daily intake of a citrus fruit for a source of vitamin C, intake of orange and dark green leafy vegetables are recommended three or four times weekly for a source of vitamin A.

V.   Grains are recommended to be obtained from whole grain, fortified, or enriched food sources.

Questions: The Basic Four Food Groups

1. What are the serving sizes suggested for the milk group:
    a. fluid milk
    b. plain yogurt
    c. On what nutrient are the servings for milk equivalents based?
    d. What is the calcium equivalent of cottage cheese for an eight ounce glass of milk?

2. What are the serving sizes suggested for the meat group:
    a. lean meat, fish, or poultry
    b. eggs
    c. On what nutrient are the servings for meat equivalents based?

3. What are the serving sizes suggested for the fruit-vegetable group:
    a. juice
    b. cut raw vegetables
    c. fresh fruit

4. a. How often is the intake of a citrus fruit recommended?
    b. Other than citrus fruits, what are three good sources of vitamin C?

5. a. How often is the intake of a good source of vitamin A recommended?
    b. What is a fruit high in vitamin A?
    c. Identify three good vegetable sources of vitamin A?

6. What are the serving sizes suggested for the grain group:
   a. bread
   b. ready-to-eat cereal
   c. cooked pasta
7. What nutrients are supplied in significant amounts by the grain group?
8. From the following list identify foods of Group Five, "Others."
   a. sugar
   b. cream
   c. tangerine
   d. lamb chop
   e. potato
   f. slice of pie
   g. glass of buttermilk
   h. dinner roll
   i. butter
   j. sour cream
9. Check Table 2-7. Plan one day's meals for an adult.
10. What are the milk servings for
    a. a teenager
    b. a child
    c. a pregnant and lactating woman

Answers: The Basic Four Food Groups

1. a. 1 cup
   b. 1 cup
   c. calcium
   d. 2 cups
2. a. 2 ounces
   b. 2 eggs
   c. protein
3. a. ½ cup
   b. 1 cup
   c. portion commonly served such as one whole medium apple or banana
4. a. daily
   b. cantaloupe, strawberries, broccoli, brussels sprouts, apples, and potatoes baked in the jacket
5. a. three or four times weekly
   b. apricots or cantaloupe
   c. broccoli, carrots, several types of dark green, leafy greens, pumpkin, sweet potatoes, tomatoes, winter squash
6. a. 1 slice
   b. 1 cup
   c. ½ cup
7. carbohydrate, thiamin, iron, and niacin
8. a, b, f, i, j
9. Day's meals should include: 2 milk servings; 2 meat servings; 4 bread/grain servings; 4 fruit and vegetable servings; a few "Other" foods.

   Example:

Breakfast	Lunch	Dinner
½ cup citrus juice	tuna fish sandwich	roast beef
1 egg	apple	gravy
1 slice toast	pickles	mashed potatoes
butter	milk	cooked, sliced, and buttered carrots
jelly		milk
		dinner roll

10. a.   4
     b.   3
     c.   4

THE MODIFIED BASIC FOUR

Some nutritionists, researchers, and dietitians believe that the Basic Four Food Groups is an inadequate guide for most Americans in terms of nutrients provided in the minimum serving recommendations, the frequency of people eating in restaurants, frequency of many persons eating processed foods, and the lack of motivation the Basic Four Food Groups seems to inspire in persons receiving nutrition education.[8] Many foods consumed in restaurants and as processed products are difficult to classify according to the Four Basic Food Groups in terms of nutrients provided.

One group of researchers has developed the Modified Basic Four which they feel fulfills at least one inadequacy of the Basic Four Food Groups: it provides significantly increased amounts of nutrients when minimum recommended servings are consumed. Amounts of serving sizes are increased for protein foods in portions which seem reasonable for adult consumption and which increase the nutrients obtained from this food group. Fruit and vegetable servings are increased to three-quarters of a cup for cooked foods. In addition to a daily source of a citrus fruit, a daily serving of a dark green vegetable is recommended. Cereal products are specified to be whole grain which increases the vitamin and mineral content obtained from this group and probably the fiber content as well. Protein is recommended to be obtained from animal, vegetable (legumes), and nut sources. One serving of fat or oil is included to provide a regular source of vitamin E.

Table 2.8.   Modified Basic Four.*

2 servings milk and milk products
4 servings protein foods:
   2 servings (3 oz each) animal protein
   2 servings (¾ cup each) legumes and/or nuts
4 servings fruits and vegetables:
   1 serving vitamin C-rich (½ cup juice or one portion commonly served such as 1 medium-size orange)
   1 serving (¾ cup cooked) dark green
   2 servings (¾ cup cooked) other
4 servings whole grain cereal products
1 serving fat and/or oil

*(*From:* King JC, Cohenour SH, Corruccini CG, and Schneeman P: Evaluation and Modification of the Basic Four Food Guide. Journal of Nutrition Education, 10, January-March 1978, pp. 27-29. Used by permission.)

Key Points: The Modified Basic Four

I.   The Modified Basic Four significantly increases the intake of nutrients above those of the traditional Basic Four Food Groups when minimum recommended servings are consumed.

II. Some daily source of vegetable protein from legumes or nuts is recommended.

III. A daily serving of a citrus fruit is recommended for a source of vitamin C and a daily source of a dark green vegetable is recommended for a source of vitamin A.

IV. Intake of whole grain food sources is emphasized.

V.   A daily source of fat or oil is recommended to provide a regular source of vitamin E.

Questions: The Modified Basic Four

1. What type of grain products are recommended?
   a. fortified
   b. enriched
   c. whole grain
2. What is the recommended portion size for animal protein? How many servings daily?
3. What other protein sources are recommended? How many servings daily?
4. What are serving sizes for fruits and vegetables?
5. What food group is added to this plan that is not specifically recommended in the Basic Four Food Groups?
6. What vitamin does the fat or oil supply in significant amount?
   a. vitamin C
   b. vitamin K
   c. vitamin E

Answers: The Modified Basic Four

1. c
2. three ounces, two
3. legumes and nuts; two servings of three-quarters of a cup each
4. One whole fresh fruit such as an apple or banana; one-half cup juice; three-quarters of a cup cooked fruits and vegetables
5. one serving fat or oil
6. c

Index of Nutritional Quality (INQ)

The index of nutritional quality expresses the ratio of a food's nutrient content to its energy (caloric) value. Food profiles are presented by bar graphs which allow visual identification of nutrient composition. Significant nutrient contribution of a particular food is very apparent by use of this bar graph. For example, whole milk is readily seen as an excellent source of protein, calcium, and riboflavin. See Figure 2-2.

The INQ numerical value is especially informative when foods are grouped according to a specific nutrient. An INQ of One indicates that a food provides approximately equivalent amounts of nutrient and energy (calories) in terms of percent of total daily recommended amounts. A value of less than One indicates that a food supplies more energy (calories) than nutrient in terms of percent of daily recommended amounts. A value greater than One indicates that a food supplies a greater amount of nutrient than energy in terms of percent of daily recommended amounts.

For example, if foods were grouped by their vitamin C content those foods with an INQ value of One or greater would be more nutrient dense for vitamin C than foods with an INQ less than One:

Food	INQ—Vitamin C content
X	10
Y	1
Z	.5

Food X supplies considerably greater amounts of vitamin C in proportion to the calorie value of that food. Food Z provides proportionally less vitamin C than calories. Therefore, food X is nutrient dense for vitamin C and food Z is calorie dense for vitamin C.

INQ is a system which helps the consumer to visualize nutritional quality of a food. It

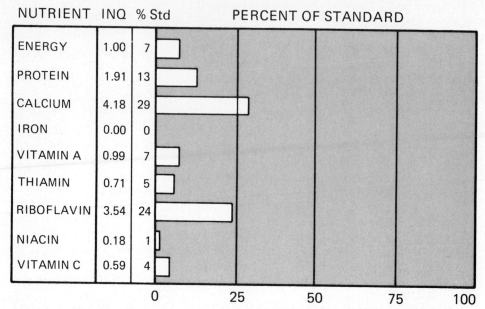

Figure 2-2. Contribution to the daily nutrient allowances by one cup of whole cow's milk. Source: Sorenson AW and Hansen RG: Index of Food Quality. Journal of Nutrition Education, 7, April-June 1975, p. 54. Used by permission.

is a method which can assist the individual requiring a calorie limited diet to identify nutrient dense foods. It visually helps the consumer to match foods of high complementation, that is, foods which mutually contribute nutrients where each is lacking (complementation is the matching of nutrient strengths to weaknesses between foods).

The developers of the INQ system feel that the consumer can make quality judgments about foods using the INQ system. They feel that a food which supplies a substantial number of nutrients with INQs of one or greater is a food of good nutritional quality.[9] These researchers also feel that INQs graphically presented on nutrition labeling would be very helpful to the consumer and that INQs are a useful tool for evaluating the nutritional quality of individual foods, meals, diets, and general food supplies.[10]

Key Points: INQ

I. The Index of Nutritional Quality (INQ) is a method of comparing the nutrient content of a specific food to the energy value of that food.

II. The INQ system can help an individual recognize nutrient dense foods.

III. Foods with an INQ of One or better are considered of good nutritional quality.

Questions: Index of Nutritional Quality (INQ)

1. What does the INQ represent?
   a. the caloric value of a food
   b. the nutrient value of a food
   c. the nutrient to energy (caloric) ratio of a food
2. How are the nutrient profiles visually presented?
3. a. An INQ of One indicates what?

    b.   An INQ of less than One indicates what?

    c.   An INQ of more than One indicates what?

4.   An INQ of ten for a particular food indicates that it is (nutrient dense/calorie dense) for a certain, identified nutrient.

5.   An individual on a limited calorie diet needs to carefully choose (nutrient dense/calorie dense) foods.

6.   INQs can be used to give nutrient profiles of individual foods, meals, diets, and general food supplies.

    a.   True

    b.   False

7.   Foods in the "Other" class noted in the Basic Four Food Groups would likely be (nutrient dense/calorie dense).

Answers: Index of Nutritional Quality (INQ)

1.   c

2.   by bar graphs

3.   a.   Nutrient and energy supplied are approximately equal in terms of percent of recommended daily amounts they supply.

    b.   More energy than nutrient is supplied in terms of percent of recommended daily amounts they supply.

    c.   More nutrient than energy is supplied in terms of percent of recommended daily amounts they supply.

4.   nutrient dense

5.   nutrient dense

6.   a

7.   calorie dense

FOOD EXCHANGE GROUPS

The food exchange system was developed as a cooperative effort between The American Diabetes Association, Incorporated and the American Dietetic Association. The use of the system allows for flexibility and variety in meal planning while including foods from recommended groupings. You do not need to memorize the calorie (energy) value of each food in order to use this system. It is informative to know the caloric as well as protein, carbohydrate, and fat values for each food group. However, the minimum necessary to remember is your total daily diet calorie limitation and the exchange pattern that fits that limitation and best suits your tastes, preferences, and life style.

You can easily plan meals using numerous food combinations after you have become familiar with the exchanges within each exchange group and you have memorized the caloric limitation and food exchange pattern of the diet best for you. The food exchange system encourages nutrients to be thought of in terms of foods; this is a valuable, practical application. Both men and women find the system easy to use even when they must frequently eat business-associated meals in restaurants. There is no need to "go off your diet" when eating in restaurants or in the homes of friends because prepared foods can be interpreted in terms of exchange groups as long as the ingredients and their relative amounts can be identified.

It is sometimes recommended to use measuring devices to portion food when using this system. However, you will soon be able to judge what one-half of a cup 125mL) of pasta looks like or what three-quarters of a cup (180-186mL) of cereal l like, especially in a familiar bowl, and you will be able to use the exchange sy successfully without actually measuring your food.

The exchange system is one of the most practical ways of teaching food selection and meal planning. The exchange system is used for many therapeutic diets. Should you ever need to follow a therapeutic diet your familiarization with the food exchange system will likely ease your diet change. One suggested way to increase familiarization with the exchange system is to tape a copy of the exchange system and suggested 1,000, 1,200, 1,500, 1,800 kcal meal plans to your refrigerator door. Then you or your other household members may easily refer to the plans.

You may not exchange foods between food groups such as between milk and meat. You may only exchange foods within each food group (exchange list). If you wish to have a snack mid-day or evening withhold one exchange from the meal plan to have at snack time. Foods appearing in bold type within the different exchange lists are generally lower in cholesterol and saturated fat than other foods within the same list.

Table 2-9.   Food Exchange Lists.

List 1.	Milk Exchanges (Includes Non-Fat Low-Fat and Whole Milk)	One exchange of milk contains 12 grams of carbohydrate, 8 grams of protein, a trace of fat and 80 calories.

This list shows the kinds and amounts of milk or milk products to use for one Milk Exchange. Those which appear in **bold type** are **non-fat.** Low-fat and whole milk contain saturated fat.

Non-Fat Fortified Milk

Skim or non-fat milk	1 cup
Powdered (non-fat dry, before adding liquid)	⅓ cup
Canned, evaporated—skim milk	½ cup
Buttermilk made from skim milk	1 cup
Yogurt made from skim milk (plain, unflavored)	1 cup

Low-Fat Fortified Milk

1% fat fortified milk (omit ½ fat exchange)	1 cup
2% fat fortified milk (omit 1 fat exchange)	1 cup
Yogurt made from 2% fortified milk (plain, unflavored) (omit 1 fat exchange)	1 cup

Whole Milk (Omit 2 fat exchanges)

Whole milk	1 cup
Canned, evaporated whole milk	½ cup
Buttermilk made from whole milk	1 cup
Yogurt made from whole milk (plain, unflavored)	1 cup

List 2.	Vegetable Exchanges	One exchange of vegetables contains about 5 grams of carbohydrate, 2 grams of protein and 25 calories.

This list shows the kinds of **vegetables** to use for one vegetable exchange. One exchange is one-half cup.

Asparagus	**Greens:**
Bean sprouts	**Mustard**
Beets	**Spinach**
Broccoli	**Turnip**
Brussels sprouts	**Mushrooms**

Table 2-9.   Food Exchange Lists (continued).

Cabbage
Carrots
Cauliflower
Celery
Cucumbers
Eggplant
Green pepper
Greens:
  Beets
  Chards
  Collards
  Dandelion
  Kale

Okra
Onions
Rhubarb
Rutabaga
Sauerkraut
String beans, green or yellow
Summer squash
Tomatoes
Tomato juice
Turnips
Vegetable Juice Cocktail
Zucchini

The following **raw vegetables** may be used as desired:

Chicory
Chinese cabbage
Endive
Escarole

Lettuce
Parsley
Radishes
Watercress

Starchy Vegetables are found in the Bread Exchange List.

List 3. Fruit Exchanges	One exchange of fruit contains 10 grams of carbohydrate and 40 calories.

This list shows the kinds and amounts of **fruits** to use for one Fruit Exchange.

Apple	1 small
Apple juice	⅓ cup
Applesauce (unsweetened)	½ cup
Apricots, fresh	2 medium
Apricots, dried	4 halves
Banana	½ small
Berries	
Blackberries	½ cup
Blueberries	½ cup
Raspberries	½ cup
Strawberries	¾ cup
Cherries	10 large
Cider	⅓ cup
Dates	2
Figs, fresh	1
Figs, dried	1
Grapefruit	½
Grapefruit juice	½ cup
Grapes	12
Grape juice	¼ cup
Mango	½ small
Melon	
Cantaloupe	¼ small
Honeydew	⅛ medium
Watermelon	1 cup
Nectarine	1 small

Table 2-9.   Food Exchange Lists (continued).

Orange	1 small
Orange juice	½ cup
Papaya	¾ cup
Peach	1 medium
Pear	1 small
Persimmon, native	1 medium
Pineapple	½ cup
Pineapple juice	⅓ cup
Plums	2 medium
Prunes	2 medium
Prune juice	¼ cup
Raisins	2 tablespoons
Tangerine	1 medium

Cranberries may be used as desired if no sugar is added.

List 4.   Bread Exchanges
(Includes Bread, Cereal, and
Starchy Vegetables)

One exchange of bread contains 15 grams of carbohydrate, 2 grams of protein and 70 calories.

This list shows the kinds and amounts of **breads, cereals, starchy vegetables,** and prepared foods to use for one bread exchange. Those which appear in **bold type** are **low-fat.**

Bread:

White (including French and Italian)	1 slice
Whole wheat	1 slice
Rye or pumpernickel	1 slice
Raisin	1 slice
Bagel, small	½
English muffin, small	½

Cereal:

Bran flakes	½ cup
Other ready-to-eat unsweetened cereal	¾ cup
Puffed cereal (unfrosted)	1 cup
Cereal (cooked)	½ cup
Grits (cooked)	½ cup
Rice or barley (cooked)	½ cup
Pasta (cooked) spaghetti, noodles, macaroni	½ cup
Popcorn (popped, no fat added)	3 cups
Cornmeal (dry)	2 tbsp
Flour	2½ tbsp
Wheat germ	¼ cup

Crackers:

Arrowroot	3
Graham, 2½" sq.	2
Matzoth, 4" x 6"	½
Oyster	20
Pretzels, 3⅛" long x ⅛" dia.	25

Plain roll, bread	1
Frankfurter roll	½
Hamburger bun	½
Dried bread crumbs	3 tbsp
Tortilla, 6"	1

Starchy Vegetables:

Corn	⅓ cup
Corn on the cob	1 small
Lima beans	½ cup
Parsnips	⅔ cup
Peas, green (canned or frozen)	½ cup
Potato, white	1 small
Potato (mashed)	½ cup
Pumpkin	¾ cup
Winter squash, acorn or butternut	½ cup
Yam or sweet potato	¼ cup

Prepared foods:

Biscuit 2" dia. (omit 1 fat exchange)	1
Corn bread, 2" x 2" x 1" (omit 1 fat exchange)	1
Corn muffin, 2" dia. (omit 1 fat exchange)	1
Crackers, round butter type (omit 1 fat exchange)	5
Muffin, plain small (omit 1 fat exchange)	1
Potatoes, french fried, length 2" to 3½" (omit 1 fat exchange)	8
Potato or corn chips (omit 2 fat exchanges)	15
Pancake, 5" x ½" (omit 1 fat exchange)	1
Waffle, 5" x ½" (omit 1 fat exchange)	1

Table 2-9.   Food Exchange Lists (continued).

Rye Wafers, 2″ x 3½″	3
Saltines	6
Soda, 2½″ sq.	4

Dried beans, peas, and lentils (omit 1
low-fat meat exchange): beans, peas,
lentils (dried and cooked)   ½ cup
Baked beans, no pork (canned)   ¼ cup

List 5. Meat Exchanges	One exchange of lean mean (1 oz) contains 7
Lean Meat	grams of protein, 3 grams of fat and 55 calories.

This list shows the kinds and amounts of **lean meat** and other protein-rich foods to use for one low-fat meat exchange.

Beef:	**baby beef (very lean), chipped beef, chuck, flank steak, tenderloin, plate ribs, plate skirt steak, round (bottom, top), all cuts rump, spare ribs, tripe**	1 oz
Lamb:	**leg, rib, sirloin, loin (roast and chops), shank, shoulder**	1 oz
Pork:	**leg (whole rump, center shank), ham, smoked (center slices)**	1 oz
Veal:	**leg, loin, rib, shank, shoulder, cutlets**	1 oz
Poultry:	**meat without skin of chicken, turkey, cornish hen, guinea hen, pheasant**	1 oz
Fish:	**any fresh or frozen**	1 oz
	canned salmon, tuna, mackerel, crab and lobster,	¼ cup
	clams, oysters, scallops, shrimp,	5 or 1 oz
	sardines—drained	3

Cheeses containing less than 5% butterfat	1 oz
Cottage cheese, dry and 2% butterfat	¼ cup
Dried beans and peas (omit 1 bread exchange)	½ cup

List 5. Meat Exchanges	For each Exchange of medium-fat meat omit
Medium-Fat Meat	one-half Fat Exchange.

This list shows the kinds and amounts of medium-fat meat and other protein-rich foods to use for one medium-fat meat exchange.

Beef:	ground (15% fat), corned beef (canned), rib eye, round (ground commercial)	1 oz
Pork:	loin (all cuts tenderloin), shoulder arm (picnic), shoulder blade, Boston butt, Canadian bacon, boiled ham	1 oz
Liver, heart, kidney, and sweetbreads (these are high in cholesterol)		1 oz
Cottage cheese, creamed		¼ cup
Cheese:	mozzarella, ricotta, farmer's cheese, neufchatel,	1 oz
	Parmesan	3 tbsp
Egg (high in cholesterol)		1
Peanut butter (omit two additional fat exchanges)		2 tbsp

List 5. Meat Exchanges	For each exchange of high-fat meat omit one
High-Fat Meat	fat exchange

Table 2-9.   Food Exchange Lists (continued).

This list shows the kinds and amounts of high-fat meat and other protein-rich foods to use for one high-fat meat exchange.

Beef:	brisket, corned beef (brisket), ground beef (more than 20% fat), hamburger (commercial), chuck (ground commercial), roasts (rib), steaks (club and rib)	1 oz
Lamb:	breast	1 oz
Pork:	spare ribs, loin (back ribs), pork (ground), country style ham, deviled ham	1 oz
Veal:	breast	1 oz
Poultry:	capon, duck (domestic), goose	1 oz
Cheese:	cheddar types	1 oz
Cold cuts		4½" x ⅛" slice
Frankfurter		1 small

List 6. Fat Exchanges	One exchange of fat contains 5 grams of fat and 45 calories.

This list shows the kinds and amounts of fat-containing foods to use for one fat exchange. To plan a diet low in saturated fat select only those exchanges which appear in **bold type.** They are **polyunsaturated.**

Margarine, soft, tub, or stick*	1 teaspoon
Avocado (4″ in diameter)**	⅛
Oil, corn, cottonseed, safflower, soy, sunflower	1 teaspoon
Oil, olive**	1 teaspoon
Oil, peanut**	1 teaspoon
Olives**	5 small
Almonds**	10 whole
Pecans**	2 large whole
Peanuts**	
Spanish	20 whole
Virginia	10 whole
Walnuts	6 small
Nuts, other**	6 small
Margarine, regular stick	1 teaspoon
Butter	1 teaspoon
Bacon fat	1 teaspoon
Bacon, crisp	1 strip
Cream, light	2 tablespoons
Cream, sour	2 tablespoons
Cream, heavy	1 tablespoon
Cream cheese	1 tablespoon
French dressing***	1 tablespoon
Italian dressing***	1 tablespoon
Lard	1 teaspoon
Mayonnaise***	1 teaspoon
Salad dressing, mayonnaise type***	2 teaspoons
Salt pork	¾ inch cube

* Made with corn, cottonseed, safflower, soy, or sunflower oil only.
** Fat content is primarily mono-unsaturated
*** If made with corn, cottonseed, safflower, soy, or sunflower oil can be used on fat modified diet

The exchange lists are based on material in the EXCHANGE LISTS FOR MEAL PLANNING prepared by Committees of the American Diabetes Association, Inc. and the American Dietetic Association in cooperation with the National Institute of Arthritis, Metabolism and Digestive Diseases and the National Heart and Lung Institute, National Institutes of Health, Public Health Service, U.S. Department of Health, Education and Welfare.

Key Points: Food Exchange Groups

I. The food exchange system emphasizes food intake and, thus, nutrient intake.

II. The food exchange system can be used effectively to plan normal as well as therapeutic diets.

III. Various food exchange patterns can be established to fit within certain caloric limitations to meet the needs and preferences of different individuals.

IV. Individual foods may be exchanged within a food group but not between different food groups.

Questions: Food Exchange Groups

1. Fill in the following values.

	Grams Carbohydrate	Grams Protein	Grams Fat	Calories
milk exchange	_____	_____	_____	_____
vegetable exchange	_____	_____	_____	_____
fruit exchange	_____	_____	_____	_____
bread exchange	_____	_____	_____	_____
meat exchange	_____	_____	_____	_____

2. The milk exchange is based upon _____ .
   a. whole milk
   b. low-fat milk
   c. skim milk

3. If you elect to drink 2 percent fat, fortified milk you must subtract how many fat exchanges from your total daily allowance for each 8 ounce glass of milk?

4. a. What is the measured amount of a vegetable in each vegetable exchange?
   b. Identify at least three raw vegetables which may be used as desired.
   c. If you add one teaspoon of margarine to one vegetable exchange, such as one-half cup of cooked carrots, how many fat exchanges must you subtract from your daily fat allowance?
   d. Are corn, potatoes, and lima beans included in the vegetable exchange?

5. The fruit exchanges provide no significant fat or protein.
   a. True
   b. False

6. Identify the amount of the following fruits in one fruit exchange.
   a. apple
   b. banana
   c. cider or apple juice
   d. grapefruit juice
   e. grape juice
   f. cantaloupe
   g. orange juice
   h. peach
   i. pineapple juice
   j. raisins

7. Biscuits, cornbread, and muffins also provide per single bread exchange one
   a. fat exchange

    b. milk exchange
    c. meat exchange

8. Identify the amount of the following bread, cereal, and starchy vegetable in one bread exchange.

a. white, whole wheat, rye, or raisin bread	f. pasta
b. English muffin	g. flour
c. hamburger or frankfurter roll	h. soda crackers
d. tortilla	i. baked beans
e. most ready-to-eat unsweetened cereal	j. corn
	k. mashed potatoes

9. Meat exchanges do not provide carbohydrate.
    a. True
    b. False

10. What amounts of the following foods provide one lean meat exchange:
    a. round steak
    b. canned tuna
    c. cottage cheese

11. How many fat exchanges must be omitted for a medium-fat meat *per meat exchange?* High-fat meat *per meat exchange?*

12. An egg is placed within the
    a. lean meat exchange
    b. medium-fat meat exchange
    c. high-fat meat exchange

13. Cheddar cheese is placed within the
    a. lean meat exchange
    b. medium-fat meat exchange
    c. high-fat meat exchange

14. What amounts of the following foods provide one fat exchange?

a. margarine or butter	f. sour cream
b. vegetable oil	g. heavy cream
c. olives	h. cream cheese
d. Spanish peanuts	i. French or Italian dressing
e. crisp bacon	j. mayonnaise

15. 1200 kcal daily diets:

Exchanges	Diet #1	Diet #2	Diet #3
milk	2	2	3
vegetable	2	2	2
fruit	4	4	3
bread	4	4	5
meat	5	7	6
fat	6	3	2

    a. Can you have some flexibility in choosing diet plans within a limited calorie level?
    b. Which food exchanges experience the greatest change between the different diet plans?
    c. Why must skim milk be used for Diet #3?
    d. Do each of the diets also fulfill the 2-2-4-4 Basic Four Food Guide pattern for an adult?

Answers: Food Exchange Groups

1.

	Grams Carbohydrate	Grams Protein	Grams Fat	Calories
milk exchange (skim)	12	8	—	80
vegetable exchange	5	2	—	25
fruit exchange	10	—	—	40
bread exchange	15	2	—	70
meat exchange (lean)	—	7	3	55

2. c
3. one fat exchange
4. a. one-half cup
   b. any of: chicory, Chinese cabbage, endive, escarole, lettuce, parsley, radishes, watercress
   c. one fat exchange
   d. No; they are included in the bread list as starchy vegetables.
5. a
6. a. 1 small
   b. ½ small
   c. ⅓ cup
   d. ½ cup
   e. ¼ cup
   f. ¼ small
   g. ½ cup
   h. 1 medium
   i. ⅓ cup
   j. 2 tablespoons
7. a
8. a. 1 slice
   b. ½
   c. ½
   d. 1-6 inches
   e. ¾ cup
   f. ½ cup, cooked
   g. 2½ tablespoons
   h. 4
   i. ¼ cup
   j. ⅓ cup
   k. ½ cup
9. a. Exception (carbohydrate source): When dried beans and peas are used to supply protein one bread exchange (carbohydrate source) must be omitted per each meat exchange.
10. a. 1 oz
    b. ¼ cup
    c. ¼ cup dry, 2 percent butterfat
11. ½ fat exchange; 1 fat exchange
12. b
13. c
14. a. 1 teaspoon
    b. 1 teaspoon
    c. 5
    d. 20 whole
    e. 1 strip
    f. 2 tablespoons
    g. 1 tablespoon
    h. 1 tablespoon
    i. 1 tablespoon
    j. 1 teaspoon
15. a. Yes; see the example of three diet plans for 1200 kcal diets.
    b. fat, meat, milk
    c. Because there are not enough fat exchanges in the diet plan to allow for use of 2 percent fat milk or whole milk which must have one fat exchange or two fat exchanges, respectively, omitted for each milk exchange.
    d. yes

REFERENCES

[1] Recommended dietary allowances revised, 1974. Dairy Council Digest, 44, May-June 1974, pp. 13-18

[2] Recommended Dietary Allowances, Ninth Revised Edition (1980). Food and Nutrition Board, National Academy of Sciences—National Research Council, Washington, DC. p. 1

[3] Leverton RM: RDA's are not for amateurs. Journal of the American Dietetic Association, 66, January 1975, p. 9

[4] Nutrition Labeling—How It Can Work For You. Bethesda, MD, National Nutrition Consortium, Inc. with Ronald M. Deutsch, 1975, pp. 67-68

[5] Nutrition Labeling—How It Can Work For You. Bethesda, MD; National Nutrition Consortium, Inc., with Ronald M. Deutsch, 1975, pp. 67-68

[6] Protein efficiency ratio (PER) is a method of expressing the quality of a protein according to how it meets the growth needs of an animal. It expresses the ratio between weight gain and protein consumed.

[7] Whitney EN, Hamilton EMN: Understanding Nutrition. St. Paul, MN; West Publishing Co., 1977, p. 418

[8] Hicks BM: Food groups—where do they belong? Food and Nutrition News, 48, February 1977

[9] Hansen RG, Wyse BW: Using the INQ to evaluate foods. Nutrition News, 42, February-March 1979

[10] Wittwer AL, et al: Nutrient density—evaluation of nutritional attributes of food. Journal of Nutrition Education, 9, January-March 1977

3
CARBOHYDRATES

Carbohydrates are the sugars and starches produced by plants and animals. *Carbohydrates normally contribute approximately one-half of the total daily caloric intake for most Americans.* Carbohydrates contain the elements carbon, hydrogen, and oxygen. The basic chemical structure of a single unit sugar is that composed of a carbon chain varying in length from three to seven carbons. Sugars composed of one of these units are known as monosaccharides. Glucose is a monosaccharide composed of six carbon units and, hence, is referred to as a hexose. The hexoses are nutritionally the most important monosaccharides.

There are three hexoses important in the human diet: glucose (also referred to as dextrose, grape sugar, corn sugar, or blood sugar), fructose (also referred to as levulose or fruit sugar), and galactose. Though they differ slightly in chemical configuration, all three of

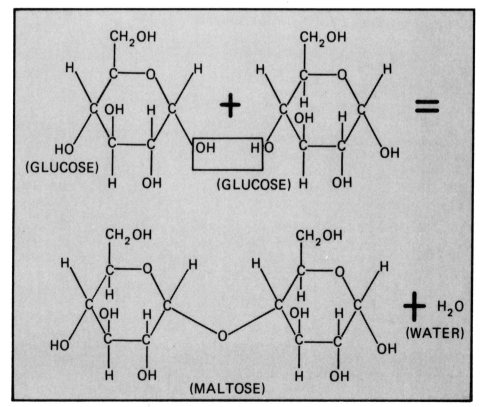

Figure 3-1.   *Condensation of two glucose molecules to form maltose.*

37

these hexoses have the same chemical formula: $C_6H_{12}O_6$. This formula reveals the 2:1 hydrogen to oxygen ratio characteristic of carbohydrates.

The chemical removal of a molecule of water (H_2O) from two monosaccharide units causes the two single units to chemically bond into a new unit termed a disaccharide. When two molecules of glucose experience a condensation reaction (removal of a molecule of water) the new disaccharide maltose is formed. The disaccharides important in human nutrition are:

Maltose (malt sugar) = glucose + glucose

Sucrose (table sugar) = glucose + fructose

Lactose (milk sugar) = glucose + galactose

The individual glucose units are also bonded together in long chains to form the group of complex carbohydrates called polysaccharides. Polysaccharides include starch (derived from plant sources), glycogen (referred to as animal starch), dextrins (an intermediary between starch and simple sugar), cellulose (found in plants but not digestible by humans), and pectins (found in ripe fruits but not digestible by humans).

The disaccharides and polysaccharides are broken down into their respective monosaccharides by the action of specific enzymes for this purpose. The appropriate enzyme splits the disaccharide where the two monosaccharides are joined and a molecule of water is taken up. The molecule of water (H_2O) splits with (-OH) going to complete the formation of one monosaccharide and (-H) going to complete the second monosaccharide. The term used for this chemical reaction involving the uptake and molecular splitting of water is *hydrolysis*. Starches and sugars are broken down to monosaccharides before they are absorbed into the blood stream.

The sweetness levels of the different sugars and polysaccharides vary a great deal. On a scale attempting to discriminate between their sweetness levels, they could be noted as shown in Figure 3-2.

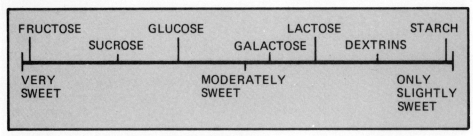

Figure 3-2. Relative sweetness scale of the carbohydrates.

Digestion, absorption, and metabolism of carbohydrates. Starch digestion begins in the mouth with the action of the salivary enzyme amylase. Salivary amylase[1] works upon the starch breaking it down to smaller units of dextrins and maltose. Further starch breakdown occurs in the small intestine with the action of the pancreatic enzyme amylopsin. Amylopsin causes the remaining starch to be broken down first to dextrins and then to maltose. Finally, the intestinal enzyme maltase completes the breakdown to monosaccharide units.

Mal*tase* acts upon mal*tose* to form glucose + glucose. The intestine also secretes necessary enzymes to complete the breakdown of the disaccharides sucrose and lactose.

Suc*rase* acts upon suc*rose* to form glucose + fructose.

Lac*tase* acts upon lac*tose* to form glucose + galactose.

The monosaccharides are absorbed from the small intestine into the portal blood system which directs them to the liver.

The liver plays an important regulatory role in the metabolism of carbohydrates. Glucose is moved from the liver into the blood stream as needed either for energy or formation of other compounds; any excess is converted to glycogen and stored in the liver or converted to fatty acids and glycerol which are synthesized into triglycerides and transported to the adipose (fat) tissue where they are stored as body fat. *The process of converting glucose to glycogen is termed glycogenesis.* Fructose and galactose are also converted by enzymatic action to glucose in the liver. The glucose in the blood can be taken up by the muscle tissue and used for energy, or a limited excess can be stored as glycogen (in muscle) to provide a ready reserve of glucose during times of increased activity.

Energy is actually produced by way of two sequential pathways. The first is an anaerobic pathway termed the Embden-Meyerhof pathway (also called glycolysis). This pathway ends with the production of pyruvic acid. The second pathway is an aerobic series of chemical reactions termed the Krebs cycle (or tricarboxylic acid cycle, TCA cycle, or citric acid cycle). Normally there is adequate oxygen to produce energy from glucose with the production of carbon dioxide and water as end-products. During exercise, an increased respiration rate (more rapid breathing) occurs causing the increased taking in of oxygen and expellation of carbon dioxide from the lungs. During heavy exercise, however, there may be a lack of adequate oxygen even with the increase in respiratory rate. Under the condition of inadequate oxygen supply an intermediate substance called lactic acid is produced from pyruvic acid. The chemical reactions leading to lactic acid formation produce a relatively small amount of energy which can sustain the individual for a period of time.

After muscular relaxation occurs the accumulated lactic acid is carried by the blood to the liver where an enzyme converts it back to pyruvic acid and it re-enters the metabolic pathway. Refer to Figure 6-5 for a diagram of this energy producing pathway. The accumulation of lactic acid in muscle tissue is thought to contribute to the feeling of muscular fatigue and achiness following strenuous muscular exertion. The above described lactic acid energy production cycle has been referred to as the Cori cycle and demonstrates the economizing ability of the body as well as another of the body's many back-up systems.

Functions of carbohydrates. The following are the main functions of carbohydrates in the body:

1. *Carbohydrate is the chief source of fuel used for energy to conduct body processes and to assist in maintenance of body temperature.* Normally, only glucose can be used by the nervous system. There is no storage of glucose or glycogen in the brain. Consequently, the blood must continually bring a supply of glucose to the brain. There is a limited storage of glycogen in the heart muscle to maintain heart muscular activity during periods of low blood glucose. Hearts damaged by various diseases may have a significantly reduced ability to form and store glycogen. Such heart conditions require a constant blood glucose supply. Herein lies one of the dangers of a low calorie, low carbohydrate diet. If such a diet is undertaken by a person with undiagnosed or borderline heart trouble, serious problems may be unnecessarily precipitated. The heat generated as a by-product of carbohydrate oxidation for production of energy is useful in assisting the maintenance of body temperature.

2. *Carbohydrate exerts a sparing action on dietary and body protein.* When carbohydrate supplies are adequate to cover all body energy needs little protein is used as an energy source. Carbohydrates also supply certain chemical elements which are needed for the manufacture of some amino acids, the basic chemical units used to form protein. Because carbohydrate food sources are generally less expensive than animal protein food sources, carbohydrates provide the most economical form of fuel for the body.

3. *Carbohydrate is needed for the complete oxidation of fat for energy production without the accumulation of undesirable end-products.* This will be discussed in greater detail in Chapter Four.

4. *Carbohydrates and/or their metabolites are necessary for the formation of certain body compounds and body tissues.* Glucuronic acid, a metabolite of glucose, is an important detoxification agent of the liver. Other carbohydrate derivatives are important for the formation of

nucleic acids, connective tissue matrix, and galactosides of nerve tissue.[2]

Carbohydrate consumption. *Carbohydrates supply 4 kcal per gram.* Approximately 50 percent of the average American diet contains carbohydrate. Thus, a diet which supplies 2000 kcal/day would derive approximately 1000 of those kcal from carbohydrate. Cereal grains, legumes, fruits, vegetables (roots and tubers), sugars, and milk supply the major portion of carbohydrate in the diet.

In the United States there has been a change in the percentage consumption of types of carbohydrate food sources since the turn of the century. Fruit and vegetable consumption has remained about the same while cereal and potato consumption has declined and refined sugar consumption has increased.[3] Significantly large amounts of simple sugars are consumed in sweets, candies, and especially soft drinks and processed foods.[4] This reduced intake of complex carbohydrate food sources is felt to contribute to the general reduction in dietary fiber intake. Scientists are currently studying the effects of these changes upon the health and disease incidence of Americans and are not yet in agreement about the consequences of these dietary changes.

Many foods supply sugar in forms not easily recognizable as sugar. Information contained in Table 3-1 will help you recognize that some foods contain large amounts of "hidden sugar." This is not to say that any one of these foods is "bad" by itself, but rather that you need to be informed in order to make rational, desirable food selections appropriate to your individual needs.

Table 3-1.   Hidden Sugar in Familiar Foods.*

	Measure	Equivalent Teaspoons sugar**
*Candies****		
Butterscotch candy	1 piece (5g)	1
Chewing gum	1 piece (3g)	½
Fudge	1 oz square (28g)	4
Hard candy	1 piece (5g)	1
Hershey candy	1 small bar (41g)	5
Peanut brittle	1 piece (25g)	3½
Cakes and Cookies		
Angel food	1/10 average cake (45g)	5½
Chocolate cake (iced)	1 piece (85g)	5½-8
Chocolate chip cookie	1 (11g)	1½
Doughnut (glazed with jelly center)	1 (65g)	6
Sandwich type cookie	1 (14g)	2
Beverages		
Beer	8 oz (240g)	2
Chocolate milk	8 oz (240g)	5-6
Chocolate milkshake	8 oz (240g)	10-12
Cola drinks	6 oz (one bottle) (180g)	3½-4
Wine, port	3½ oz (100g)	3
Desserts		
Apple pie	1 slice (160g)	12
Cherry pie	1 slice (160g)	12
Hot fudge sundae	1 dish (266g)	16-17
Chocolate pudding	½ cup (144g)	6-7
Custard	½ cup (112g)	4
Gelatin (sweetened)	½ cup (120g)	4½

Table 3-1.   Hidden Sugar in Familiar Foods (continued).

Ice cream	½ cup (67g)	3
Lemon meringue pie	1 piece (140g)	10½
Sherbet	½ cup (96g)	5-6
Strawberry shortcake	1 serving (175g)	12
Syrups, Sugars, Snacks		
Brown sugar	1 tablespoon (14g)	2½-3
Honey	1 tablespoon (20g)	3½
Jam, jelly	1 tablespoon (20g)	3
Maple syrup	1 tablespoon (20g)	2½
Sweet pickle	1 large (100g)	7½
Fruits		
Apricots, dried	4 to 5 halves (25g)	3
Dates, pitted	5 (50g)	7
Figs, dried	2 small (30g)	4
Grape juice (unsweetened)	½ cup (120g)	4
Grapefruit juice (unsweetened)	½ cup (125g)	2
Orange juice	½ cup (124g)	2½
Prunes, dried	2 large (20g)	3
Prune juice	½ cup (120g)	4-4½
Raisins	1 tablespoon (10g)	1½
Bread and Cereals		
Cinnamon bun	1 average (97g)	10½
Cheerios	1 cup (25g)	3½
Cornflakes, Wheaties	1 cup (22-28g)	4-4½
Hamburger bun	1 whole bun (30g)	3
Hot dog bun	1 whole bun (36g)	3½
White bread	1 slice (23g)	2½

* (Sugar content estimated from values listed for carbohydrates in the various foodstuffs *from:* Pennington JAT and Church HN: Bowes and Church's Food Values of Portions Commonly Used, 13th edition, 1980, Philadelphia, J. B. Lippincott Company.)

** Each teaspoon is equivalent to about 5 g white granulated sugar.

*** Candy is generally composed of more than 75 percent sugar.

Key Points: Carbohydrates

I. Important nomenclature involved with the study of carbohydrates:
hex = 6
-ose = refers to carbohydrate (sugar)
mono- = refers to single or one
saccharide = sugar
di- = 2
poly = many
glyco = glycogen
genesis = creating; building
-lysis = breaking down

II. Hexose monosaccharides especially important to human nutrition:

Glucose   (dextrose, blood sugar, corn sugar, grape sugar)
Fructose   (fruit sugar, levulose)
Galactose (component of milk sugar, lactose)

III. Disaccharides especially important to human nutrition:
Maltose   (malt sugar) + H_2O = glucose + glucose
Sucrose   (table sugar) + H_2O = glucose + fructose
Lactose   (milk sugar) + H_2O = glucose + galactose

IV. Fructose is the sweetest tasting of the various sugars.

V. Carbohydrates are absorbed as monosaccharides which are carried by the portal blood system to the liver. Appropriate enzymes in the liver convert fructose and galactose to glucose. From the liver glucose enters the blood stream as needed, for energy or as a precursor for other products, or, if in excess, converts to glycogen for storage in the liver, or, if this is in excess, converts to fat for storage in adipose tissue.

VI. Energy is basically produced from glucose by way of two sequential pathways:
A. Embden-Meyerhof pathway (also called glycolysis), an anaerobic pathway.
B. Krebs cycle (also called the tricarboxylic acid cycle, the TCA cycle, or the citric acid cycle), an aerobic pathway.

VII. During heavy exercise there may be inadequate oxygen for the complete oxidation of glucose to produce energy, CO_2 and H_2O.
A. Some energy is then derived from the chemical reactions converting glucose to lactic acid. These chemical reactions do not require oxygen.
B. Later, lactic acid is reconverted to pyruvic acid in the liver by the necessary enzyme; then pyruvic acid may continue along the glucose metabolic pathway for energy production (The Cori cycle).

VIII. Important functions of dietary carbohydrate include serving as the chief source of body energy, sparing protein from use as body fuel, enabling the complete oxidation of fat for energy production without the build-up of undesirable end-products, and forming other body compounds and tissues.

IX. Approximately half of the average American diet contains carbohydrate from such food sources as grains, vegetables, fruits, milk, and sugars.

X. Carbohydrates supply 4 kcal/gram.

Questions: Carbohydrates

1. The most important monosaccharides in human nutrition contain how many carbon atoms?

2. Match the items on the right to the terms on the left which they best represent:

_____ 1. a hexose   a. contain C, H, O, with H:O ratio of 2:1
_____ 2. fruit sugar   b. glucose
_____ 3. hex   c. means single or one
_____ 4. mono   d. $C_6 H_{12} O_6$
_____ 5. galactose   e. means six
_____ 6. -ose   f. fructose
_____ 7. carbohydrates   g. refers to carbohydrate (sugar)
_____ 8. blood sugar   h. a component of milk sugar, lactose

3. The chemical removal of a molecule of water from two individual units, which causes the formation of one more complex unit, is termed a _____ reaction.

4. The term used for the chemical reaction which involves the uptake and molecular splitting of water is _____ .

5. The suffix -ose refers to carbohydrate (sugar). To what does the suffix -ase refer?
6. Define the following terms:
    a. Glyco refers to glycogen and genesis refers to creating. What is the meaning of the term glycogenesis?
    b. The suffix -lysis means dissolution or breakdown. What is the meaning of the term glycogenolysis?
7. Match the disaccharides on the right to their appropriate monosaccharide components on the left:
    _____ 1. glucose + glucose   a.   sucrose
    _____ 2. glucose + fructose   b.   lactose
    _____ 3. glucose + galactose   c.   maltose
8. Identify the enzymes produced at the following points which act upon the saccharides:

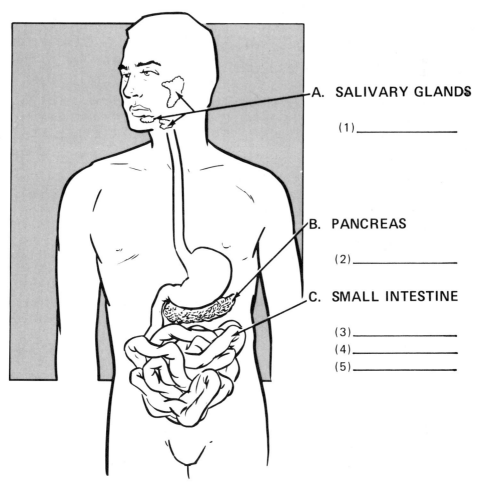

A. **SALIVARY GLANDS**

(1)_____

B. **PANCREAS**

(2)_____

C. **SMALL INTESTINE**

(3)_____
(4)_____
(5)_____

Figure 3-3.

9. The portal blood system carries the newly absorbed monosaccharides to what organ?

10. Name three of the pathways glucose may take after it reaches the liver.
    a. _____
    b. _____
    c. _____

11. When the body is undergoing exercise it attempts to provide the necessary oxygen for energy production by increasing the _____ rate.

12. When the body is undergoing heavy exercise and insufficient oxygen is available for energy production, a series of chemical reactions occur which provide some energy capable of sustaining the individual for a period of time. What intermediary product is produced by these chemical reactions?

13. Check Figure 3-2 to examine the relative sweetness levels of the various carbohydrates. Even though all carbohydrates provide 4 kcal per gram, fructose is being presented by some food producers as a "low calorie" sugar. Can you deduce the theory behind this claim?

14. If a 2000 kcal/day diet derives approximately 1000 kcal from carbohydrates, how many grams of carbohydrate does that diet contain?

15. Two very important functions of carbohydrate are to provide fuel for body energy needs (along with the by-product of heat to maintain body temperature) and to spare protein from use as a body fuel. Which is the most economical form of fuel for the body, carbohydrate or protein?

16. Identify two additional functions (other than those given in question 15) of carbohydrate in the body.

17. The brain is able to store glycogen which may be used to supply glucose to the brain during periods of low blood sugar.
    a. True
    b. False

18. Low carbohydrate diets are not recommended for persons with a damaged heart condition.
    a. True
    b. False

19. Identify the trend in food consumption in the U.S. which has occurred since the turn of the century.
    a. Potato consumption has continued to increase.
    b. Refined sugar and processed sugar products consumption has increased.
    c. Fruit and vegetable consumption has greatly decreased.

20. Carbohydrate consumed in excess of body energy needs is converted for storage to glycogen and/or _____ .

21. The liver stores approximately 100g of glycogen and the muscle tissues store approximately 200g glycogen.
    a. Disregarding current blood glucose how much energy in kcal is available from glycogen stores?
    b. What approximate percentage of a 2000 kcal/day would this provide?

22. The alcohol in alcoholic beverages provides approximately 7 kcal/g. In addition, there is significant carbohydrate content in beer, wine, and many mixed drinks. Approximately how many kcal due to carbohydrate are there in (refer to Table 3-1):
    a. 8 oz of beer

b.   3½ oz port wine
Approximately how many grams of white granulated sugar does each value for beer and wine represent?

23.   Port is a very sweet wine. Would you expect a dry table wine to contain more or less sugar than port?

24.   Compare grape juice with grapefruit juice. What is the ratio of sugar values for these two juices?

25.   Compare sugar values for ice cream and sherbet. Which of these two desserts is generally higher in sugar content? What other ingredient in ice cream adds to its generally higher caloric content? Just because it is lower in fat content can sherbet reasonably be considered a low calorie dessert? Many people erroneously equate low fat as meaning low calorie. Does this example as well as question number 22 help you recognize the various sources of energy (calories) in food?

26.   Compare the sugar content of custard and gelatin. What is their approximate sugar ratio? What forms of sugar would you expect to find in custard? In gelatin?

27.   What food groups supply significant amounts of carbohydrates? What foods supply large amounts of simple sugars?

Answers: Carbohydrates

1.   6
2.   1.   d
      2.   f
      3.   e
      4.   c
      5.   h
      6.   g
      7.   a
      8.   b
3.   condensation
4.   hydrolysis
5.   enzyme
6.   a.   The process of creating or building glycogen.
      b.   The chemical process of glycogen breaking down by enzymatic hydrolysis into dextrins and finally to glucose.
7.   1.   c
      2.   a
      3.   b
8.   a.   1—salivary amylase (ptyalin)
      b.   2—amylopsin
      c.   3—maltase, 4—sucrase, 5—lactase
9.   the liver
10.   a.   to the blood
      b.   converted to glycogen and stored in the liver
      c.   converted to fatty acids and transported via blood to adipose (fat) tissue
11.   respiration
12.   lactic acid
13.   Because fructose (under certain conditions such as temperature and form) is so much sweeter tasting than other sugars, less of it is required to sweeten a food product to the desired level of sweetness. Hence, total calories from sugar in that foodstuff are lower than those of a comparable product sweetened with another

sugar such as sucrose.
14. $1000 \div 4 = 250$ grams carbohydrate
15. carbohydrate (for example, bread or beans compared to ground beef, lamb chops, or beefsteak)
16. a. Carbohydrate is necessary to allow the complete oxidation of fat.
    b. Carbohydrate is necessary for the formation of certain body compounds and body tissues.
17. b
18. a
19. b
20. fat
21. a.   200g
          +100g
          —————
          300 g carbohydrate
          $300g \times 4 \text{ kcal} = 1200 \text{ kcal}$
    b. $1200 \div 2000 = $ only 60 percent of one day's kcal needs
22. a. approximately 10g white granulated sugar (2 teaspoons) $\times 4 \text{ kcal/g} = 40 \text{ kcal}$
    b. approximately 15g white granulated sugar (3 teaspoons) $\times 4 \text{ kcal/g} = 60 \text{ kcal}$
23. less
24. 2:1. Grape juice has almost twice as much sugar as grapefruit juice.
25. sherbet; cream (fat); no
26. 1:1; lactose and sucrose in custard; sucrose in sweetened gelatin.
27. cereal grains, legumes, fruits, vegetables, sugar, and milk; sweets, candies, soft drinks, and many processed foods

AN IMPORTANT CARBOHYDRATE: CELLULOSE

Cellulose is a major contributor to the fiber in foods. Since cellulose is undigestible by humans, of what value is it in the human diet? Cellulose, nondigestible carbohydrates, and lignin are all contained in plant foods and generally proceed through the human digestive system in bulk without being digested or absorbed. *This bulk stimulates intestinal motility and aids in establishing regularity of bowel movements.* This bulk also tends to draw and hold water thus easing its movement through the intestines.

The decreased consumption of high fiber foods such as cereal and potatoes by Americans since the turn of the century has been accompanied by an increase of low fiber foods such as meat, dairy products, and highly refined carbohydrate processed foods. This diet trend has led to a general decrease in the fiber consumption of Americans. Some scientists have correlated the occurrence of diseases such as cancer of the colon and rectum, hemorrhoids, and diverticulosis to the low fiber consumption of the American population. These correlations are basically founded upon the data obtained from various epidemiological studies.[5] These studies contrast differences between the low fiber diets of Americans and certain disease incidence with the higher fiber diets of other societies and their disease incidence. The correlations, however, remain drawn from observed associations and are not yet predictable or demonstrable of cause and effect relationships.

The fiber bulk is thought to aid in the prevention of disease by:

1. Accelerating intestinal transit time, thereby decreasing the intestinal exposure time to fecal carcinogens (cancer-causing agents).
2. Binding bile salts and certain drugs, chemicals, and food additives thereby reducing their concentration and the concentration of possible metabolic carcinogenic or toxic by-products.

3. Interfering with intestinal flora responsible for degrading bile salts thereby reducing possible carcinogen production.

4. Diluting the concentration of intestinal carcinogens and, consequently, their effect.[6]

It is also possible that fiber may bind essential nutrients in the intestine causing their increased fecal loss. This may be a negative aspect of high fiber diets and would be of increased importance to persons on an already nutritionally marginal diet.[7] At the present time, however, it seems advisable to consume some sources of high fiber foods daily. These foods are also generally good sources of other essential nutrients. Good selections can be made from whole grain products, legumes, nuts, seeds, fruits, and vegetables.

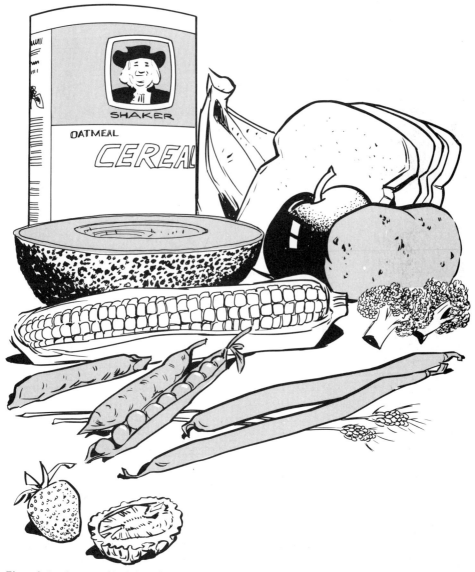

Figure 3-4.   Sources of high fiber foods.

Key Points: Cellulose

I.   Cellulose is a nondigestible plant fiber that increases bulk and water content of feces, thus influencing the stimulation of intestinal motility and the establishment of regular bowel movements.

II. *Epidemiological* studies have demonstrated an association between low fiber diets and the occurrence of such diseases as cancer of the colon and rectum, hemorrhoids, and diverticulosis.

III. Good selections of fiber-containing foods can be made from whole grain products, legumes, nuts, seeds, fruits, and vegetables.

Questions: An Important Carbohydrate: Cellulose

1. Cellulose is a _____ carbohydrate.
   a. digestible
   b. nondigestible

2. Identify two actions of cellulose and other food fiber.

3. Choose the three food groups containing the greatest amounts of cellulose and other food fiber:
   a. meat and dairy products
   b. whole grain cereals
   c. fruit juices
   d. raw fruits and vegetables
   e. highly processed carbohydrate foods
   f. potatoes, peas, and beans

4. Which food source do you identify with food fiber?
   a. animal
   b. plant

5. Which health condition is *known* to be alleviated with the increased addition of dietary fiber?
   a. cancer of the colon
   b. constipation
   c. diverticulosis

6. The relationship of fiber to the prevention of such diseases as colon cancer, hemorrhoids, and diverticulosis, however reasonable, is best described as presently:
   a. hypothetical
   b. factual

Answers: An Important Carbohydrate: Cellulose

1. b
2. a. provides bulk which increases intestinal motility.
   b. draws fluid into the intestine which eases movement of intestinal bulk.
3. b, d, f
4. b
5. b
6. a

BLOOD GLUCOSE LEVELS

Blood glucose levels are indicators of various body conditions. Normal blood glucose levels range between approximately 70 to 120 mg per 100 mL of blood. Normal fluctuations within this range occur daily within all persons. Toward the lower range of normal (near 70 mg/100 mL), you probably begin to experience the sensations of hunger. Shortly after eating a rise in blood sugar levels begins. The beta cells of the pancreas respond to this rise by secreting the hormone insulin. Insulin causes the liver, muscle, and fat cells to increase their uptake of the sugar from the blood thereby again reducing the blood sugar level to within the normal range. The glucose absorbed is converted to glycogen or fat, or used for energy according to body needs.

Irregularities can occur in the above system of blood sugar level maintenance. *Hyperglycemia* is the term used to describe the blood glucose level when it is above the upper limits of the normal range. The normal body response is to produce insulin and effect the lowering of blood glucose levels. However, in the disease diabetes mellitus not enough insulin activity occurs (either through lowered production, unavailability, or inactive form) to cause the adequate uptake of glucose from the blood. Consequently, blood sugar levels stay high and hyperglycemia occurs. The glucose tolerance test is used as a diagnostic tool for diabetes. An abnormal diabetic response to this test shows blood glucose levels still very high four to five hours after a measured amount of glucose is consumed. This is why supplementary insulin is given to many diabetic individuals in an effort to control their blood sugar levels.

Blood sugar levels may also fall too low. If you do not respond to the sensation of hunger by eating, then your blood sugar level drops below normal as blood glucose and glycogen stores are depleted. *Hypoglycemia* is the term used to describe blood sugar levels below normal. Hypoglycemia produces symptoms of weakness, dizziness, hunger, trembling, and mental confusion. If blood sugar levels fall very low convulsions and unconsciousness may even occur.[7] This can happen to a diabetic individual when he or she has taken too much insulin. This person needs a ready supply of simple carbohydrate to take when hypoglycemia occurs. A glucose tolerance test is necessary to identify a true hypo-

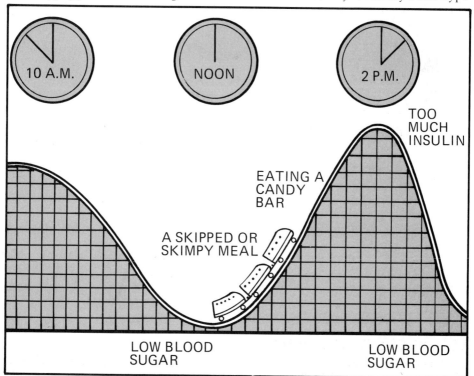

Figure 3-5.   Roller coaster effect of blood sugar levels.

glycemic condition.

Normally, when hypoglycemia occurs the glycogen reserves in the liver are converted back to glucose and released into the blood in an attempt to raise the blood sugar level back into the normal range. Liver glycogen converts to glucose directly and can enter the bloodstream quickly. Muscle glycogen can only be used to produce energy. However, the lactic acid produced when muscle glycogen is used as an energy source is returned to the liver and converted into pyruvic acid which may be used to form additional glucose. This glucose can be released into the blood (Cori Cycle). The hormone glucagon secreted by the alpha cells of the pancreas promotes the conversion of glycogen to glucose, especially that of the glycogen in liver. In this way the body attempts to provide a back-up system for the regulation of the blood sugar level.

However, some people have a roller coaster pattern of response with their blood glucose levels. This seems to occur when high carbohydrate foods, especially those of simple sugars, are frequently consumed as a response to hunger. If a concentrated sweet, such as candy or soda, is eaten in order to quickly relieve the symptoms of hypoglycemia the large amount of glucose from this snack is rapidly absorbed into the bloodstream. There is an over-reaction by the beta cells of the pancreas and too much insulin is produced. So much glucose is removed from the blood as a result of excess insulin that hypoglycemia recurs. This cycle may repeat itself several times throughout the day producing highs and lows in such an individual's feeling of physical well-being and emotional behavior. A better snack choice for a person with this response would be a protein or complex carbohydrate food such as peanut butter and crackers. *The best diet therapy for persons especially sensitive to changes in blood sugar levels is the development of regular, balanced meal habits.*

Key Points: Blood Glucose Levels

I. Important nomenclature regarding blood glucose:
    hyper = excess
    hypo = too little
    glycemia = glucose in the blood

II. Normal blood glucose levels range between 70 to 120 mg per 100 mL of blood.

III. Blood glucose levels are influenced by a variety of factors, some of which are:
    A. Effective insulin production (lowers blood glucose level)
    B. Glucagon production (raises blood glucose level)
    C. Rapid absorption of simple sugars (raises blood glucose level).
    D. Increased exercise which utilizes muscle glycogen and blood glucose (lowers blood glucose level).

IV. A glucose tolerance test is necessary to confirm a diagnosis of diabetes mellitus or reactive hypoglycemia.

V. Persons especially sensitive to changes in blood glucose levels need to develop regular, balanced meal habits and to choose snacks containing a minimum of simple sugars.

Questions: Blood Glucose Levels

1. Which of the following represent blood sugar levels within the normal range:
    a. 30-60 mg per 100 mL
    b. 70-120 mg per 100 mL
    c. 140-160 mg per 100 mL

2. Insulin is secreted by the:
    a. alpha cells of the pancreas
    b. beta cells of the pancreas
    c. alpha and beta cells of the pancreas

3. Match the phrases on the right to the terms on the left which they best describe:
    _____ 1. insulin
    _____ 2. hyperglycemia
    _____ 3. glycemia
    _____ 4. hypoglycemia
    _____ 5. glucagon

    a. hormone which causes the release of glucose into the blood
    b. means glucose in the blood
    c. means low blood glucose levels
    d. means high blood glucose levels
    e. hormone which effects the take-up of glucose from the blood into various body cells

4. The lack of effective insulin production results in what disease?
5. Why are complex carbohydrate or protein foods good snack choices for the hypo-glycemic person?
6. Which of the following graphs most accurately represents:

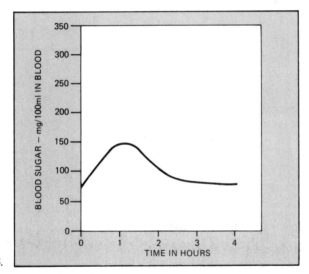

Figure 3-6.

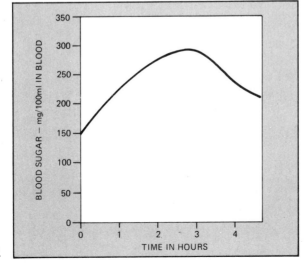

Figure 3-7.

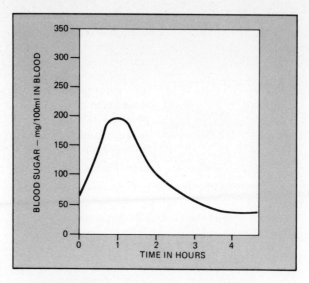

Figure 3-8.

   a.   a diabetic response to a glucose tolerance test?
   b.   normal response to a glucose tolerance test?
   c.   a hypoglycemic response to a glucose tolerance test?

7.   Normally, only glucose can be used by the brain as an energy source. This glucose is carried to the brain by the blood. With this information, can you explain the basis for some of the symptoms of hypoglycemia?

Answers: Blood Glucose Levels

1.   b
2.   b
3.   1. e
      2. d
      3. b
      4. c
      5. a
4.   diabetes mellitus
5.   Because there is no rapid absorption and release of glucose into the blood system to cause an over-production of insulin with a resulting hypoglycemic reaction.
6.   a.   Figure 3-7
      b.   Figure 3-6
      c.   Figure 3-8
7.   With a sharply decreased blood glucose supply the brain cannot function properly resulting in trembling, dizziness, mental confusion, and possibly even convulsions and unconsciousness.

DENTAL HEALTH AND CARBOHYDRATE INTAKE

Dental caries is one health problem affecting millions of persons which is generally agreed upon by nutritionists, dentists, and scientists to be diet related. *A causative relationship has been shown between the intake of certain types of high carbohydrate foods and in the increased incidence of dental caries, as well as between the frequency of such intake and the increased incidence of dental caries.* Dental caries, or tooth decay, is the result of the dissolving of surface tooth enamel and the subsequent erosion into the softer dentin layer, even to the pulp, which contains blood vessels and nerves. Inflammation of the pulp area leads to the familiar toothache.

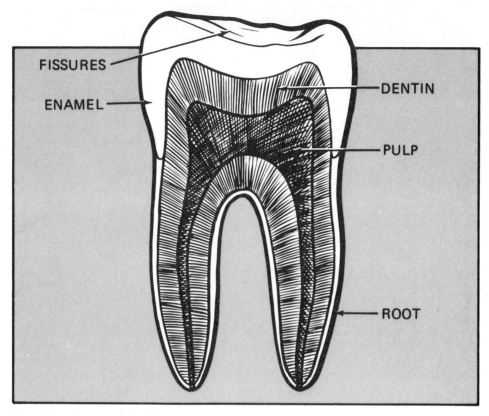

Figure 3-9.   Diagram of a tooth.

There are three factors which interact together to produce tooth decay:

1.   The host which is the tooth itself
2.   The agent which is the oral microflora (bacteria found within the mouth)
3.   The substrate which is the diet.[9]

Various conditions regarding any one or all of these factors can greatly enhance the possibility of caries development. The health and action of the salivary glands also play an important role in dental health.

Some individuals may have a genetic predisposition to caries susceptibility. However, the host or tooth may be more susceptible to caries development if the individual was malnourished during tooth formation. This implies the need for good maternal nutritional habits during pregnancy since teeth are formed in utero, although they do not normally begin to erupt until several months after birth.

Numerous nutrients are needed for healthy tooth formation. Vitamins A, D, and C are necessary as well as the minerals calcium and phosphorous along with other trace minerals and nutrients. The mineral fluoride exhibits special abilities to protect the teeth against dental caries by increasing enamel hardness and decreasing enamel solubility. Fluoridation of public water supplies to levels of one part per million (1 ppm, or 1 mg per liter) has demonstrated under rigid scientific controls effective caries reducing benefits. Fluoridation has been shown to be medically safe and economically reasonable. Fluoride is never absorbed in great amounts—but it's greatest absorption occurs during tooth formation. However, even mature teeth are capable of taking up some fluoride from food and fluids in the mouth.[10]

Active bacteria located in the mouth harbor in large numbers within dental plaque, a complex, gelatinous material. These bacteria have the ability to convert certain carbohydrates to a sticky adhesive material which aids in holding the plaque to the teeth. These bacteria also convert carbohydrates to various acids of which lactic acid is predominant. This acid is largely responsible for the dissolution of tooth enamel leading to tooth decay.[11]

The substrate or nutrient environment is important to the action of the plaque bacteria. It appears that sucrose, table sugar, is especially implicated as a caries producing nutrient. It is not only the amount of sugar which is detrimental, however, but also the frequency of its consumption. Lactic acid production occurs with carbohydrate consumption. If this consumption is frequent then the length of time the teeth are exposed to the lactic acid is increased. Thus, the possibility of tooth enamel erosion is increased.

Especially potent in caries formation are the sticky carbohydrate foods such as sweetened pastries, caramels or other chewy candies, jelly, cake with icing, and even dried fruits.[12] The clinging nature of these foods causes increased adhesion to the teeth. Though not providing a direct source of sugar, starchy foods create an additional unique set of problems associated with tooth decay. *Starchy foods stick between the teeth and in the fissures of molars where they can trap bacteria and absorb other sugars which are taken into the mouth.* Brushing the teeth after meals and snacks is effective in removing much of the food particles and plaque from the mouth, as is the use of dental floss or tape and even toothpicks. The simple rinsing of the mouth with water when other tools are not available may be helpful in reducing plaque formation and exposure of the teeth to the otherwise accumulating lactic acid.

Some foods are helpful in reducing adhesion of food particles and plaque to the teeth. *Fat can reduce the clinging ability of some foods.* The addition of butter, margarine, sour cream and cheeses on bread, potatoes, rice, pasta, and crackers can reduce the cariogenic (caries-producing) properties of these carbohydrate foods. Fresh fruits and vegetables may help to cleanse the teeth through the possible abrasive action of food fibers.

Saliva also has a protective influence against caries formation. Besides diluting the food contents in the mouth, *saliva contains buffers* which can reduce the acid level *as well as minerals* necessary for tooth maintenance.[13] People who have experienced a loss of their salivary gland function are soon plagued by general tooth decay.

One problem unique to inducing dental caries at the infant and toddler ages is the use of a nap or nighttime feeding bottle containing milk, juice, or water with a sweetener such as honey. These fluids contain carbohydrates. When they are used in a sleeptime bottle, the carbohydrate accumulates around the teeth and remains for a long time during a period of reduced saliva production. This bottle habit frequently leads to the decay of upper front and back teeth.[14] Such decay of first teeth can lead to negative effects on the health of the second, permanent teeth.

Good diet habits along with maintenance of healthy oral hygiene will undoubtedly assist most individuals in reducing the incidence of dental caries. Choosing snack foods low in carbohydrates and reducing the frequency of eating times will also aid the maintenance of healthy teeth. (Refer to Table 3-1 for a list of some foods and their "hidden sugar" content.) In view of the high cost of dental repair, it makes sense to cleanse the mouth frequently as advised, choose foods wisely, and to have dental check-ups regularly. Following such a dental health care plan can possibly help avoid the development of dental caries or at least allow for the early detection and treatment of dental caries in order to avoid more costly and painful problems later.

Key Points: Dental Health and Carbohydrate Intake

I.   Development of dental caries is a diet related problem. Causative relationships have been demonstrated between the *type* of carbohydrate intake and the *frequency* of such carbohydrate intake.

II.   Lactic acid is largely responsible for the dissolution of tooth enamel leading to tooth decay. Lactic acid is produced by the microflora in dental plaque from nutrients ingested, especially simple sugars.

III.   Fluoride exerts protective abilities against the development of dental caries by increasing tooth enamel hardness and decreasing tooth enamel solubility.

IV.   Especially potent cariogenic foods are sticky carbohydrates and those containing sucrose, table sugar.

V.   Use of sleeptime feeding bottles filled with carbohydrate-containing fluids such as milk, juice, or sweetened water increases the incidence of dental caries involving upper front and back teeth of infants and toddlers.

VI.   Oral hygiene techniques helpful in reducing the incidence of tooth decay are the use of dental floss, dental tape, toothbrush, and/or toothpicks. Other techniques which may be helpful include rinsing the mouth with water following ingestion of food and the chewing of fresh fruits and vegetables high in fiber content and coarse in texture.

VII.   General recommendations for reducing the incidence of dental caries include:
   A.   practice of healthy oral hygiene
   B.   reduction in frequency of eating times
   C.   reduction in intake of carbohydrate-containing foods, especially simple sugars and sticky sweets and fruits.

Questions: Dental Health and Carbohydrate Intake

1.   The two general causative factors for dental caries which are diet related are summarized as (1.) consumption of certain types of carbohydrates, and (2.) _____ .

2.   The dissolving of tooth enamel by acids leads to _____ .

3.   The following are the three factors which interact together to produce tooth decay: the host, the agent, and the substrate. Match the appropriate items on the right to the term on the left which they best describe.

   _____ 1.   host   a.   saliva
   _____ 2.   agent   b.   diet
   _____ 3.   substrate   c.   enamel
                                          d.   oral microflora
                                          e.   tooth

4. Tooth buds are formed:
   a.   before birth (in utero)
   b.   after birth

5.   Match the phrases on the right to the most appropriate term on the left.

   _____ 1.   fluoride   a.   vitamins necessary for proper tooth de-
   _____ 2.   plaque   velopment
   _____ 3.   oral microflora   b.   harbor within plaque and produce lac-
   _____ 4.   calcium and phos-   tic acid
               phorous   c.   a gelatinous material containing active
   _____ 5.   A, D, C   bacteria
   _____ 6.   cariogenic   d.   increases enamel hardness
                                          e.   major minerals necessary for tooth
                                                formation
                                          f.   means "caries-producing"

6.   List the following from the greatest to the least according to known cariogenic properties:

a. starch
b. sucrose
c. fat

7. Complete the following:
   The longer teeth are exposed to lactic acid the greater the possibility of
   _____ .

8. Patients who undergo irradiation therapy frequently experience a reduction or stoppage of salivary gland functions. What is the dental consequence of this condition?

9. Milk left in the mouth for long periods of time can induce tooth decay in small children, especially in the upper front and back teeth. How can this type of tooth decay be reduced or eliminated?

10. Match the phrases on the right to the terms on the left which they most correctly describe:

    _____ 1. pulp   a. the softer, inner layer of the tooth
    _____ 2. dentin   b. the hard, outer layer of the tooth
    _____ 3. enamel   c. portion of tooth below the gum line
    _____ 4. fissures   d. contains blood vessels and nerves for
    _____ 5. root   the tooth
                               e. dental surface cracks where starches
                                  can accumulate and trap bacteria

11. Choose from the items below the snacks which are the least caries-producing:

    a. plain popcorn   g. dill pickles
    b. taffy   h. hard cooked eggs
    c. apple   i. candy-coated nuts
    d. noodles with butter   j. raisins
    e. sweetened soft drinks   k. celery sticks
    f. sherbet   l. caramel popcorn

12. Identify four simple oral hygiene techniques thought to be helpful in preventing or reducing the incidence of tooth decay.

Answers: Dental Health and Carbohydrate Intake

1. frequency of such carbohydrate consumption
2. tooth decay
3. 1. e
   2. d
   3. b
4. a
5. 1. d
   2. c
   3. b
   4. e
   5. a
   6. f
6. b, then a, then c
7. tooth enamel erosion
8. greatly increased incidence of dental caries
9. by eliminating sleeptime bottles of milk or any sweetened fluid
10. 1. d
    2. a

3. b
4. e
5. c
11. a, c, d, g, h, k
12. 1. use of toothpicks
      2. use of dental floss or tape
      3. use of toothbrush
      4. rinsing the mouth with water after eating

LACTOSE INTOLERANCE

Some persons have an inability to produce sufficient lactase, the enzyme necessary to digest (break down) the sugar in milk, lactose. There are three types of lactase deficiency:

1. Congenital lactose intolerance which is the absence of lactase from birth. This is a relatively rare condition.

2. Secondary lactose intolerance which is frequently experienced as a consequence of intestinal disease, surgery upon infants, surgery for gastric disorders, and malnutrition.

3. Primary lactose intolerance which is the gradual decline in lactase activity in susceptible individuals as they grow older.[15] This is the most common form of lactose intolerance.

Lactase breaks down lactose into the monosaccharides glucose and galactose. This breakdown must occur *before* absorption from the intestines can take place. Consequently, when lactase is deficient the lactose cannot be broken down or absorbed. This condition is termed lactose intolerance and produces symptoms of bloating, abdominal discomfort, nausea, vomiting and explosive, acidic diarrhea following the ingestion of lactose.[16] The lactose remains undigested in the intestines, causes water to be drawn into the intestines by osmotic action, and ferments due to the action of the bacteria in the colon producing the symptoms of lactose intolerance.

Decreased lactase production is the most common form of lactose intolerance and seems to have a direct relationship to age and ethnic origin. Incidence of lactose intolerance is higher for American Negroes, Orientals, Southern Europeans, and African populations.[17]

The best diet therapy is to remove milk from the diet to the degree necessary to relieve symptoms. Infants who are lactose intolerant must be placed on a milk-free formula such as a soy-based formula. Other persons who are lactose intolerant may be helped by consuming milk and milk products in which the lactose has already been fermented to lactic acid such as cultured buttermilk, yogurt, and acidophilus milk. Many children and adults may benefit from moderate milk consumption, even if they are lactose intolerant due to low lactase levels.[18]

Table 3-2.   Comparison of nutrients in human and cow's milk.

Nutrient	Human	Cow's (Whole, 3.3% Fat)
	100g	100g
Kcal	77	61
Protein (g)	1.1	3.3
Fat (g)	4.0	3.3

Table 3-2.   Comparison of nutrients in human and cow's milk (continued).

Nutrient	Human	Cow's (Whole, 3.3% Fat)
	100g	100g
Carbohydrates (g)	9.5	4.7
Calcium (mg)	33	119
Phosphorus (mg)	14	89
Iron (mg)	0.1	Trace
Sodium (mg)	16	50
Potassium (mg)	51	152
Vitamin A (I.U.)	240	126
Thiamin (mg)	0.01	0.03
Riboflavin (mg)	0.04	0.17
Niacin (mg)	0.2	0.08
Ascorbic acid (mg)	5	0.82

From: Bowes and Church's Food Values of Portions Commonly Used, 13th edition. Revised by Pennington JAT and Church HN, Philadelphia, J. B. Lippincott Company, 1980

Key Points: Lactose Intolerance

I.   Lactose intolerance occurs when an individual is unable to produce sufficient active lactase to digest the sugar in milk, lactose.

II.   Breakdown of lactose into its monosaccharide components of glucose and galactose must occur *before* absorption from the intestine can take place. Therefore, a deficiency in lactase results in the malabsorption of lactose, the sugar in milk.

III.   The most common form of lactose intolerance is the decrease in lactase production that occurs in some individuals with increased age.

IV.   Ethnic origin is also associated with the occurrence of lactose intolerance; incidence of lactose intolerance is increased for American Negroes, Orientals, Southern Europeans, and African populations.

V.   Infants who are lactose intolerant must be placed on a milk-free diet; adults and older children are benefited by milk intake as tolerated.

Questions: Lactose Intolerance

1.   Which is the most common form of lactose intolerance?
    a.   inherited lactase deficiency
    b.   secondary low lactase activity
    c.   primary low lactase activity

2.   The symptoms of lactose intolerance including bloating, nausea, abdominal discomfort, and explosive diarrhea are created by what conditions?

3.   Choose from the following list those milk products which may be best tolerated by the lactose intolerant individual:
    a.   cheddar cheese
    b.   skim milk
    c.   buttermilk
    d.   ice cream

e.   yogurt
f.   acidophilus milk

4.   Refer to Table 3-2. Would breast feeding an infant prevent the occurrence of symptoms for an infant with inherited lactase deficiency?

5.   What is the best diet therapy for a middle-aged man with primary low lactase activity?
a.   Remove all milk and milk products from his diet.
b.   Allow only fermented milk products in the diet.
c.   Allow milk and milk products as tolerated without distressful symptoms.

6.   What is the best diet therapy for a newborn infant with inherited lactase deficiency?
a.   goat milk formula
b.   milk-free formula
c.   human breast milk

Answers: Lactose Intolerance

1.   c
2.   fermentation of the lactose by intestinal bacteria; and water drawn into the intestine by osmotic action
3.   a, c, e, f
4.   No, human milk is even more concentrated in lactose than is cow's milk which is most frequently used for infant feeding formulas.
5.   c
6.   b

REFERENCES

[1] Salivary amylase was formerly called ptyalin.

[2] Krause MV and Mahan LK: Food Nutrition and Diet Therapy. Philadelphia, W. B. Saunders Company, 1979, pp. 41 and 44

[3] Friend B: Nutrients in US food supply. American Journal of Clinical Nutrition, 20, 1967, p. 908

[4] Hama MY: "Household Food Consumption, 1977 and 1965." Family Economics Review, Spring, 1980, p. 9.

[5] **Epidemiological studies** are those which examine the factors influencing the frequency and distribution of disease within a population.

[6] Nutrition, diet and cancer. Dairy Council Digest, 46, September-October 1975, p. 29

[7] Weininger J and Briggs GM: Nutrition Update, 1976. Journal of Nutrition Education, 8, October-December 1976, p. 173

[8] A critique of low carbohydrate ketogenic weight reduction regimens. Journal of the American Medical Association, 224, June 4, 1973, pp. 1415-19

[9] Morhart RE and Fitzgerald RJ: Nutritional determinants of the ecology of the oral flora. Dental Clinics of North America, 20, July 1976, pp. 473-74

[10] An excellent discussion of fluoride and fluoridation is presented in the following article: Richmond VL: Health effects associated with water fluoridation. Journal of Nutrition Education, 11, April-June 1979, pp. 62-64
Various comments on that article which illustrate the political controversy over fluoridation are presented in:
Letters, Journal of Nutrition Education, 11, October-December 1979, pp. 162-68

[11] Brown AT: The role of dietary carbohydrates in plaque formation and oral disease. In Present Knowledge in Nutrition, 4th ed. New York and Washington, D.C.; The Nutri-

tion Foundation, Inc., 1976, p. 492

[12] Joseph L: Foods and drinks that will cause you the fewest cavities. Today's Health, October 1973, p. 27

[13] Enwonwu CO: Nutrition and dental health. Nutrition News, 39, February 1976, p. 4

[14] Skalka P: Solving the mystery of the decaying teeth. Today's Health, January 1974, p. 27

[15] Garza C and Scrimshaw NS: Relationship of lactose intolerance to milk intolerance in young children. American Journal of Clinical Nutrition, 29, February 1976, p. 192

[16] Kretchmer N: Lactose and lactase. Scientific American, 227, October 1972, p. 72

[17] Bayless TM: Disaccharidase deficiency. Journal of the American Dietetic Association, 60, June 1972, p. 479

[18] Perspective on milk intolerance. Dairy Council Digest, 49, November-December 1978, p. 31

4
LIPIDS

Lipids are the plant and animal substances which include fats, fatty acids, phospholipids, oils, waxes and steriods, such as cholesterol, vitamin D, and some hormones. Most lipids are oily, greasy to the touch, and insoluble in water, but they are usually soluble in alcohol, ether, benzene or chloroform. This chapter will focus on those lipids with properties of significant nutritional importance.

Fats are built from two major types of components: *glycerol* (an alcohol) and *fatty acids*. When an alcohol and an acid are chemically combined with the resultant removal of a molecule of water, a compound termed an *ester* is formed. *When glycerol combines with three fatty acids a triglyceride is formed.* Triglycerides are sometimes called simple lipids or neutral lipids. Most fatty acids in our diet contain 16 or 18 carbon atoms, although some contain more and those found in butterfat contain much less. Figure 4-1 shows the formation of a triglyceride which contains three long-chain fatty acids. Where each molecule of water is removed an ester linkage[1] results. See Figure 4-2. *When all the fatty acids are the same, the triglyceride is called a simple triglyceride.* See the example in Figure 4-2. *When each of the three fatty acids is different the triglyceride is called a mixed triglyceride.* See Figure 4-3. When the glycerol portion has only one or two fatty acids attached, a monoglyceride or diglyceride is formed, respectively. See Figures 4-4 and 4-5.

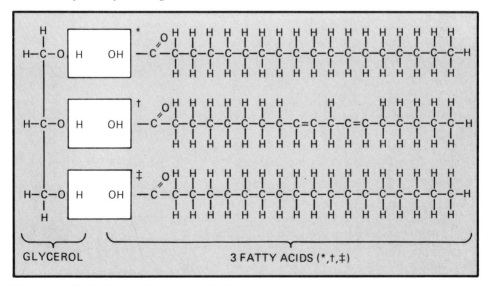

Figure 4-1. *H is hydrogen, C is carbon, and O is oxygen. As you can see, fatty acids and triglycerides contain relatively small amounts of oxygen compared to carbon and hydrogen. (* and ‡ are a stearic acid and † is linoleic fatty acid.)*

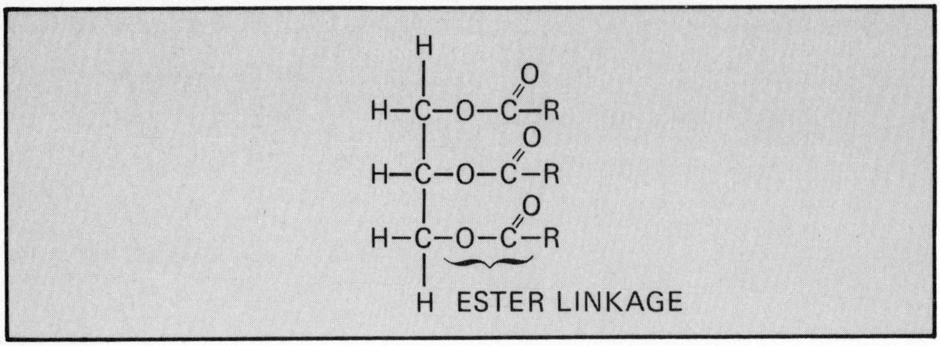

Figure 4-2. A simple triglyceride. R *represents the remainder of that molecule.*

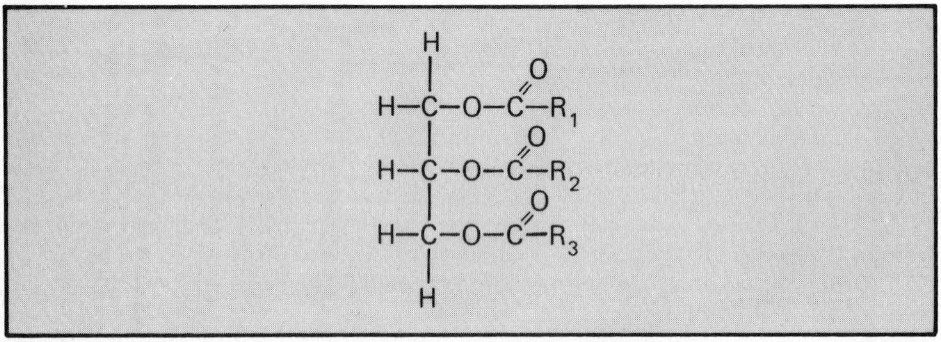

Figure 4-3. A mixed triglyceride. Each R factor represents a different fatty acid.

Unsaturated fats and saturated fats are terms which refer to the chemical form of the fatty acids. Fatty acids are chains of carbon atoms with hydrogen attached and with an acid group ($C-OH$) at one end. Carbon has a valence number of four which means up to four atoms may attach to a single carbon atom when carbon compounds are formed. *When all four bonding positions are filled the molecule is said to be saturated.* Sometimes a hydrogen atom may be missing in one bonding position in each of two adjacent carbon atoms within a fatty acid. In this case the two carbon atoms fill the vacant bonding positions between themselves forming a double bond. *When double bonding occurs the fatty acid is said to be unsaturated.* When two or more double bonds occur within one fatty acid, that fatty acid is said to be polyunsaturated.[2] See the middle fatty acid in Figure 4-1.

Hydrogenation is the process of adding hydrogen to the double bonds within the fatty acid, turning them into saturated fatty acids. Hydrogenation causes the solidification of liquid oils so they can be used as vegetable shortenings or margarine and reduces the possibility of their rancidity as well.

Rancidity is the development of foul odor and taste due to the breaking of the double bonds in unsaturated fatty acids through oxidation.

Rancidity usually occurs slowly by oxygenation to aged fats and oils exposed to air. Additives called antioxidants are added to commercially processed foods to reduce the occurrence of rancidity. Vitamin E occurs naturally in many plant oils which contain unsaturated fatty acids. Vitamin E acts as an antioxidant protecting the double bonds.

The length of the fatty acid chains and the degree of saturation affect the solidarity of a fat. Generally, the greater the degree of unsaturation and the shorter the fatty acid

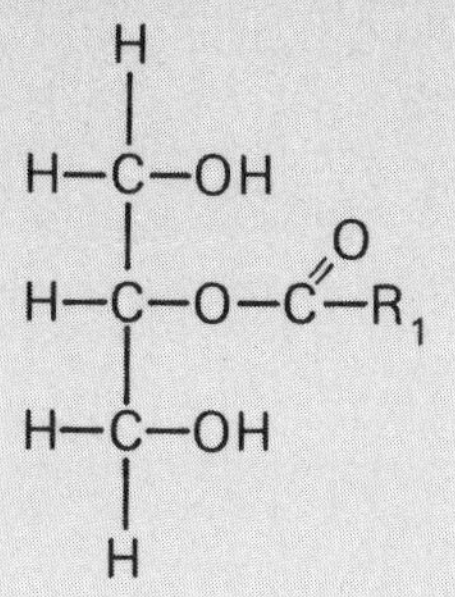

$$
\begin{array}{c}
\text{H} \\
| \\
\text{H--C--OH} \\
| \quad\quad \text{O} \\
\text{H--C--O--C--R}_1 \\
| \\
\text{H--C--OH} \\
| \\
\text{H}
\end{array}
$$

Figure 4-4. A monoglyceride.

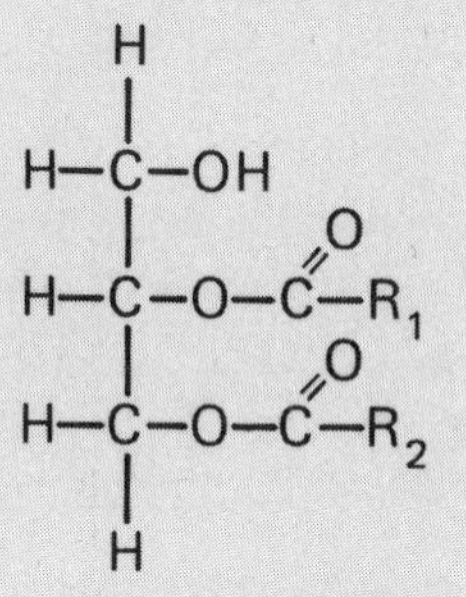

$$
\begin{array}{c}
\text{H} \\
| \\
\text{H--C--OH} \\
| \quad\quad \text{O} \\
\text{H--C--O--C--R}_1 \\
| \quad\quad \text{O} \\
\text{H--C--O--C--R}_2 \\
| \\
\text{H}
\end{array}
$$

Figure 4-5. A diglyceride.

chain length, the lower the melting point of the fat. However, most fats and oils are mixtures of different fatty acids and it is the predominance of one characteristic over another which determines the degree of solidarity and melting point in any one fat. Consequently, beef suet (hard fat), a relatively saturated fat with long-chain fatty acids, is solid at room temperature and vegetable oils which contain a large number of relatively long-chain, polyunsaturated fatty acids, are liquid at room temperature. Fish fats though polyunsaturated are composed of very long-chain fatty acids so they are somewhat firm at room temperature. Coconut oil is liquid at room temperature though it is saturated because it is composed of medium- and short-chain fatty acids.

Food fats are actually mixtures of both saturated and unsaturated fats. *A food fat is termed saturated or unsaturated according to the type of fatty acids which predominate in the fat.* A better way of expressing the degree of saturation is through the use of a ratio which gives the proportion of unsaturated fatty acids to saturated fatty acids. This is the P/S ratio. A P/S ratio of 2 to 1 would indicate a polyunsaturated fatty acid content twice that of saturated fatty acid content within one food fat source.

Linoleic acid, a fatty acid with 18 carbon atoms and two double bonds, is found predominately in seed oils. Linoleic acid cannot be produced in the body. However, our bodies are able to convert the linoleic acid which we consume in our diet to other necessary fatty acids, which are more difficult to obtain through our diet and are needed to prevent certain deficiency disease symptoms. *Consequently, linoleic acid is termed an essential fatty acid (EFA) as it must be supplied in our diet and is needed for proper body functioning.*

The phospholipids are similar to triglycerides in that they are composed of glycerol and two fatty acids. But they have a phosphorus-containing acid bonded to a nitrogen-containing compound in place of the third fatty acid. Lecithin is a phospholipid. *Phospholipids are good emulsifying agents*[3] *and aid in the absorption and transport of fatty acids in the body*. They are also important components of cell membranes. Phospholipids are especially abundant in brain and nerve cells.

The steroids are lipid-related compounds which have carbon atoms arranged in a basic ring structure. The steroids include sex hormones, bile acids, sterols, and vitamin D. The sterols contain a single alcohol group and are fat-soluble. Cholesterol is an important animal source sterol. See Figure 4-6 for the "picture" of cholesterol as well as the similar structure to cholic acid, a bile acid.

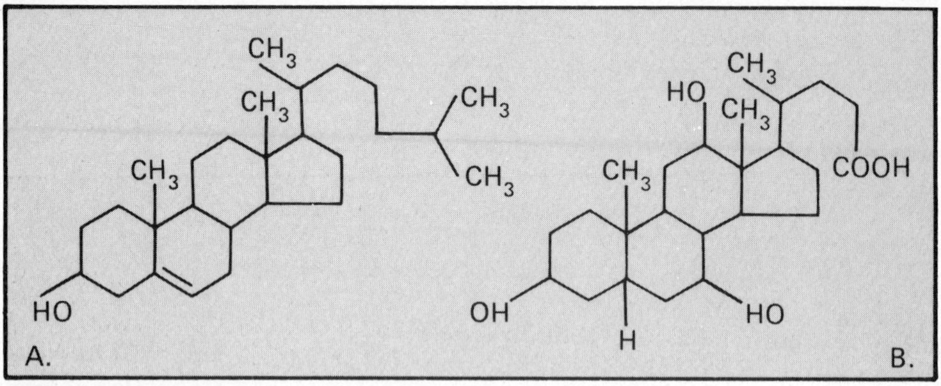

Figure 4-6.   A. Chemical structure of cholesterol.
B. Chemical structure of cholic acid, a principal bile acid.

Digestion, absorption, and metabolism of fats. The digestion of fat begins with its mechanical breakdown during mastication[4] and peristalsis[5] of the stomach. Fats do not mix with water and the contents of the intestine are water-based. *However, fats are emulsified by the bile salts which are produced by the liver*. Bile salts are held in storage by the gallbladder and are released when fat enters the intestine. The following section of this text is an amplification of the composition and functions of bile salts and some physiological complications involving bile salts. The emulsification of fats by bile salts allows for their more even disbursement throughout the intestinal contents (chyme) and their greater surface exposure to the action of *fat digestive enzymes, lipases.*

Lipases are released from the pancreas. The lipases hydrolyze the fats into glycerol, fatty acids, di-, and monoglycerides. The enzymatic hydrolysis of fats is essentially the reversal of the action of esterification presented in Figure 4-1. However, lipases generally hydrolyze one fatty acid at a time from the triglyceride molecule. The rate of hydrolysis of triglycerides is dependent upon the chain length of the fatty acids and their degree of saturation. Generally, the longer the chain length and the greater the degree of saturation the longer the rate of hydrolysis. Glycerol, unesterified acids (free fatty acids: FFA's) of short-and medium-chain length, and medium-chain triglycerides may be absorbed directly into the portal vein, complexed with albumin, and carried to the liver.[6]

Table 4-1.   Summary of factors affecting the absorption of fat.

Approximately 95 percent of dietary fats are absorbed. The following are factors which affect the absorption of fat:

1.   Increased motility of the gastrointestinal tract reduces absorption by reducing the time in which fat is in contact with the digestive juices and the absorbing area of the intestinal wall.
2.   Reduced amounts or absence of bile salts.

Table 4-1.   Summary of factors affecting the absorption of fat (continued).

---

3.   Reduced amounts or absence of the fat-splitting enzymes, lipases.
4.   Diseases of the pancreas which reduce its ability to form and release lipase.
5.   Reduction of the absorbing surfaces of the intestine due to disease conditions or as a consequence of surgery on the small intestine.
6.   Fatty acid chain length:
     Longer-chain fatty acids are not absorbed as well as shorter-chain fatty acids.
7.   Degree of saturation of fatty acids:
     Saturated fatty acids are not absorbed as well as unsaturated fatty acids.
8.   Intestinal calcium:
     Although optimal absorption of fat requires the presence of some calcium, high intestinal calcium levels reduce the absorption of fat.

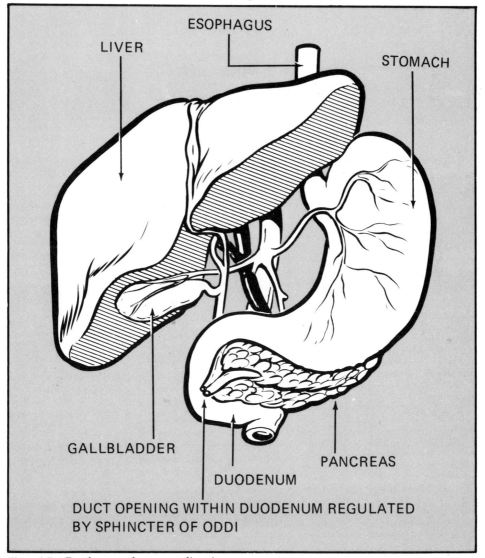

Figure 4-7.   Duodenum and accessory digestive organs.

The monoglycerides, diglycerides, and long-chain fatty acids remaining after lipase hydrolysis are taken to the intestinal mucosa as micellar complexes (bile salt plus lipid compounds). The bile salts separate from the lipids and the lipids are absorbed. It is here in the intestinal mucosa where the final products of fat digestion are formed: some fatty acids,

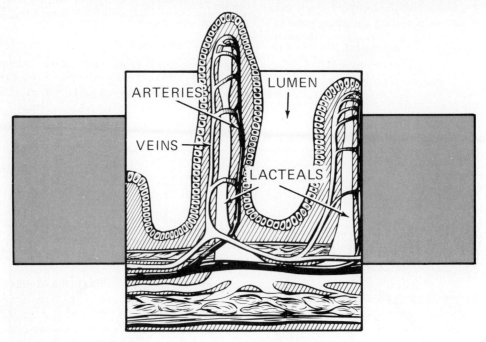

Figure 4-8.   Intestinal villi.

phospholipids, free cholesterol, cholesterol esters, and triglycerides. These end-products then combine with very small amounts of protein to form *chylomicrons*. It is this protein complex which enables the fat to be emulsified again in the watery solution of the blood and lymph systems and, thus, able to be further transported. *The chylomicrons are then absorbed into the lacteals* and are carried by the lymphatic system to the thoracic duct. The thoracic duct connects to a large vein which goes directly to the heart, finally emptying the chylomicrons into the blood system.

Lipoprotein lipase is the enzyme which hydrolyzes the triglycerides of chylomicrons. This enzyme quickly clears chylomicrons from the blood and is sometimes referred to as the *clearing factor*. Lipoprotein lipase is found especially in heart muscle and in the blood capillaries within adipose (fat) tissue. The tri-, di-, and monoglycerides and fatty acids at this point are available for utilization for energy needs, storage,[7] or synthesis into other lipid body compounds. The glycerol portion is carried back to the liver and is the only portion of fat which can be used to help form glucose.[8] This is a small though significant contribution to blood glucose since only about 10 percent of dietary fat is glycerol.[9] In addition, the 3-carbon glycerol molecule supplies only half of the carbon atoms needed to form a 6-carbon glucose molecule.

The lipid factions left after lipoprotein lipase hydrolysis not immediately stored or used for energy needs are carried to the liver.[10] In the liver they are resynthesized to triglycerides and combined with protein to form *lipoprotein complexes* necessary for body needs. Lipoproteins are relatively large aggregates and provide the main transport form of lipid substances in the blood. Plasma lipoproteins contain cholesterol, phospholipids, triglycerides, unesterified fatty acids, and traces of other related materials such as fat-soluble vitamins and the steroid hormones.[11]

Functions of fat. The functions of fat in the diet and the body are varied.

1. *The most important function of dietary fat is as an energy source.* Fats provide 9 kcal/gram. Therefore, fats contribute more than twice the calories per gram than do either carbohydrates or protein.

2. *Dietary fat facilitates the absorption of fat-soluble vitamins A, D, E, and K.*

3. *Fats in the diet increase satiety.*[12] This means, fat delays the feeling of hunger because it stimulates the production of the hormone *esterogastrone,* which slows down the motility of the intestine. Enterogastrone is produced by glandular cells in the duodenum, the portion of the small intestine that is located just after the stomach (see Figure 4-7).

4. *Fats contribute to the flavor, aroma, and palatability of foods.*

Body fat provides insulation against temperature variations and cushions many delicate organs against damage due to physical shock. Body fat is also the concentrated storage form of energy for body needs. The body seems to have an unlimited ability to store fat. All cells store some fat, and there are also specialized cells for storing fat. Fat tissue composed of the specialized fat storing cells is referred to as *adipose tissue.* Adipose tissue is a dynamically active tissue which continually and simultaneously undergoes fat build-up, breakdown, and resynthesis. Excess intake of carbohydrate and protein, as well as fat beyond body needs, is converted to and stored as body fat.

Consumption of fat. The current consumption of fat in American diets is slightly more than 40 percent.[13] This represents an increase of almost 30 percent since the turn of the century in our national fat intake. Sources of the largest increases in fat intake are edible fats and oils, ice cream, and red meat.[14] Many highly processed food products and so-called "fast foods" are especially high in fat content. Fat in foods is apparent when you can see the oil or hard animal fat, margarine, or butter. However, "hidden fats" are those which you cannot see but are present in foods such as milk, egg yolk, the marbeling in meats, and the oil in nuts. Consumers need to be aware of the fats and oils in food even though such fats are not visible.

As previously mentioned, fats increase the palatability of foods. A medium-sized baked potato contains approximately 100 kcal. One tablespoon of fat in the form of margarine or butter increases the favorable aroma and taste appeal of the baked potato but also increases the caloric value over 100 percent. Because of the high caloric value of fat, it is the single most effective nutrient to decrease in the diet when attempting to control the caloric level of the diet.

Key Points: Lipids

I.   Important nomenclature involved with the study of lipids:
antioxidants = compounds which delay or prevent oxidation
EFA = essential fatty acid: linoleic fatty acid
FFA = free (unesterified) fatty acid
ester = compound formed from an alcohol and acid
glyceride = glycerol + fatty acid
lipo = refers to fat
long-chain fatty acid = 14-26 carbon atoms
medium-chain fatty acid = 8-12 carbon atoms
micelles = bile salts + lipid compounds
short-chain fatty acid = six or less carbon atoms
P/S ratio = polyunsaturated to saturated fatty acid ratio

polyunsaturated = fatty acid containing two or more double bonds between its carbon atoms

saturated = fatty acid composed of carbon atoms with all four possible chemical combining positions filled with other carbon atoms or hydrogen atoms

sterol = lipid compounds of the sterol group having one alcohol group and their carbon atoms arranged in basic ring structures such as cholesterol.

II.   Glycerol esters:
   A.   Monoglyceride = glycerol + one fatty acid
   B.   Diglyceride = glycerol + two fatty acids
   C.   Triglyceride = glycerol + three fatty acids (also called neutral fats)
      1.   Simple triglyceride = glycerol + three identical fatty acids
      2.   Mixed triglyceride = glycerol + three different fatty acids
   D.   Phospholipids = glycerol + fatty acids + phosphoric acid + a nitrogen-containing compound. Phospholipids are good emulsifying agents.

III.   Digestion, Absorption, and Metabolism of Fats
   A.   Lipids must be emulsified in the intestine by bile salts produced in the liver and stored in the gallbladder.
   B.   Lipids are hydrolyzed in the intestine by lipases, fat-splitting enzymes, produced by the pancreas.
   C.   Glycerol, short-, medium-chain FFA's, and triglycerides do not form micelles; are hydrolyzed by intestinal lipase; complexed with albumin for blood transport. Are absorbed into the portal vein and carried directly to the liver.
   D.   Monoglycerides, diglycerides, and long-chain fatty acids and triglycerides are carried to the intestinal mucosa as micellular complexes.
      1.   Bile salts split off; travel to ileum; absorb into portal blood.
      2.   Lipids absorbed; recombined to triglycerides; complex with protein forming chylomicrons; absorbed into lymph system.
      3.   Lipoprotein lipase (the clearing factor) hydrolyzes triglycerides of chylomicrons in different tissues, especially adipose tissue.
      4.   Fatty acids are then used for energy or carried with glycerol to the liver to form lipoprotein complexes.

IV.   Function of Fat
   A.   Dietary fat is an important source of energy; facilitator for absorption of the fat-soluble vitamins A, D, E, and K; contributor to the feeling of satiety; and contributor to the flavor, aroma, and palatability of foods.
   B.   Body fat (adipose tissue) insulates the body against temperature variations, cushions body organs, and provides a storage form for an energy source.

V.   American diets consist of over 40 percent fat. Some fats are readily visible such as butter or margarine and some fats are "hidden" such as those in egg yolk and the marbling in meat.

VI.   Fat contributes 9 kcal/gram, more than twice the kcal contributed per gram than either carbohydrates or protein.

Questions: Lipids

1.   Lipids form the group of plant and animal substances which includes
   _____ , _____ , _____ , _____ ,
   _____ , and _____ .
2.   Lipids are insoluble in _____ .
3.   Match the phrases on the right to the terms on the left which they best describe:
   _____ 1.   an ester   a.   all carbon atom bonding positions are
   _____ 2.   an alcohol   filled

      _____ 3. saturated
      _____ 4. polyunsaturated
      _____ 5. triglyceride
      _____ 6. hydrogenation
      _____ 7. rancidity

b. solidifies oils such as those for use as margarine
c. glycerol
d. an alcohol + an acid
e. two or more double bonds
f. oxidation of double bonds in fats and oils
g. glycerol + three fatty acids

4. Identify the following chemical configurations:

a.

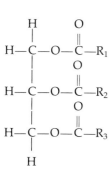

b.

$$H-\underset{|}{\overset{H}{C}}-OH$$
$$H-\underset{|}{C}-O-\overset{O}{\overset{||}{C}}-R_1$$
$$H-\underset{|}{\overset{|}{C}}-OH$$
$$H$$

c.

$$H-\underset{|}{\overset{H}{C}}-OH$$
$$H-\underset{|}{C}-O-\overset{O}{\overset{||}{C}}-R_1$$
$$H-\underset{|}{C}-O-\overset{O}{\overset{||}{C}}-R_2$$
$$H$$

d.

$$H-\underset{|}{\overset{H}{C}}-O-\overset{O}{\overset{||}{C}}-R_1$$
$$H-\underset{|}{C}-O-\overset{O}{\overset{||}{C}}-R_1$$
$$H-\underset{|}{C}-O-\overset{O}{\overset{||}{C}}-R_1$$
$$H$$

5. A fat with a large percentage of highly saturated, long-chain fatty acids would probably be solid at room temperature.
    a. True
    b. False

6. A fat with a large percentage of polyunsaturated, medium-chain fatty acids would probably be _____ at room temperature.
    a. solid
    b. liquid

7. A P/S ratio of 1.5:1 states:
    a. the percent of polyunsaturated fat to saturated fat is 50 percent
    b. the percent of polyunsaturated fat to saturated fat is 15 percent
    c. the percent of polyunsaturated fat to saturated fat is 150 percent

8. A certain type of dermatitis involving red and irritated skin in infants is symptomatic of a deficiency of arachidonic fatty acid.
    a. What essential nutrient needs to be added to the infant's diet to alleviate this dermatitis?
    b. Why?

9. What are the important functions of phospholipids?

10. What is the structural difference between a sterol molecule and other lipid molecules?
    a. it is polyunsaturated
    b. it is formed in a ring instead of chains or branches
    c. it is saturated

11. What substances emulsify fats in the intestines?

12. The fat-splitting enzymes are:
    a. bile salts
    b. fatty acids
    c. lipases

13. Lipases are secreted by the:
    a. gallbladder
    b. liver
    c. pancreas

14. What chemical reaction is essentially the reversal of esterification of glycerol and fatty acids?

15. The shorter the chain length and the greater the degree of unsaturation, the longer the rate of hydrolysis of fatty acids.
    a. True
    b. False

16. The following questions refer to the sequences involved in fat absorption:
    a. How is fat emulsified by bile salts within the watery intestinal contents?
    b. At what location are bile salts released from the lipid molecule within the intestine?
    c. What path do bile salts take for reabsorption into the body? What path do the newly formed chylomicrons take?

17. Glycerol, unesterified fatty acids (free fatty acids) of short- and medium-chain length, and medium-chain triglycerides are absorbed into the portal blood system and carried to the liver.
    a. With what substance are they complexed to for blood transport?
    b. Into what form are the remaining fats complexed for transportation?

18. Match the phrases on the right to the items on the left which they best describe:

    _____ 1. thoracic duct
    _____ 2. lipoprotein
    _____ 3. chylomicrons
    _____ 4. gluconeogenesis
    _____ 5. lipoprotein lipase

    a. formation of glucose from noncarbohydrate sources such as glycerol released during lipid hydrolysis
    b. clearing factor
    c. entrance place of the chylomicrons of the lymph system into the blood system
    d. long-chain triglycerides
    e. give a milky appearance to blood after a fat-rich meal

19. How many kcal does 35 grams of fat supply?
    a. 140
    b. 245
    c. 315

20. Which meal provides the greatest satiety? Why?
    a. apple juice, toast with jelly, two poached eggs, coffee
    b. cereal with skim milk and sliced bananas, grape juice

c. orange juice, toast with peanut butter, two eggs scrambled in one tablespoon margarine

21. What hormone is produced by cells in the intestinal wall upon stimulation by the presence of fat in the duodenum and then causes the slowing of intestinal motility?

22. Identify three functions of body fat.

23. Fat tissue is referred to as _____ tissue.

24. Which foods contain hidden fat?

a.	lard	f.	cheese
b.	egg yolk	g.	bacon
c.	whole milk	h.	olives
d.	butter	i.	pastry crust
e.	coconut	j.	peanut butter

25. One teaspoon of fat weighs approximately five grams. Three teaspoons equal one tablespoon. How many calories does one tablespoon of margarine contain?

26. Which conditions delay or interfere with fat absorption (refer to Table 4-1)?
  a. diarrhea
  b. small amounts of calcium in the intestine
  c. blockage of the ducts or disease of the gallbladder or pancreas
  d. consumption of salad dressing made with polyunsaturated oil
  e. consumption of heavily larded beef

27. A 2000 kcal daily diet containing 42 percent fat provides how many grams of fat?

Answers: Lipids

1. fats, fatty acids, phospholipids, oils, waxes, steroids
2. water
3. 1. d
    2. c
    3. a
    4. e
    5. g
    6. b
    7. f
4. a. mixed triglyceride
    b. monoglyceride
    c. diglyceride
    d. simple triglyceride
5. a
6. b
7. c
8. a. linoleic acid
    b. the infant can manufacture arachidonic acid from linoleic acid within his or her body
9. as emulsifying agents; aiding and transporting fatty acids in the body; components of cell membranes
10. b
11. bile salts
12. c
13. c
14. enzymatic hydrolysis of fat (glycerides)

15. b
16. a. By formation of micelle complexes in the intestine.
     b. At the intestinal mucosa.
     c. Bile salts enter the blood stream and transfer to the liver by way of the portal
         blood system; chylomicrons enter the lacteals of the lymph system.
17. a. the protein albumin
     b. chylomicrons
18. 1. c
     2. d
     3. e
     4. a
     5. b
19. c
20. c (#c meal contains some dietary fat)
21. enterogastrone
22. cushions body organs; provides a concentrated storage form of energy; insulates
     the body against temperature changes
23. adipose
24. b, c, e, f, h, i, j
25. 5 grams × 3 teaspoons = 15 grams × 9 kcal/gram = 135 kcal
26. a, c, e
27. 2000 kcal × .42 = 840 kcal from fat
     840 kcal ÷ 9 kcal/g = 93.3 g

BILE SALTS AND SOME MALFUNCTIONS INVOLVING LIPID DIGESTION AND ABSORPTION

Bile is composed of water and other compounds including bile acids and salts, phospholipids, cholesterol, and bile pigments. Bile is formed in the liver then drained into the gallbladder and concentrated and stored. Salts are formed in the liver from cholesterol but the main portion are products of reabsorption and recirculation in an efficient and conservative system termed the *enterohepatic circulation.*

When fats enter the duodenum they stimulate the secretion of *cholecystokinin* into the bloodstream from glands located in the walls of the intestine. When this hormone reaches the gallbladder it stimulates that organ to contract. Contraction of the gallbladder forces its bile contents into the duodenum. It also helps to initiate the relaxation of the sphincter of Oddi which is at the base of the common bile duct. This sphincter assists in the regulation of bile flow into the duodenum. Here the alkaline bile neutralizes the acid chyme[15] from the stomach and the bile salts perform their important function of fat emulsification.

Emulsification of fat occurs because the bile salts form a shell around individual tiny lipid droplets in chyme. *This bile salt-lipid complex is called a micelle.* One end of a bile salt molecule has an affinity or attraction for lipids and one end has an affinity for water. The fat-loving end associates with the oil droplet and the water-loving end extends into the water-based solution. Thus, the micelles enable lipids to become dispersed and suspended in a watery medium (see Figure 4-9). Bile salts also lower the surface tension of the finely dispersed and suspended fat globules which allows easier penetration by fat-splitting enzymes, lipases.[16]

Bile provides the alkaline environment necessary to activate the lipases secreted by the pancreas. Lipases, and other contents of the pancreas, and bile from the gallbladder are secreted simultaneously into the intestine and mixed with the chyme.[17] *Secretin,* a hormone produced by certain intestinal cells of the duodenum, is released into the bloodstream when acid chyme enters the duodenum. Upon reaching the pancreas, secretin stimulates that organ into secreting its enzymes and alkaline fluid into the intestine.

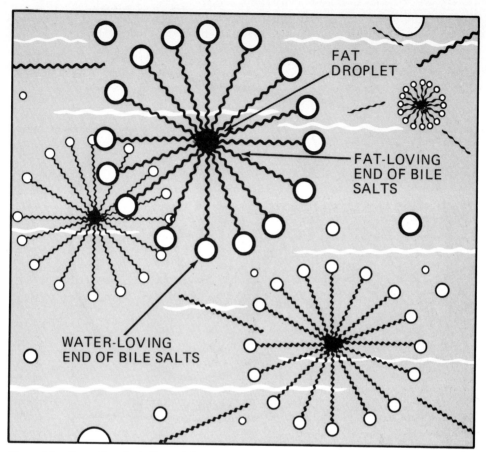

Figure 4-9.   Formation of micelles and their emulsification action in water-based solution.

In the intestinal wall, bile salts are released from the lipid complex. *About 98 percent of bile salts are reabsorbed in the small intestine after their release and are returned directly to the liver via the portal blood.* In the liver the bile salts are extracted and resecreted into bile, completing one enterohepatic circuit.[18] Reabsorption of the different bile salts occurs principally in the ileum portion of the small intestine. See Figure 4-10.

A small percentage of bile salts is not reabsorbed and is excreted in the feces. When bile salt malabsorption occurs in the small intestine, the concentration of bile salts in the colon may become quite high. An abnormally high concentration of bile salts in the colon interferes with the sodium and water reabsorption that should occur there and results in a watery diarrhea.[19]

When inflammation occurs to the gallbladder or gallstones[20] form, the gallbladder may need to be surgically removed. A person can live without a gallbladder though some dietary adjustments involving the reduction of fat consumption *according to individual tolerance* may be necessary. There may also be a need to take food in smaller, more frequent meals. The bile produced by the liver backs up into the common bile duct which to some degree takes over the storage function of the gallbladder. The sphincter of Oddi may still function to assist in the control of bile release into the intestine.

Cystic fibrosis. Cystic fibrosis is an inherited disease that affects the exocrine glands[21] as well as other tissues and organs. There is an overproduction of thick mucus which becomes blocked in ducts such as those of the pancreas, liver, and lungs. Large amounts of sodium chloride (components of ordinary table salt) are excreted in perspiration. This fact gave rise to the Cystic Fibrosis Foundation's national campaign slogan, "Kiss Your Baby." The advice is: if your baby tastes salty when you kiss him, you should have him checked by a physician for the possible presence of cystic fibrosis.

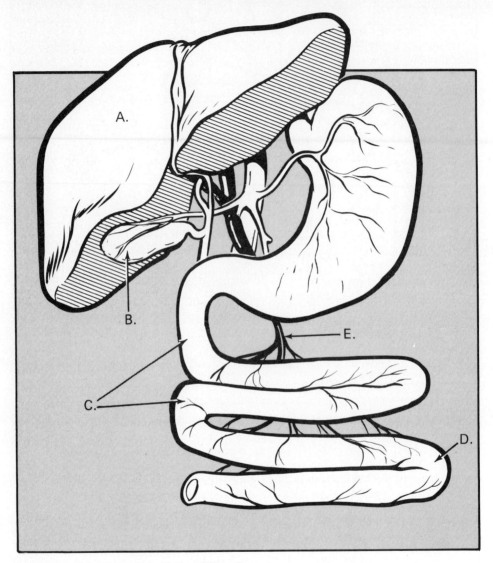

Figure 4-10. *Enterohepatic circulation of bile salts.*
A. Formation of bile salts in the liver.
B. Concentration and storage of bile salts in the gallbladder.
C. Emulsification of fat by bile salts within the small intestine.
D. Reabsorption of bile salts in intestinal wall, especially in the ileum.
E. Transport of reabsorbed bile salts in portal blood system to liver.

When pancreatic ducts are blocked, as in cystic fibrosis, the pancreatic enzymes cannot enter the duodenum. Lipid digestion as well as starch and protein digestion is impaired and severe malabsorption results. Foul, foamy, greasy, and bulky stools are produced. *Steatorrhea is the name given to the condition of excessive fats in feces.* Steatorrhea is symptomatic of a serious disorder and requires proper medical care as well as a special diet.

Pancreatitis. Pancreatitis is the inflammation of the pancreas. Any disease of the pancreas interferes with the normal production of pancreatic enzymes. The digestion of fats as well as that of starches and proteins is impaired as in cystic fibrosis. Fat-soluble vitamins are poorly absorbed and the same foul stools which occur in cystic fibrosis are produced.[22] Pancreatitis is a painful, grave condition in which the backed-up digestive enzymes actually begin to digest the pancreas itself. During the attack, foods cannot be taken orally as contents in the intestine stimulate more pancreatic and bile secretion. Fluids and electrolytes are replaced parenterally (intravenously). The occurrence of pancreatitis is frequently associated with alcoholism.

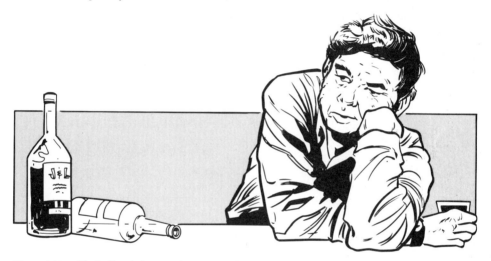

Figure 4-11.   Alcoholism is frequently associated with the development of cirrhosis of the liver and pancreatitis.

Key Points: Bile Salts and Some Malfunctions Involving Lipid Digestion and Absorption

I. Bile contains water, bile salts, bile acids, phospholipids, cholesterol, and bile pigments.
  A. Bile formed in the liver; concentrated and stored in gallbladder.
  B. Bile salts formed in liver from cholesterol.
  C. Bile salts are efficiently recirculated within the body in a conservative system called the enterohepatic circulation.
  D. Bile is released from the gallbladder into the duodenum by the stimulation of the hormone cholecystokinin.
  E. Functions of bile include emulsifying fat within the intestine and the neutralizing of acid chyme.
    1. Fat is emulsified by the formation of bile salt-lipid complexes called micelles.
    2. The alkaline environment of the duodenum is necessary to activate lipases, fat-splitting enzymes, secreted there by the pancreas.

II.   Bile salt malabsorption leads to increased concentration of bile salts in the colon with resultant diarrhea and interference with sodium and water reabsorption.

III.   Individuals may survive comfortably following gallbladder removal providing individual diet adjustments are made regarding fat intake and the frequency of meals.

IV.   Interference with the secretion of digestive enzymes impairs lipid digestion and absorption.
   A.   Blockage of the pancreatic duct by thick mucus occurs with cystic fibrosis, an inherited disease.
   B.   Blockage of pancreatic ducts and impaired production of pancreatic enzymes occurs during pancreatitis, inflammation of the pancreas.
   C.   Malabsorption of lipids results in steatorrhea, excessive fats in feces.

Questions: Bile Salts and Some Malfunctions Involving Lipid Digestion and Absorption

1.   Bile salts are formed in the liver from _____ .

2.   What are the two basic functions of the gallbladder?

3.   The efficient and conservative reabsorption and recirculation system for bile salts within the body is called the _____ .

4.   Match the phrases on the right to the terms on the left which they best describe:

   _____ 1.   micelle
   _____ 2.   secretin
   _____ 3.   cholecystokinin
   _____ 4.   lipases
   _____ 5.   emulsify

   a.   stimulates the pancreas to secrete its contents
   b.   fat-splitting enzymes
   c.   to disperse and suspend lipids in a watery medium
   d.   tiny bile salt-lipid complex
   e.   stimulates the gallbladder to release bile

5.   A person can live without a gallbladder should it become diseased and require surgical removal.
   a.   True
   b.   False

6.   An abnormally high concentration of bile salts in the colon interferes with the reabsorption of what nutrients?
   a.   sodium
   b.   protein
   c.   fat
   d.   water
   e.   carbohydrate

7.   What percentage of bile salts is reabsorbed in the ileum portion of the small intestine?
   a.   about 25 percent
   b.   about 50 percent
   c.   over 90 percent

8.   What sphincter aids in regulating bile release?

9.   Which disease is characterized by blockage of exocrine gland ducts with thick mucus?
   a.   pancreatitis
   b.   fatty liver
   c.   cystic fibrosis

10. How can "kissing your baby" be helpful in identifying the possible occurrence of cystic fibrosis?

11. The condition of excessive fats in feces is termed:
    a. diarrhea
    b. steatorrhea

12. Pancreatitis causes the digestive enzymes to accumulate in the pancreas causing extreme pain and the _____ of the organ itself.

13. What type of vitamins are largely unabsorbed in cystic fibrosis and pancreatitis:
    a. water-soluble
    b. fat-soluble

14. Why can a person suffering from pancreatitis not take food orally?

15. The occurrence of pancreatitis is frequently associated with what condition?

Answers: Bile Salts and Some Malfunctions Involving Lipid Digestion and Absorption

1. cholesterol
2. concentrating and storing bile from the liver
3. enterohepatic circulation
4. 1. d
   2. a
   3. e
   4. b
   5. c
5. a
6. a and d
7. c
8. sphincter of Oddi
9. c
10. It provides the opportunity to detect a salty taste of the skin characteristic of the excessive sodium chloride in the perspiration of a baby with cystic fibrosis.
11. b
12. digestion
13. b
14. Because food entering the duodenum will stimulate further pancreatic enzyme production compounding the effects of the current attack.
15. alcoholism

SOME MALFUNCTIONS INVOLVING LIPID METABOLISM

Ketosis. The oxidation of fat and carbohydrate occurs simultaneously in the body. An intermediary substance called oxaloacetic acid, formed during carbohydrate metabolism, is necessary to completely oxidize the fatty acids to carbon dioxide and water, the so-called "clean wastes" of energy metabolism. They are referred to as clean wastes because carbon dioxide and water can be efficiently excreted from the body through perspiration, urine, and respiration.

Oxaloacetic acid may be in short supply when a high rate of fatty acid metabolism occurs. When this condition occurs the chemical substances *ketones* and *acetones* are produced *(ketone bodies).* When ketone bodies are not oxidized sufficiently by the liver, they diffuse into the circulation where they are extracted by other tissues and are oxidized in preference to other fuels.[23]

Ketone bodies are acid products. When they accumulate in the body faster than the body can oxidize or excrete them the body goes into *ketosis (acidosis)*. Acidosis interferes with many body functions and can lead to coma and death if left unchecked. Ketosis can be a severe complication of uncontrolled diabetes mellitus. Ketosis also occurs during lengthy fasting periods, starvation, and while "dieting" for weight loss using any one of many low carbohydrate, high fat, high protein fad diets.

   Fatty liver. The liver does not normally store deposits of fat. Lipotropic factors help to transfer fatty acids from the liver by way of the circulatory system to other tissues. *Lipotropic factors are compounds which have an affinity or attraction for fat.* The vitamin-like compound choline is an important lipotropic agent. Choline is a part of lecithin, a phospholipid. Choline can be synthesized in the body as well as attained from dietary sources. Choline as well as available protein is needed for formation of lipoproteins in the liver. Lipoproteins promote movement of lipids from the liver to other tissues.

   Fatty acids accumulate in the liver when their production exceeds that of the liver's capacity to produce lipoproteins. It also occurs when fatty acid synthesis is increased or fatty acids are not being adequately used for fuel. Fat that accumulates in the liver interferes with blood flow from capillaries to the cells. As the fat infiltration increases and the condition becomes chronic, the liver cells which are deprived of blood die from a lack of nutrients and oxygen. Fibrocytic changes occur where the cells have died resulting in the formation of scars. This condition can progress to impaired liver function and the disease state called *cirrhosis of the liver*. Ingested alcohol increases total fat production in the liver.[24] Alcohol also depresses protein synthesis. Therefore, fatty liver and its progression to cirrhosis is often a consequence of alcoholism.[25]

Key Points: Some Malfunctions Involving Lipid Metabolism

   I.   Ketosis is a condition of acidosis resulting when lipids are unable to be oxidized completely to CO_2, H_2O, and energy.

      A.   Ketosis occurs when there is a shortage of oxaloacetic acid, an intermediary of carbohydrate metabolism.

      B.   A shortage of oxaloacetate may occur during uncontrolled diabetes, fasting, starvation, or adherence to a low carbohydrate, high fat, high protein fad diet.

      C.   Acidosis is a serious condition which interferes with many body functions and can lead to coma and death.

   II. Fatty liver occurs when fats accumulate in the liver.

      A.   Movement of fat out of the liver is facilitated by lipotropic agents which have an affinity for fat such as choline along with adequate protein for lipoprotein formation.

      B.   Fat deposits in the liver interfere with blood flow in that organ causing cellular death, scar formation, and impaired liver function: cirrhosis of the liver.

      C.   Chronic and excessive alcohol intake favors development of fatty liver and cirrhosis.

Questions: Some Malfunctions Involving Lipid Metabolism

   1.   What substance is necessary to completely oxidize fatty acids to carbon dioxide and water?

   2.   What are the so-called clean waste products of energy metabolism?

   3.   Ketone bodies are:
      a.   acetones
      b.   acid products
      c.   ketones

   4.   Accumulation of ketone bodies in the human body leads to the condition of _____ .

5. Identify three conditions which can lead to ketosis.
6. What is one good reason for drinking plenty of fluids while going on a weight reduction diet?
7. Why is it desirable to consume some carbohydrate even while on a weight reduction diet?
8. A substance which has an affinity or attraction for fat is called a _____.
9. Identify a specific lipotropic agent from the following:
   a. acetones
   b. ketones
   c. choline
10. The continued synthesis of what compound is necessary for mobilization and transportation of fatty acids from the liver?
11. What condition is a risk factor for the development of cirrhosis of the liver?
12. The fat infiltration and scar tissue in cirrhosis of the liver interferes with what function?
13. Malnutrition involving insufficient protein intake can cause the development of fatty liver.
    a. True
    b. False

Answers: Some Malfunctions Involving Lipid Metabolism

1. an intermediary of carbohydrate metabolism, oxaloacetic acid
2. water; carbon dioxide
3. a, b, c
4. ketosis (acidosis)
5. uncontrolled diabetes mellitus, fasting periods, starvation, adherence to a low carbohydrate, high fat, high protein diet
6. to help flush from the body undesirable products such as ketone bodies formed during energy metabolism
7. To provide sufficient oxaloacetic acid from carbohydrate metabolism necessary for complete oxidation of *body fat* to carbon dioxide and water. This helps avoid the accumulation of ketone bodies with resultant acidosis.
8. lipotropic agent
9. c
10. lipoproteins
11. alcoholism
12. blood circulation within the liver
13. a

ATHEROSCLEROSIS AND DIET—A CONTROVERSY

Arteriosclerosis is a broad and general term which encompasses various types of degeneration of the arteries. This degeneration usually results in the thickening and hardening of the arterial walls. *Atherosclerosis is one type of arteriosclerosis and is associated with an accumulation of various lipids including cholesterol, triglycerides, and phospholipids in arterial walls.*[26] Nearly half the deaths in the United States are due to coronary heart disease (CHD) and a large percentage of those deaths can be attributed to atherosclerosis.[27]

It appears that lipids in the blood stick and accumulate in the walls of arteries. The deposits occur as spots or streaks along the interior blood vessel and are referred to as *plaques.* When these plaques build up to a point where they extend into the cavity of the blood vessel they cause a disturbance in the flow of blood. As additional lipid material accumulates at the plaque site the plaque becomes soft. The plaque eventually breaks down forming ragged edges and some fibrous scar tissue. The blood vessel then begins to lose its necessary interior smoothness and general elasticity.

The disturbances in the flow of blood by these plaque areas may trigger the physical and chemical reactions which initiate blood clotting. If a *clot (thrombus)* becomes lodged in a vessel it cuts down the flow of blood past the clot. A clot may even break loose (or part of one) and travel until an artery or arteriole narrows sufficiently to stop its passage. In this case the blood clot obstructs further blood flow. See Figure 4-12.

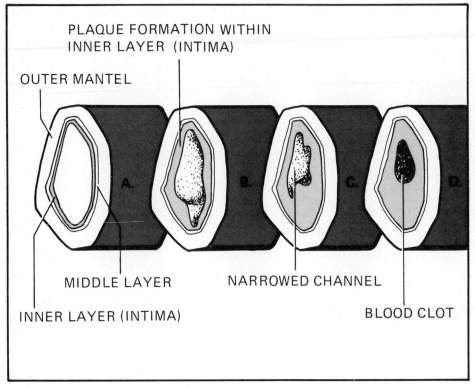

PLAQUE FORMATION WITHIN
INNER LAYER (INTIMA)

OUTER MANTEL

A.   B.   C.   D.

MIDDLE LAYER

NARROWED CHANNEL

INNER LAYER (INTIMA)

BLOOD CLOT

Figure 4-12.   Progression of plaque formation leading to atherosclerosis and thrombosis.
A. Normal blood vessel.
B. Development of plaque within the inner layer (intima).
C. Hardening of plaque deposits.
D. Blood clot (thrombus) in narrowed vessel.

The death of cells supplied by a blood vessel that becomes blocked occurs rapidly due to a lack of nutrients and oxygen. *Cellular death is referred to as necrosis. Myocardial infarction is the localized death (necrosis) of heart muscle cells. Myocardial ischemia* is the temporary deficiency of blood supply to heart muscle due to an obstruction such as a thrombus or the constriction of a blood vessel. *Angina pectoris* is the severe chest pain which can also extend up the neck and down the left arm that is associated with sudden myocardial ischemia. *Coronary thrombosis* is the sudden blockage of a major branch of one of the coronary arteries resulting in a deprivation of blood to a large section of the heart's muscular wall. A thrombus blocking a vessel in the brain results in a stroke *(cerebral thrombosis).* Unfortunately, it appears that by early middle age many persons in the U.S. and Western Europe have extensive and severe lesions of atherosclerosis in their coronary arteries, aorta, arteries of the legs, and cerebral arteries.[28]

When the chemical analyses of plaques showed that they were largely composed of lipids, especially cholesterol, and high blood serum cholesterol levels were shown to be associated with persons who suffered coronary heart disease, the controversial "lipid/diet hypothesis" was developed. The crux of this hypothesis is that the elevated levels of blood serum cholesterol associated with CHD can and should be altered by a diet reduced in saturated fat and cholesterol in order to lower the risk of CHD. The hypothesis can be summarized by the scheme: Diet→Hypercholesteremia→Atherosclerosis→Coronary Disease.[29]

Many comparisons have been made between different social and ethnic groups consuming different types of diets. It does appear that atherosclerosis is prevalent in more prosperous countries such as the United States, Canada, Australia, and those of Western Europe where people can afford more costly meat, shellfish, and dairy products which are the foods especially high in saturated fat and cholesterol. However, when comparisons are made between specific smaller groups of people, one of which has a high fat/cholesterol intake, and one of which has a moderately low fat/cholesterol intake, the *serum cholesterol levels* frequently do not correlate with the *fat/cholesterol intakes.* Some researchers have even suggested that a very high fat diet may not raise cholesterol levels if caloric (energy) intake is in balance with caloric (energy) needs.[30]

Serum cholesterol levels of the American population associated with dietary changes have fluctuated only slightly since the turn of the century. During this time period there occurred a large substitution of unsaturated fat for saturated fat in American diets. Interestingly, this occurred during the same period of time in which the *incidence* of CHD increased markedly.[31] This is in direct contrast to the lipid/diet hypothesis. More recently, the total *mortality* from CHD has been shown to be decreasing on an age-adjusted basis. This leaves open the argument that CHD is a disease of old age. Since Americans on a whole are living longer the incidence of CHD would be expected to rise.

The best known study of cardiovascular disease in the U.S. is the Framingham study which ended in 1970. Over 5,000 men and women were involved in this study for a 20-year period. The Framingham population sample was statistically typical of the general U.S. population in food consumption patterns. After all results were carefully studied, the scientists found no significant relationship between animal fat and dietary cholesterol *intake* and blood serum cholesterol levels.[32]

Results from other dietary trials have been contradictory. Some trials have shown simple sugars raise the triglyceride/cholesterol levels of the blood serum. Other trials have shown that certain food fibers have a lowering effect on serum cholesterol levels. Several trials have found that an intake involving a higher polyunsaturated fat/saturated fat ratio (P/S ratio) will lower serum cholesterol levels.[33] Another relationship has been demonstrated between hard water (versus soft water) consumption and lowered serum cholesterol levels. Still another relationship has been discovered between high zinc to copper ratio intakes and elevated serum cholesterol levels. Results of other studies have shown that while blood cholesterol levels may decrease due to dietary changes total body cholesterol may not. This suggests that cholesterol is simply being taken from the blood into the various tissues.[34] A critical review of the relationships between diet, blood lipids, and the incidence of atherosclerosis by one scientist led to his conclusion that many diet constituents, through different mechanisms, may affect some degree of variation of blood lipids but not enough to be clinically significant.[35]

Elevated serum cholesterol levels do appear to have a strong relationship to the occurrence of the first coronary event in CHD, but evidence of the ability to reduce further attacks by lowering serum cholesterol levels seems to be lacking. Perhaps this is because CHD becomes apparent in middle age but the processes leading to it are begun in childhood and are, consequently, well advanced by middle age. If the high fat/cholesterol intake of most Americans does raise serum cholesterol levels over a long period of time, and an elevated serum cholesterol level is found to be causative rather than symptomatic of CHD, then dietary modification of fat and cholesterol might be warranted and even prove necessary to begin in childhood. Long-term, well-documented scientific trials need to be conducted to further examine such relationships. Most scientists at the present time agree that more convincing evidence is needed to demonstrate that restriction of dietary fat and cholesterol significantly lowers blood cholesterol, which in turn significantly lowers the incidence of CHD before dietary modifications can be advised for the general population.

Total blood serum cholesterol levels have been shown recently to be an incomplete picture of the risk factor associated with development of CHD. It appears that it is much more informative to measure serum cholesterol according to its association with various lipoprotein carriers. It seems that the percentage of cholesterol in low density lipoprotein factions (LDL) is more indicative of CHD risk than that amount found associated with high density lipoproteins (HDL).[36] It is generally agreed that more research is warranted in investigating this approach to risk as represented by elevated serum cholesterol levels.

Elevated serum cholesterol level is not the only risk factor associated with diet and involved with the development of CHD. Being overweight and obesity due to excessive caloric intake seem to be associated with a higher risk of developing elevated serum lipid levels and CHD. Hypertension (high blood pressure) seems clearly established as a risk factor for the development of coronary heart disease. Hypertension is also closely related to obesity and salt intake. The presence of diabetes is also related to the increased risk of CHD and is related to diet because of its association with obesity. Low fiber diets have been implicated in the development of CHD as well as the increased intake of simple sugars (perhaps in part because diets high in refined sugars are also low in fiber content).

There are numerous other risk factors which have no connection to diet and which many researchers are now beginning to feel may have far more significance than any single dietary factor.[37] Cigarette smoking, lack of physical activity, and even certain personality types have shown to be strongly associated with the development of CHD. Even these risk factors are interrelated. It may be that certain personality types are the ones who participate less fully in physical exercise and are prone to smoke cigarettes. There is an increased recognition of genetic predisposition toward CHD regardless of the presence or absence of other risk factors. Many researchers are also looking at stress as an important risk factor for CHD.

The Report of the Advisory Panel of the British Committee on Medical Aspects of Food Policy (Nutrition) on Diet in Relation to Cardiovascular and Cerebrovascular Disease stated that the presence of two or more risk factors in any one individual may raise the risk of CHD greater than the sum of the occurrence of the risk factors singly.[38] It is also generally recognized that the risk factors are more aptly applied to population groups than to specific individuals.[39]

In the absence of unequivocal proof that controlling any one or more of the risk factors will prevent, mitigate, cure, or reduce mortality due to CHD, what recommendations can be given to the general public? The expressed feeling of researchers and representative organizations involved with the study and research of CHD seems more and more to be that specific changes in diet and environment should be made on an individualized basis, and that drastic changes cannot yet be advised for the *general population.*[40] However, it seems *that certain guidelines aimed toward attaining and maintaining good health can be given:*[41-42]

1. Consume an adequate diet at a caloric level sufficient to maintain desirable body weight.
2. Take measures to correct hypertension.
3. Reduce or eliminate cigarette smoking.
4. Participate in a program of regular exercise.

5. Avoid unnecessary stress and frustration.
6. Have regular medical examinations.

Key Points: Atherosclerosis and Diet—A Controversy

I. Almost half of the deaths in the U.S. are due to coronary heart disease (CHD) and many of those deaths can be attributed to atherosclerosis in particular.

II. High blood serum cholesterol levels have been shown to be associated with the incidence of CHD, especially with the occurrence of the first coronary event.

III. Through epidemiological studies, atherosclerosis appears to be most prevalent in prosperous countries where consumption of foods elevated in saturated fat and cholesterol such as meat, shellfish, and dairy products is high. However, correlations between fat/cholesterol intake and serum cholesterol levels often cannot be made between specific, smaller societies.

IV. Establishment of a specific relationship between diet, serum lipids, and the incidence of CHD is difficult because various dietary trials have shown that many different diet constituents act in different ways to affect some change in blood lipids.

V. Additional diet-related risk factors for CHD are hypertension, obesity, diabetes, and possibly low fiber diets and the increased intake of simple sugars.

VI. Significant non-diet risk factors for CHD are genetic predisposition, stress, cigarette smoking, certain personality types, and physical inactivity.

Questions: Atherosclerosis and Diet—A Controversy

1. Match the phrases on the right to the terms on the left which they best describe:

_____ 1.	arteriosclerosis	a.	cellular death
_____ 2.	plaques	b.	temporary deficiency of blood supply to heart muscle
_____ 3.	atherosclerosis		
_____ 4.	thrombus	c.	blood clot blockage of a major coronary artery branch
_____ 5.	necrosis		
_____ 6.	coronary thrombosi	d.	blood clot
_____ 7.	stroke	e.	blood clot in cerebral blood vessel
_____ 8.	myocardial infarction	f.	sharp pain associated with myocardial ischemia
_____ 9.	angina pectoris		
_____ 10.	myocardial ischemia	g.	general term describing degeneration of the arteries
		h.	arterial thickening and hardening due to deposits of lipids and cholesterol
		i.	lipid deposits in interior arterial walls
		j.	localized death of heart muscle cells

2. The processes involved in development of CHD begin in childhood.
    a. True
    b. False

3. Plaques are deposits within arterial walls which are largely composed of _____ including _____ .

4. The lipid/diet hypothesis is best described as:
    a. a now proven relationship between saturated fat/cholesterol intake and the development of CHD
    b. controversial and warranting further research
    c. totally unproven

5. Atherosclerosis seems to be most prevalent in:

a. third world countries
b. most countries
c. prosperous countries

6. Which food group contains high amounts of cholesterol:
   a. fruits and vegetables
   b. shellfish, meats, dairy products
   c. grains

7. Increased intake of polyunsaturated fat has consistently corresponded with decreased *incidence* of CHD according to U.S. vital statistics since the early 1900s.
   a. True
   b. False

8. The Framingham study showed a positive relationship between the *intake* of saturated fat and cholesterol and increased *serum levels* of cholesterol.
   a. True
   b. False

9. Considering the results of various diet trials, the association of dietary factors to the incidence of CHD can best be described as:
   a. varied and contradictory
   b. multi-faceted and interrelated
   c. both of the above

10. It is the cholesterol complexed in the low density lipoprotein factions (LDL) which appears implicated within the elevated serum cholesterol risk factor.
    a. True
    b. False

11. Correcting obesity and hypertension would appear to _____ the risk of developing CHD.
    a. increase
    b. decrease

12. List three nondietary risk factors associated with CHD.

13. The risk factors for CHD are best applied to:
    a. individuals
    b. population groups
    c. people over 65 years of age

14. The presence of two or more risk factors in any individual raises the risk of CHD _____ .

15. A five-foot four-inch woman who is 25 years-old weighs 130 pounds. She is an office worker and normally rides to work. This woman is consuming 2500 kcal per day. Her weekend hobbies include sewing, cooking, and reading. Is she developing risk factors associated with CHD? (Hint: refer to Table 2-4.)

16. Use Table 4-2 to answer the following questions:
    a. Which portion of the egg contains cholesterol?
    b. Which type of seafood contains large amounts of cholesterol?
    c. Which type of meat is highest in cholesterol content, flesh or organ meats?
    d. Why are cheese and ice cream higher in cholesterol content than fluid milk?

Answers: Atherosclerosis and Diet—A Controversy

1. 1. g
    2. i
    3. h
    4. d

5. a
6. c
7. e
8. j
9. f
10. b

2. a
3. lipids; cholesterol
4. b
5. c
6. b
7. b
8. b
9. c
10. a
11. b
12. cigarette smoking, lack of physical exercise, personality type, genetic predisposition, stress
13. b
14. greater than the sum of the occurrence of the risk factors separately
15. It appears that she is. She is presently overweight and seems sedentary. She is consuming kcal above the upper range for her weight and age and seems headed for obesity if her eating and energy expenditure patterns are not brought into balance. Obesity is implicated as a risk factor in CHD as well as lack of physical exercise.
16. a. egg yolk
    b. shellfish
    c. organ
    d. because cheese and ice cream are more concentrated forms of milk and milk-fat

Table 4-2. Fat and cholesterol content of some foods.

Food	Fat content per common portion	Cholesterol mg per 100 g portion	Cholesterol mg per common portion
Brains	7.3g/3oz	2100	2100/3½oz (100g)
Egg yolk, fresh	5.2g/1 med.	1602	272/1 med. (17g)
Egg white	tr/1 med.	0	0
Liver, calf, fried	13.2g/3½oz	438	438/3½oz (100g)
Oysters, canned	2.2g/3½oz	230	230/5-8 med. (100g)
Lobster, raw	.5g/3½oz	200	200/3½oz (100g)
Shrimp, canned	1.1g/3½oz	150	150 3½oz (100g)
Cheese, cheddar	9.1g/oz	106	30/oz (28g)
Beef, cuts*		70	70/3½oz (100g)
Chuck roast, braised	23.9g/3½oz		
Hamburger, med. fat			
cooked patty	14.5g/3oz		
Tenderloin, broiled			
lean	9.2g/3½oz		
Fish, sticks, frozen	8-9g/3½oz	70	70/4-5 sticks (100g)
Chicken, flesh only	2.7g raw or		
	7.8g fried/3½ oz	60	60/3½oz (100g)

Table 4-2.   Fat and cholesterol content of some foods (continued).

Food	Fat content per common portion	Cholesterol mg per 100 g portion	Cholesterol mg per common portion
Ice cream (12% fat)	16.4g/1 cup	60	80/cup (133g)
Milk, fluid, whole	8.1g/1 cup	14	34/cup (244g)
Milk, fluid, skim	.4g/1 cup	2	5/cup (246g)
Sherbet, orange	4g/1 cup	7	14/cup (200g)

* Though cholesterol content stays approximately the same for various beef cuts, note the large variation in fat content between different beef cuts. *From:* Bowes and Church's Food Values of Portions Commonly Used, 13th edition. Revised by Pennington JAT and Chuch HN, Philadelphia, J. P. Lippincott Company, 1980

REFERENCES

[1] **Ester linkage** is the chemical bond that occurs between an alcohol and an acid. A glycerol/ fatty acid bond is frequently referred to as a *glyceride linkage.*

[2] **PUFA** is frequently used to designate a polyunsaturated fatty acid.

[3] **Emulsify** means to distribute relatively and uniformly, and to stabilize lipid droplets in a water-based solution.

[4] **Mastication** is the biting and chewing of food which breaks the food into smaller particles.

[5] **Peristalsis** is the wave-like contraction and relaxation movement of muscles in the esophagus, stomach, and intestines which causes their contents to be propelled along the alimentary tract and helps to mechanically break down and mix those contents.

[6] Williams SR: Nutrition and Diet Therapy, 3rd ed. St. Louis, The C. V. Mosby Company, 1977, p. 36

[7] These compounds are recombined as triglycerides for storage.

[8] **Gluconeogenesis** is the term used to describe the formation of glucose from noncarbohydrate sources such as glycerol.

[9] Suitor CW and Hunter MF: Nutrition: Principles and Application in Health Promotion. Philadephia, J. B. Lippincott Company, 1980, p. 155

[10] Krause MV and Mahan LK: Food, Nutrition and Diet Therapy, 6th ed. Philadelphia, W. B. Saunders Company, 1979, p. 63

[11] Williams SR: Nutrition and Diet Therapy, 3rd ed. St. Louis, The C. V. Mosby Company, 1977, p. 31

[12] **Satiety** is the feeling of fullness or satisfaction after eating. It is the absence of hunger contractions or the desire to eat.

[13] Recommended Dietary Allowances, Ninth Revised Edition, 1980. Food and Nutrition Board, National Academy of Sciences-National Research Council, Washington, D.C.; p. 31

[14] Kreutler PA: Nutrition in Perspective. Englewood Cliffs, NJ; Prentice-Hall, Inc., 1980, p. 107

[15] **Chyme** is the semi-liquid material produced in the stomach after enzymatic and mechanical action on ingested food. Chyme is passed from the stomach into the duodenum and proceeds down the small intestine.

[16] Williams SR: Nutrition and Diet Therapy, 3rd ed. St. Louis, The C. V. Mosby Company, 1977, p. 35

[17] McNutt KW and McNutt DR: Nutrition and Food Choices. Chicago, Science-Research Associates, Inc., 1978, p. 64

[18] Cholesterol metabolism. Dairy Council Digest, 50, November-December 1979, p. 34

[19] Holt P: Fats and bile salts. Journal of the American Dietetic Association, 60, June 1972, 494

[20] Gallstones form from bile constituents and may remain in the gallbladder. If they move into the biliary duct they block the flow of bile into the duodenum.

[21] **Exocrine glands** are glands that excrete their substances out of the body. They are the glands with ducts. These glands do not excrete their hormones directly into the bloodstream.

[22] Robinson CH: Basic Nutrition and Diet Therapy, 3rd ed. New York, Macmillan Publishing Co., Inc., 1975, pp. 287-88

[23] Harper HA: Review of Physiological Chemistry. Los Altos, California; Lange Medical Publications, 1973, p. 298

[24] Boeker EA: Metabolism of ethanol. Journal of the American Dietetic Association, 76, June 1980, p. 551

[25] An excellent explanation of fatty liver and its relation to alcohol consumption can be found in:
Whitney EN and Hamilton EMN: Understanding Nutrition. St. Paul, MN; West Publishing Company, 1977, pp. 304-305

[26] Sherman WC: Atherosclerosis—Part I, Diet in Disease Series, Food and Nutrition News, 46, December-January, 1974-5, p. 3

[27] 1978 Information Please Almanac and Monthly Vital Statistics, U.S. Dept. of Health and Human Services, August 7, 1980

[28] McGill HC and Mott GE: Diet and coronary heart disease. In Present Knowledge in Nutrition, 4th ed. New York and Washington, D.C.; The Nutrition Foundation, Inc., 1976, p. 377

[29] Mann GV: The saturated vs. unsaturated fat controversy. *In* Labuza TP(ed): The Nutrition Crisis—A Reader. St. Paul, MN; West Publishing Co., 1975, p. 341

[30] Sherman WC: Atherosclerosis—Part II, Diet in Disease Series, Food and Nutrition News, 46, February 1975, p. 3

[31] Speckmann EW: Coronary heart disease—a scientific imbalance. Nutrition Today, 10, January-February 1975, p. 31

[32] Mann GV: The saturated vs. unsaturated fat controversy. *In* Labuza TP(ed): The Nutrition Crisis—A Reader. St. Paul, MN: West Publishing Co., 1975, p. 343

[33] An increased P/S ratio has been advocated by some scientists for a number of years. A 1:1 to 2:1 ratio has been recommended for heart patients. However, some tests now suggest that increased polyunsaturated fat intake itself may lead to complicating problems of gallstone formation, premature aging, increased requirement for other nutrients, and possibly cancer.

[34] Speckmann EW: Coronary heart disease: A scientific imbalance. Nutrition Today, 10, January-February 1975, p. 31

[35] Reiser R: Diet and blood lipids: An overview. Food and Nutrition News, 51, December 1979-January 1980, p. 4

[36] Weininger J and Briggs GM: Nutrition update, 1977. Journal of Nutrition Education, 9, October-December 1977, p. 174

[37] It is important to emphasize that the risk factors have been determined through epidemiological studies and, therefore, are recognized as associations and not yet as cause and effect relationships.

[38] Diet and Coronary Heart Disease. Report of the Advisory Panel of the British Committee on Medical Aspects of Food Policy (Nutrition) on Diet in Relation to Cardiovascular and Cerebrovascular Disease, Nutrition Today, 10, January-February 1975, p. 18

[39] A good review of risk factors associated with CHD is:
Kannel WB: Status of coronary heart disease risk factors. Journal of Nutrition Education, 10, January-March 1978, pp. 10-14

[40] Weininger J and Briggs GM: Nutrition update, 1977. Journal of Nutrition Education, 9, October-December 1977, pp. 174-175

[41] Newer concepts of coronary heart disease. Dairy Council Digest, 45, November-December 1974, p. 34

[42] Sherman WC: Atherosclerosis—Part IV. Food and Nutrition News, 46, May-June 1975, p. 3

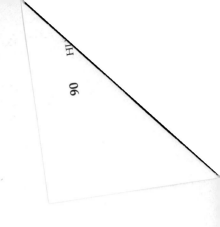

5
PROTEINS

Protein shares a common classification with carbohydrates and lipids (fats): it is an organic substance. All three energy nutrients contain carbon, hydrogen, and oxygen in their chemical structures. One major characteristic that distinguishes proteins from carbohydrates and lipids is the *presence of nitrogen atoms in all protein*. About 16 percent of protein is nitrogen.[1] Protein may also contain other elements such as sulfur. The complex protein molecules are constructed from *amino acids, the building blocks of protein*. The amino acids occur in a specific pattern within an individual protein.

Proteins are built from approximately 20 different amino acids. It is the difference in the chemical arrangement and composition of the individual amino acids, and their pattern within each type of protein, that enables each protein to perform its special functions. Amino acids also give each protein its special characteristics. These 20 plus amino acids can be combined in an almost infinite variety of patterns.

Protein synthesis (creation) and breakdown occur simultaneously in a dynamic state within the body. The "metabolic pool" of amino acids represents those amino acids available throughout the body for use as needed, whether obtained from the diet, various body chemical reactions, or tissue breakdown. The "metabolic pool" is not symbolic of a designated place. There is no extended storage area for proteins (that is, amino acids) within the body. Dietary protein must be supplied continuously and in sufficient quantity to cover maintenance of existing tissues. These dietary protein needs are increased during periods of growth and new tissue development.

Some of the amino acids can be manufactured by the body providing the basic elements are available. These amino acids are called *nonessential (dispensable) amino acids*. However, eight amino acids which are necessary for making body proteins cannot be manufactured within the body. These are methionine, threonine, tryptophan, isoleucine, leucine, lysine, valine, and phenylalanine. Another amino acid, histidine, may be essential for infants and even some adults. These amino acids must be obtained in completed form from the diet. *Amino acids which must be supplied by the diet are called essential amino acids.*

Protein foods which supply all the essential amino acids in proportions closely approximating the body's requirement for making body proteins with which to construct new tissue, are called *complete proteins*. Proteins which lack enough of one or more essential amino acids to adequately meet body needs for tissue maintenance and new tissue growth are called *incomplete proteins*. Complete proteins are generally of animal origin: meat, fish, poultry, milk, eggs, and cheese. These proteins are said to be of high biological value.

Incomplete proteins are generally of plant origin: cereals, grains, vegetables, and fruits. Incomplete proteins are of lesser biological value than complete proteins. Wheat is deficient in lysine. Zein, the protein in corn, is deficient in lysine and tryptophan. Gelatin is an exception to the high quality of animal protein rule as it is very deficient in tryptophan. The amino acid of lowest quantity in a given food source is referred to as the *limiting amino acid*. Gelatin and zein are so deficient in their limiting amino acids that they are incapable of supporting life if eaten singly as a sole source of protein.

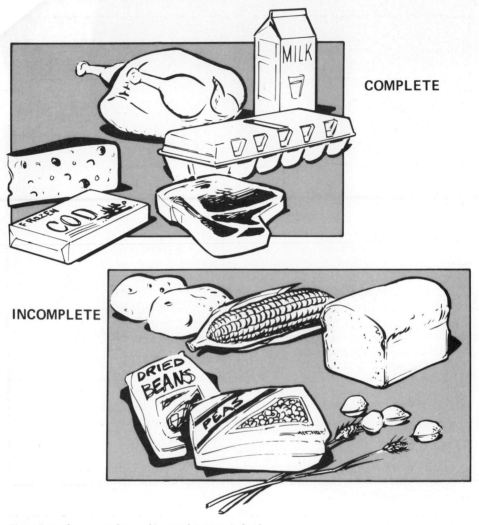

COMPLETE

INCOMPLETE

Figure 5-1. Some complete and incomplete protein foods.

Structure of amino acids and proteins. Amino acids have a central carbon atom between an acid group and an amino group (base). It is the presence of both an acid and a base component which gives amino acids and, therefore, proteins their *buffering*[2] capacity. The amino acid illustrated in Figure 5-2 is the simplest amino acid, glycine. The hydrogen within the shaded square designates the location where side chains are attached for the various amino acids.

When amino acids bond together they form the characteristic peptide bond of proteins. When this reaction occurs between many amino acids a long chain is formed. This chain is called a *peptide*. Very long chains of several hundred amino acids are called *polypeptides*.

The polypeptides of proteins are not just long chains, but have four general structural arrangements. The *primary structure* is the peptide bonding which causes the amino acids to combine in long chains. *Secondary structure* results in a helix shape due to various types of chemical bonding between elements within the chain. *Tertiary structure* is the folding back

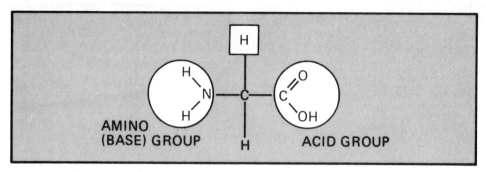

Figure 5-2. Glycine.

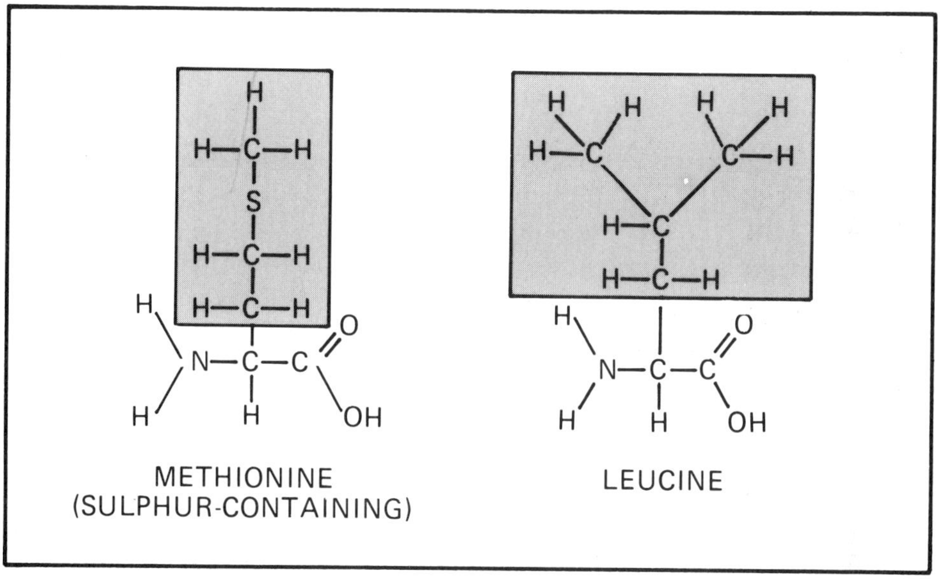

METHIONINE
(SULPHUR-CONTAINING)

LEUCINE

Figure 5-3. Two amino acids.

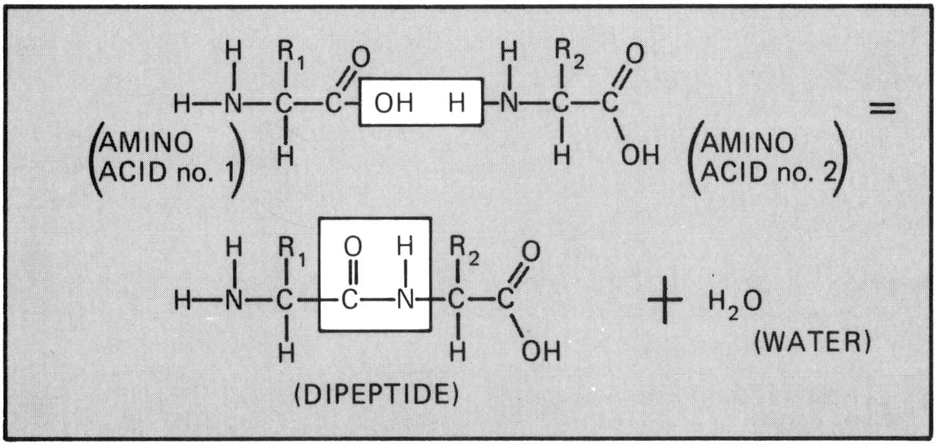

$$\left(\begin{matrix}\text{AMINO}\\\text{ACID no. 1}\end{matrix}\right) \quad \left(\begin{matrix}\text{AMINO}\\\text{ACID no. 2}\end{matrix}\right) =$$

(DIPEPTIDE)

$+ H_2O$ (WATER)

Figure 5-4. Condensation reaction forming a peptide bond.

and forth of the long helix strand upon itself. Finally, if several of these twisted polypeptide helixes become attracted to one another they form the large, globular aggregate characteristic of *quaternary structure*. See Figure 5-5. The structures of protein molecules can be altered or changed by environmental agents such as heat or acid. This change of protein structure is referred to as *denaturation*.

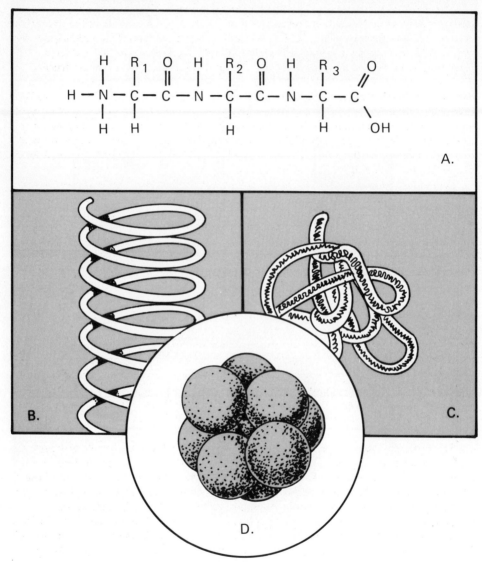

Figure 5-5.   Structures of protein.
        A. Primary (peptide bond).
        B. Secondary (helix).
        C. Tertiary (twisted coil-globular).
        D. Quaternary (globular aggregate).

Digestion, absorption, and metabolism of proteins. The digestion of proteins involves their hydrolysis to their basic components, amino acids. Digestion begins in the mouth with the mechanical action of chewing. Chewing helps to break up the food particles which exposes more of the food surface area to the action of digestive enzymes in the stomach and small intestine. The saliva does not contain a digestive enzyme for protein as it does for carbohydrate (starch). Mechanical churning due to peristalsis of the stomach and intestine is also necessary to break up food particles. This releases protein from carbohydrate and fat with which it is commonly associated in a food source.

The chemical digestion of protein begins in the stomach. The sight, smell, or anticipation of food, as well as the actual presence of food in the stomach, stimulates the stomach's secretion of *hydrocholoric acid (HCl).*[3] *HCl is necessary to convert the precursor pepsinogen to the active enzyme pepsin which activates the hydrolysis of protein in the stomach. HCl, a strong acid, is also responsible for the denaturation of proteins.* This denaturation results in the destruction of certain chemical bonds and uncoils the protein molecule. The uncoiled protein molecule is more susceptible to enzymatic action on its remaining chemical bonds.[4] See Figure 5-5. Infants and children have a special gastric[5] enzyme, rennin. In the presence of calcium rennin coagulates (denatures) milk protein, casein. Note that calcium is inherently supplied within milk. The coagulation of casein into curds causes it to remain in the stomach for a longer period of time than it would as a liquid. Therefore, casein is exposed for a greater length of time to the digestive action of pepsin.

Pepsin breaks protein down at specific chemical bond linkages to proteoses (smaller polypeptides). *Trypsinogen* is an inactive *protein enzyme (protease)* which is produced by the pancreas. Trypsinogen (the precursor) is activated to *trypsin* by *enterokinase, an enzyme* produced in the intestinal wall. Trypsin requires an alkaline medium for its activity. (Remember, the gallbladder and pancreatic secretions neutralize the gastric acid and help to make the intestinal contents more alkaline.) Another inactive pancreatic enzyme (precursor), *chymotrypsinogen,* is actually activated by the presence of trypsin to *chymotrypsin.*[6] *Carboxypeptidase* is a third active pancreatic protease which further hydrolyzes the polypeptides.

Certain cells of the intestinal wall produce other peptidases (enzymes which hydrolyze the smaller peptides). Peptidases produce the end-products of protein digestion: amino acids. Amino acids are then absorbed into the blood system. Absorption of amino acids appears to be accomplished largely by an active transport system which requires an energy source. Some amino acids are absorbed by simple diffusion. It is interesting to note the contribution of nondietary protein sources for digestion and absorption at this point. Sloughed-off intestinal cells and some enzymes are degraded (digested) to their component amino acids which are also absorbed in the intestine. These amino acids are indistinguishable within the "metabolic pool" of amino acids from the amino acids obtained from dietary sources.

The absorption rate of amino acids seems to be coordinated with the rate of digestion. This conservative mechanism prevents undue loss of amino acids through the feces as well as the overloading of amino acids in the blood system, even after the consumption of a high-protein meal. The amino acids are then absorbed into the portal blood system and transported to the liver, the dynamic regulator of amino acid/protein metabolism.

Sometimes whole proteins or polypeptides are absorbed through the intestinal mucosa into the blood system. It is thought that these large fragments set up sensitivity responses by the body which are expressed as allergic reactions to those proteins.[7] An example of this action is the apparent crossing of an immature intestinal mucosal wall of an infant by milk proteins, establishing an allergic reaction to proteins in milk distinguishable from the symptoms of lactose intolerance.

The fate of amino acids and the direction of their metabolism depends largely upon body needs and condition at the time of their absorption, and the availability of amino acids in terms of presence and proportion. The adult person not diseased or experiencing an abnormality in metabolism uses absorbed amino acids for general tissue repair and maintenance. Even as adults we lose and replace worn out body cells, grow hair and fingernails, undergo healing of small cuts, and form antibodies in response to exposure to disease agents and viruses. All these conditions require protein. However, a person in the process of tissue growth, such as a child or pregnant woman, is using even greater amounts of protein in order to build new body tissue.

Functions of proteins. Proteins are constituents of all living matter and are necessary in the diet of all animal organisms. Due to the marvelous versatility of proteins they can perform a great variety of functions. Generally, the functions of proteins can be divided into three major categories:

1. Growth and maintenance of body tissue
2. Regulation of body processes
3. Production of energy.

More specifically, proteins lend structure to the body in the bones, connective tissue, and cartilage; proteins assist in the maintenance of body neutrality through their buffering action; proteins assist the production of body movement through the action of contractile proteins in muscle cells; proteins detoxify certain toxic and poisonous substances; and proteins are transporters of various substances within the circulatory system as well as through cellular membranes. Some proteins are antibodies which protect the body by attacking disease agents such as viruses and bacteria. Many important proteins are enzymes which catalyze[8] chemical reactions within the body. Some proteins are hormones which influence various activities of the body.

Protein is vital to the circulatory system as a constituent of hemoglobin which carries oxygen to and carbon dioxide from the various cells. Protein is also a constituent of the blood clotting factors and is a major influence in controlling water balance. Protein can also be used as an energy source. *Proteins supply 4 kcal/gram.*[9]

Measurements of protein quality. As evidenced by the previous discussion on complete and incomplete proteins and the concept of the limiting amino acid, *the quality of various proteins is not nutritionally equal.* Protein quality is also dependent upon its ability to be absorbed. A protein food source which is poorly digested and/or absorbed is inferior in quality to an equal amount of another food protein source which is easily digested and efficiently absorbed. The more complete the protein source the better it is absorbed. This is thought to be due to the fact that it more adequately meets body needs. Also, it is thought that fiber in plant food protein sources may decrease the absorption of those proteins. Absorption is also affected by methods of preparation and cooking. Overheating and over-cooking protein foods generally decreases digestibility and absorption of their protein. There are several ways of measuring or comparing quality of protein.

Biological value (BV) expresses the utilization by the body of protein that is absorbed. This involves a nitrogen-based measurement. The biological value is assessed by determining the nitrogen in the food intake and the urinary and fecal excretions.[10] It can be summarized as:

$$BV = \frac{\text{Nitrogen retained}}{\text{Nitrogen absorbed}} \times 100$$

The greater the proportion of nitrogen retained, the higher the biological value (quality) of the protein being tested. The highest biological values are obtained from protein foods containing optimal quantities and proportions of all the essential amino acids plus adequate amounts of nonessential amino acids. Consequently, protein foods of animal origin have the highest biological values with eggs topping the list.[11] Because this method is based only upon absorbed nitrogen (not the amount consumed), it does not indicate the digestibility of a specific protein food source.

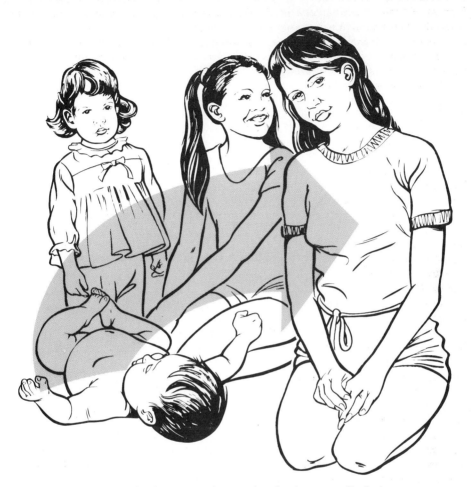

Figure 5-6.   Protein is absolutely necessary for growth and maintenance of body tissues.

Net protein utilization (NPU) is an expression of both the digestibility of a food protein source and its biological value. NPU represents the proportion of protein *retained* compared to the amount of food protein source *consumed.* NPU is expressed by the formula:[12]

$$P = \frac{BW \times N}{1000}$$

P   =   protein utilization
BW   =   body weight change in grams per day
N   =   nitrogen retention in mg per kg per day

Protein efficiency ratio (PER) expresses the ratio of weight gain in a growing animal in relation to its protein intake. Caloric intake needs to be adequate for this calculation to be valid. This method was devised to simplify calculations from feeding experiments using small laboratory animals. This is the measurement used for determining protein requirement in the U.S. RDAs.

Consumption of Protein. Consumption of protein per person in this country is generally more than needed. In addition, a large percentage of the protein comes from sources of high biological value. The adult RDA for protein is based upon .8g protein/kg desirable body weight. (Refer to Chapter Two, The RDAs—What Are They?, for an explanation of how the RDA for protein was set.) For an adult healthy male between the ages of 23 to 50 years weighing 154 pounds (70kg) that amounts to 56g of protein/day. A three ounce portion of meat (an average serving) contains approximately 21g of protein. One cup of milk supplies approximately 8g of protein. Consequently, just two servings of meat and two servings of milk in any one day's time provide this adult man with more than enough protein to meet his daily allowance.

Many people have the opinion that athletes require a very large daily protein allowance in order to build and maintain larger muscles. However, a normal varied diet contains sufficient protein to allow for growth and maintenance of muscle tissue even for an athlete in training.[13] What the athlete does need is increased caloric intake from carbohydrates and some fat to cover the higher physical energy expenditure for training and competition. *A very high protein intake places stress on the liver and kidneys and increases calcium excretion.*

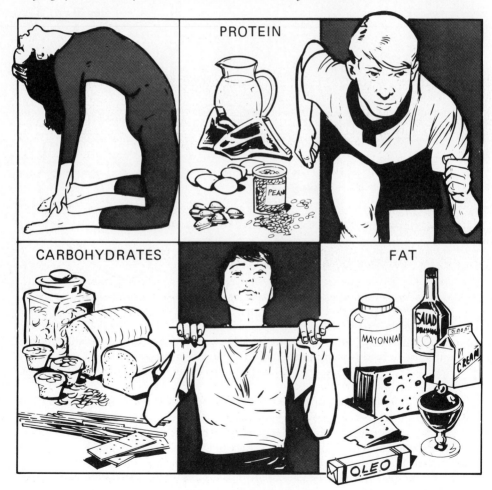

Figure 5-7.   An athlete's nutritional needs are similar to the healthy nonathlete's needs for a varied diet. It is not extra protein which athletes require but increased total calories, especially from carbohydrates and some fat, to cover their increased energy expenditures for training and competition.

Key Points: Proteins

I. Important nomenclature involved with the study of proteins:
acid group:

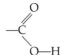

amino group (base):

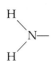

complete proteins: food proteins which supply all the essential amino acids in proportions similar to the body's requirement for making body proteins; generally of animal origin

essential amino acids: must be consumed in the diet

incomplete proteins: food proteins which appreciably lack one or more essential amino acids; generally of plant origin

limiting amino acid: amino acid of lowest quantity in a given food

"metabolic pool" of amino acids: conceptual term for amino acids available throughout the body for use as needed; not representative of a specific location

nonessential (dispensable) amino acids: can be manufactured by the body provided the basic elements are available

peptide bond: characteristic chemical bond of proteins =

$$-\overset{\overset{\textstyle O}{\|}}{C}-\overset{\overset{\textstyle H}{|}}{N}-$$

polypeptide: long chain peptides

II. Proteins are: organic, built from amino acids, 16 percent nitrogen-containing.
   A. Dietary protein must be supplied throughout life to maintain body tissues.
   B. Dietary protein needs are increased during periods of growth and new tissue development.

III. Essential amino acids are amino acids which cannot be manufactured by the body so they must be consumed in completed form from the diet.
   A. They are: methionine, threonine, tryptophan, isoleucine, leucine, lysine, valine, and phenylalanine.
   B. The amino acid histidine may be essential for infants and some adults.

IV. High quality proteins are complete proteins containing all the essential amino acids in favorable proportions for body protein synthesis and are, generally, of animal origin.

V. Protein polypeptides have four general structural arrangements.
   A. Primary structure is due to peptide bonds which cause peptide chain formation.
   B. Secondary structure is due to chemical bonding between elements within the peptide chain and results in helical formation.
   C. Tertiary structure is due to additional chemical bond formation between more

widely spaced elements within the peptide chain and results in the helical peptide folding back and forth upon itself.

 D. Quaternary structure of some proteins is due to bonding between two or more polypeptides with tertiary structure and results in a clumping or globular aggregate formation.

VI. Digestion of protein begins in the stomach.

 A. HCI is necessary for denaturation of protein and activation of pepsinogen to pepsin.

 B. Rennin, another gastric enzyme, is present in infants for the purpose of coagulating milk protein, casein.

 C. Major pancreatic proteases are:

  1. trypsinogen $\xrightarrow{\text{enterokinase}}$ trypsin
   (precursor)

  2. chymotrypsinogen $\xrightarrow{\text{trypsin}}$ chymotrypsin
   (precursor)

  3. carboxypeptidase

 D. Intestinal peptidases hydrolyze smaller peptides to amino acids.

VII. Amino acids are absorbed into the blood system.

 A. The absorption rate of amino acids is coordinated with the rate of digestion.

 B. Under some circumstances whole proteins are absorbed into the blood system. These proteins probably set up a sensitivity response which is expressed as an allergic reaction.

VIII. Functions of proteins can be categorized generally as:

 A. Growth and maintenance of body tissues

 B. Regulation of body processes

 C. Production of energy: proteins supply 4 kcal/gram

IX. More common methods of quantifying protein quality are:

 A. Biological value (BV)

 B. Net protein utilization (NPU)

 C. Protein efficiency ratio (PER)

X. The adult RDA for protein is based upon .8g protein/kg desirable body weight.

 A. Americans generally consume greater amounts of protein than needed.

 B. Even athletes are able to obtain adequate protein from a normal varied diet, providing their increased caloric needs are met.

Questions: Proteins

1. Besides carbon, hydrogen, and oxygen what other element is found in all proteins?

2. Identify the three general functions of protein.
 a. maintenance and growth of body tissue
 b. insulation of body against temperature changes
 c. regulation of body processes
 d. provide a source of energy

3. Upon analysis, a certain food source is found to contain 2g of nitrogen. How many grams of protein does this food source contain?

4. Nitrogen is found in the air we breathe. Nitrogen crosses the membranes of the lungs and enters the circulatory system where it is carried to the liver and is incorporated into newly synthesized proteins.
 a. True
 b. False

5. The basic building blocks of proteins are:
    a. fatty acids
    b. keto acids
    c. amino acids

6. Specificity of a given protein's characteristics and functions is due to:
    a. its dietary source: animal or plant
    b. its amino acid composition and pattern sequence
    c. its degree of "completeness"

7. Why are some amino acids termed "essential?"

8. What does the "metabolic pool" of amino acids represent?
    a. the storage area for amino acids
    b. the amino acids excreted in urine
    c. the total amino acids available for meeting body needs at any given time.

9. Which equation best represents the "metabolic pool" of amino acids.
    a. intake + excretion
    b. intake + products of body processes
    c. products of body chemical reactions + products of tissue breakdown

10. Choose the two statements which most correctly identify complete proteins:
    a. complete proteins have high biological value
    b. complete proteins contain all essential amino acids in the approximate pro-
        portions required to make body protein
    c. complete proteins are severely deficient in one limiting amino acid

11. Sources of incomplete proteins are generally of:
    a. plant origin
    b. animal origin

12. Which two foods contain proteins that are so incomplete they will not support life
    if eaten alone with no other added source of protein?
    a. meat, eggs
    b. fish, cheese
    c. gelatin, corn

13. Match the phrases on the right to the items on the left which they best describe:
    _____ 1. nonessential amino   a. must be obtained in completed form
                acids   from the diet
    _____ 2. incomplete proteins   b. meat, milk, eggs, cheese
    _____ 3. essential amino acids   c. building blocks of protein
    _____ 4. complete proteins   d. dispensable amino acids
    _____ 5. amino acids   e. grains, vegetables, fruit

14. Very long chains of several hundred amino acids are called _____ .

15. Hydrolysis of protein proceeds to → proteoses → polypeptides → peptides →
    dipeptides → _____ .

16. Chewing and _____ help to break up food and release protein from
    carbohydrate and fat associations.

17. What acid is needed for the activation of pepsinogen to pepsin?

18. Why does protein denaturation make a protein more "digestible?"

19. Describe the factors which contribute to the digestibility of milk protein (casein)
    for infants.

20. Indicate the activator for each of the following reactions:
    a. trypsinogen ⇌ trypsin
    b. chymotrypsinogen ⇌ chymotrypsin
    c. peptides ⇌ amino acids

21. Identify the following protein structures:

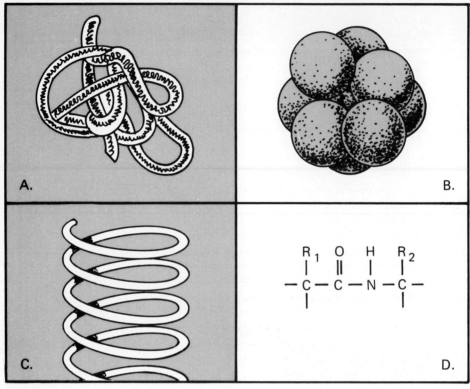

Figure 5-8.

a. _____
b. _____
c. _____
d. _____

22. What nondietary sources of protein provide significant sources of amino acids for absorption?

23. The absorption rate of amino acids is a constant factor regardless of the amount within the intestine to be absorbed.
     a. True
     b. False

24. Amino acids are absorbed into the:
     a. lymph system
     b. lacteals
     c. portal blood system

25. Sometimes the absorption of whole proteins or polypeptides occurs. This condition is thought to trigger the production of antibodies against those proteins with the resulting symptoms of an _____ .

26. The direction of amino acid metabolism depends upon:
     a. body needs and condition at the time of absorption
     b. availability of amino acids
     c. presence of pepsin in the stomach

27. Anemia results from a deficiency of hemoglobin and/or red blood cells in the circulating blood. Can protein deficiency cause anemia?
     a. Yes
     b. No
28. Which proteins protect the body by attacking disease agents such as viruses and bacteria?
     a. enzymes
     b. antibodies
     c. hormones
29. Dietary protein is generally an efficient and economic source of energy (body fuel).
     a. True
     b. False
30. Which proteins are catalysts?
     a. antibodies
     b. hormones
     c. enzymes
31. Proteins supply the same kcal/g as what other nutrient?
     a. carbohydrate
     b. fat
32. The following is an approximate indication of the percentage of amino acid content in wheat. Which amino acid is the "limiting amino acid?"

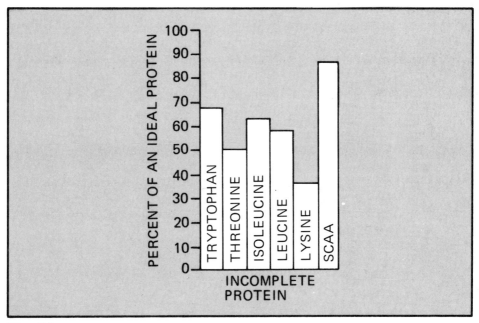

Figure 5-9.

33. Explain what happens to an egg when it is hard-boiled.
34. The quality of various proteins is not nutritionally equal.
     a. True
     b. False

35.   High heat and/or heat for an extended period of time generally _____ the digestibility and the absorbability of protein in a food source.
      a.   increases
      b.   decreases

36.   Match the items on the right to the phrases which they best represent on the left.
      _____ 1.   expresses both digesti-   a.   biological value (BV)
                 bility and BV   b.   net protein utilization (NPU)
      _____ 2.   expresses   utilization   c.   protein efficiency ratio (PER)
                 of absorbed protein
      _____ 3.   used in U.S. RDAs for
                 estimating protein re-
                 quirement   according
                 to the quality of pro-
                 tein consumed
      _____ 4.   represents protein re-
                 tained   and   utilized
                 compared to protein
                 consumed
      _____ 5.   very useful in small
                 animal feeding experi-
                 ments
      _____ 6.   determined from ni-
                 trogen measurements
                 of food intake and
                 urinary and fecal ex-
                 cretions

37.   American diets normally provide more than enough protein to meet body re-
      quirements.
      a.   True
      b.   False

38.   What is the protein RDA for a 30 year-old woman who is five-foot four-inches tall
      and weighs 120 pounds (55kg)?

39.   Approximately how many average servings of three ounce portions of meat
      would the woman in question 38 need to consume to meet her RDA for protein?

40.   Why is the RDA for protein based upon desirable body weight for body height?

41.   An athlete in training interested in building and maintaining larger muscles
      needs to:
      a.   consume large amounts of protein foods daily
      b.   needs to eat a variety of foods daily
      c.   needs to increase caloric intake to cover increased energy expenditure in
           exercise

42.   Why does a high protein intake place stress on the liver and kidneys?

Answers: Proteins

1.   nitrogen
2.   a, c, d
3.   2g N X 6.25 = 12.5g protein
4.   b; nitrogen must be obtained from dietary protein
5.   c
6.   b

7. They must be obtained from the diet because the body cannot manufacture them.
8. c
9. b
10. a and b
11. a
12. c
13. 1. d
    2. e
    3. a
    4. b
    5. c
14. polypeptides
15. amino acids
16. peristalsis of the stomach and intestine
17. hydrochloric acid (HCl)
18. Because it uncoils the polypeptide and exposes more of its chemical bonding to the action of various proteases and peptidases (enzymes).
19. The gastric secretion of rennin coagulates casein and causes it to remain for an extended period in the stomach, which increases exposure time of casein to the digestive action of pepsin.
20. a. enterokinase
    b. trypsin
    c. peptidases
21. a. tertiary   c. secondary
    b. quaternary d. primary
22. degraded intestinal cells and enzymes
23. b
24. c
25. allergic reaction
26. a and b
27. a. Protein is a constituent of hemoglobin. If protein intake is deficient hemoglobin production is reduced and anemia can result.
28. b
29. b
30. c
31. a; CHO at 4 kcal/gram
32. lysine
33. its protein is coagulated (denatured)
34. a
35. b
36. 1. b
    2. a
    3. c
    4. b
    5. c
    6. a
37. a
38. 44g
39. 1 oz meat = 7g protein
    3 oz portion (one average serving) = 21g

2 servings = 42g
answer: approximately two servings

40. Because it is the lean tissue of the body rather than the adipose tissue (fat) with which protein is most metabolically active and necessary for proper maintenance, growth, and functioning.

41. b and c

42. The liver must work harder to catabolize amino acids and metabolize their nitrogenous waste products; the kidneys must work harder to filter and excrete urea in urine. Also, both the liver and kidneys are exposed to the toxicity of ammonia as it accumulates faster than it can be metabolized.

PROTEIN SYNTHESIS AND BREAKDOWN

Efficient use of protein for both maintenance and building of new tissue requires two important conditions:

1. All necessary amino acids are available proportionally and simultaneously to meet tissue synthesis needs.

2. Energy intake is adequate to cover energy expenditure thus sparing protein from use as an energy source.

Anabolism is the term used to designate a building-up process like that of protein synthesis. Protein synthesis is a complex and beautifully orchestrated process. *Proteins are synthesized according to each cell's needs.* A detailed explanation of protein synthesis is not warranted here but a familiarization with the process and terms involved is necessary.

Deoxyribonucleic acid (DNA) is the substance containing genetic codes in each cell of your body. DNA contains your architectural and operational blueprint, so to speak, which makes each individual unique. *DNA is contained in the chromosomes of the cell nucleus.* However, protein synthesis occurs in the cell cytoplasm. (See footnote 4, Figure 1-4, Chapter One for illustration and explanation of the major cellular parts.) Consequently, the code must be carried from the nucleus to the site of protein synthesis. *Messenger ribonucleic acid (mRNA)* performs this function. The mRNA is a substance very similar (though not identical) to DNA. Messenger RNA copies the DNA configuration (its blueprint for the protein it wants to produce and then moves to the site in the cytoplasm (most frequently the ribosomes) where the protein synthesis will occur. Another substance called *transfer ribonucleic acid* (tRNA)[14] then carries individual amino acids to the points alongside the mRNA strand where each amino acid is to be located in the chain of the new protein. Once tRNA has brought all the necessary amino acids to their designated locations, peptide bonding occurs along the amino acid chain. This bonding action requires an energy source. The new polypeptide is released and tRNA is freed to again perform its pick-up and delivery function.

If there is a shortage of any one amino acid necessary for the production of a given protein then that protein's duplication process is limited. The term used to represent the amino acid in the smallest quantity in any one food source is *limiting amino acid.* An analogy to protein synthesis can be made to a weaver working at copying a fabric from the design he has set upon his loom. His ability to produce that fabric in that color design can be continued only as long as he has all the colors and varieties of yarn needed. As soon as the weaver runs out of one color or variety he can no longer produce that fabric or that specific color design, regardless of how many other yarns he has left in his supply basket. His production of identical fabrics is "limited" by the total amount of required yarns he has.

There are times when amino acids are broken down and the end-products of their breakdown are oxidized for energy or are excreted. *Catabolism* is the term used to designate the metabolic breakdown of complex substances to simpler substances. Catabolism involving protein can occur during extreme fasting and starvation as well as in uncontrolled diabetes. This catabolism involves body protein from tissue breakdown. It also occurs when there is an excess intake of protein above body protein synthesis needs. This catabolism involves dietary protein.

The catabolism of amino acids begins with the removal of the nitrogenous group of the molecule. This process is called *deamination* and occurs chiefly in the liver. Deamination results in the formation of *ammonia*, which is toxic to the body. Normally, however, it is converted to *urea* within the liver through a special chemical change cycle. Urea is then released from the liver into the circulatory system and carried to the kidneys where it is filtered and excreted within urine. A small amount of the released nitrogenous groups is used to produce other nitrogen-containing compounds including the nonessential amino acids. This reaction is called *transamination* because the nitrogenous group is transferred from one amino acid to another compound to form a new amino acid. Enzymes facilitating transamination reactions are called transaminases.

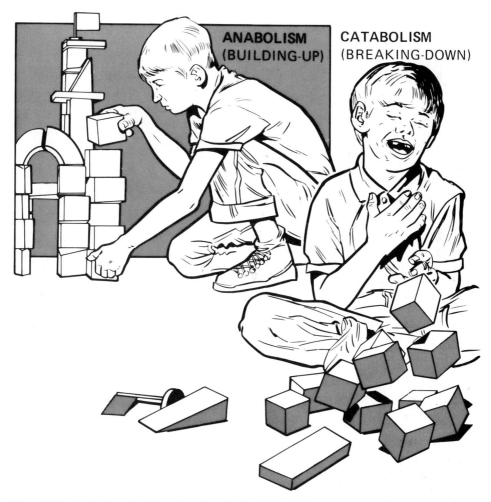

Figure 5-10.   Anabolism (building up) and catabolism (breaking down).

The non-nitrogenous portion of the catabolized amino acid is referred to as a *keto-acid*. Keto-acids can enter the energy producing cycle ultimately forming the end-products of energy, carbon dioxide and water. Keto-acids are further subdivided into two classifications: glucogenic and ketogenic. Glucogenic keto-acids have a greater potential to form glucose and glycogen when they are not used for energy.

Because of the relatively constant nitrogen factor in protein structure, the measurement of nitrogen intake versus products of excretion can give a good indication of the amount of protein retained in the body, and can give insight into what is happening to it during metabolism. Nitrogen balance studies help to determine whether a person is in an anabolic, catabolic, or homeostatic[15] state. When measured nitrogen intake is greater than measured nitrogen excretion the body is in *positive nitrogen balance (protein anabolism)*. Positive nitrogen balance indicates a growth state of new tissue, as in childhood and pregnancy. When nitrogen intake equals nitrogen excretion, nitrogen balance is in *equilibrium (homeostasis)* and is a sign that the body is obtaining sufficient amino acids to repair and replace those cells lost through normal aging and "wear and tear." When nitrogen intake is less than nitrogen excretion the body is in *negative nitrogen balance (protein catabolism)*. Negative nitrogen balance indicates the breaking down of body protein and is characteristic of such states as starvation, injury, immobilization, disease, and consumption of poor quality proteins.

Certain hormones influence amino acid/protein metabolism. A little analysis of the role of each hormone reveals whether it will have an anabolic or catabolic influence on amino acid metabolism. *Generally, those hormones which stimulate growth such as the pituitary growth hormone and sex hormones, estrogens and androgens, have an anabolic effect.* In addition, insulin is known to promote anabolism two ways. It provides for the absorption and utilization of available glucose. Glucose is used as an energy source conserving amino acids for other uses such as protein synthesis. This is a protein sparing process. Insulin also promotes protein synthesis because it facilitates the transportation of amino acids across cellular membranes. Thyroxine, hormone of the thyroid gland, stimulates growth when released in normal amounts so it has an anabolic effect.

Those hormones which stimulate the production of glucose for use as an energy source generally have a catabolic effect on protein/amino acid metabolism. The adrenocortical hormones[16] stimulate glucose production from the products of body protein breakdown (gluconeogenesis). An excess of thyroxine greatly increases the metabolic rate which results in a faster rate of energy production requiring an increased energy source. Both of these processes have a catabolic effect on protein metabolism.

Key Points: Protein Synthesis and Breakdown

I.   The maintenance and synthesis of new tissue requires that food intake provide all necessary amino acids and adequate calories to cover energy expenditures.

   A.   Anabolism is a term meaning a "building up" process such as protein synthesis.

   B.   DNA is the substance containing the genetic codes for each cell and is located in the chromosomes within the nucleus of the cell.

   C.   The codes are carried from the nucleus to the cytoplasm where they are replicated during protein synthesis with assistance of the substances messenger RNA and transfer RNA.

   D.   The amino acid in smallest quantity in any one food source is referred to as the limiting amino acid.

II. Protein broken down to amino acids can be ultimately metabolized for energy or the products of metabolism can be excreted.

   A.   Catabolism is the term which designates the metabolic breakdown of complex substances to simpler substances such as protein breakdown.

B. Body (tissue) protein is catabolized during fasting, starvation, and uncontrolled diabetes.

C. Dietary protein is catabolized when the intake is in excess of protein synthesis needs.

D. Catabolism includes:

1. Deamination: the removal of the nitrogenous group of the amino acid resulting in the formation of ammonia. In the liver, ammonia is converted to urea. Urea is then carried by the blood to the kidneys which filter urea into urine for excretion from the body.

2. Transamination: the transference of a nitrogenous group from an amino acid to another compound which can result in the formation of nonessential amino acids.

3. Non-nitrogenous portions of amino acids remaining after catabolization are called keto-acids.

III. The measurement of body nitrogen balance is a good indicator of the direction of current protein metabolism.

A. Positive nitrogen balance occurs when nitrogen intake is greater than nitrogen excretion and indicates a state of tissue growth.

B. Negative nitrogen balance occurs when nitrogen excretion is greater than intake and indicates a state of tissue breakdown.

IV. Hormones influence amino acid/protein metabolism. Generally:

A. Hormones which stimulate growth have an anabolic effect.

B. Hormones which stimulate glucose production for energy use have a catabolic effect.

Questions: Protein Synthesis and Breakdown

1. Identify the two conditions most favorable to efficient use of protein for body tissue synthesis.

a. adequate energy intake

b. negative nitrogen balance

c. intake of all necessary amino acids in proportions most favorable for protein tissue synthesis

2. Match the phrases on the right to the terms they best describe on the left.

_____ 1.	anabolism	a.	converted to urea in liver
_____ 2.	keto-acid	b.	means breaking down
_____ 3.	transamination	c.	removal of the nitrogenous group
_____ 4.	glucogenic	d.	means building up
_____ 5.	catabolism	e.	transfer of a nitrogenous group to form a new amino acid
_____ 6.	deamination	f.	glucose-forming
_____ 7.	ammonia	g.	non-nitrogenous portion of a catabolized amino acid

3. Identify the following conditions as either in positive nitrogen balance (p) or negative nitrogen balance (n).

a. healthy, growing infant

b. a healthy woman seven months pregnant

c. adult woman with a high fever

d. adult man bedridden and in traction with two broken legs

e. healthy adolescent girl

f. starving adult man

4. Identify the following participants in protein synthesis:

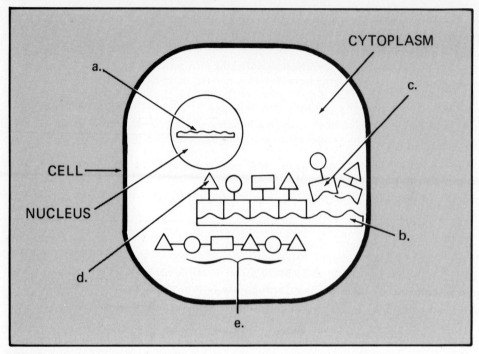

Figure 5-11.

   a. _____
   b. _____
   c. _____
   d. _____
   e. _____

5. Generally, those hormones which stimulate growth have an _____ effect on protein metabolism; and those hormones which stimulate production of glucose have a _____ effect on protein metabolism.

Answers: Protein Synthesis and Breakdown

1. a and c
2. 1. d
    2. g
    3. e
    4. f
    5. b
    6. c
    7. a
3. a. p
    b. p
    c. n
    d. n
    e. p
    f. n

4. a. DNA
    b. mRNA
    c. tRNA
    d. amino acids
    e. newly formed and released polypeptide
5. anabolic; catabolic

PROTEIN DEFICIENCY

The lack of an adequate quality and quantity of protein food is a problem of international concern. The number of children and adults with clinical and sub-clinical signs of protein deficiency worldwide is considerable. Protein deficiency is most common in tropical and subtropical countries. Protein deficiency in the United States is presently most often a result of neglect or ignorance of good nutrition principles rather than the inability to obtain protein foods.[17]

A diet deficient in protein but adequate in energy (calories) results in the disease termed *kwashiorkor*. Kwashiorkor is frequently found in association with another deficiency disease, *marasmus*. Marasmus is the wasting condition which results from a lack of adequate energy (calorie) intake. In reality, an individual frequently shows clinical symptoms for deficiencies falling somewhere between these two extremes. In addition, both diseases are usually accompanied by vitamin and/or mineral deficiencies. Because of the close association between protein and calorie deficiencies, the diseases are most often grouped together in a class called *protein-calorie (energy) malnutrition* (PCM). For study purposes, an attempt to separate the symptoms between these two conditions follows.

Marasmus occurs at any age in childhood when the total food intake falls below body needs. Marasmus generally results in a "little old man" appearance: the child's face has sunken cheeks and eyes. Though the abdomen may be swollen, the child's extremities are terribly thin showing the wasting of his or her body. Body height is retarded. The child is irritable during the first stages of hunger. Later, apathy and listlessness begin to characterize the starving child's behavior. This quieter, unemotional behavior requires less effort and caloric expenditure and may be the body's way of trying to conserve energy.

Kwashiorkor most frequently appears between the ages of two and four years. *The consistency of kwashiorkor occurring between these ages is related to the fact that this condition occurs in the child who is weaned from the breast of his or her nursing mother in order that a new sibling arrival may be put to the mother's breast.* The name of the disease, according to the language of the society in which it was first noted, literally means "the sickness the older child gets when the next baby is born."[18] Adequate intake of human breast milk prevents kwashiorkor because it is an excellent source of protein as well as other nutrients. Unfortunately, foods very low in protein, though high in carbohydrates, generally become the staple diet of the child after weaning.

Causes of kwashiorkor are multifaceted with a basis on poor economics, poor nutrition knowledge and infant feeding practices, poor sanitation practices, poor health care facilities, and even disturbed psychological/emotional relationships. The abrupt weaning of the first child may break or interfere with the formation of the necessary maternal-child bond. The child probably interprets the loss of maternal nurturance as rejection and reacts by refusing to eat. The mother who is engrossed with her own stressful problems gives up trying to coax the child to eat. As a result, the child fails to thrive.

Nutritional edema is observed in kwashiorkor. Edema is the condition of body tissues swelling with fluid. The edema may make a child appear normal in weight. The face even appears round and full. If pressure of a finger is applied to the skin of a person with edema a pit will form and remain for an extended time after the finger is lifted. The edema is a result of a dramatic decrease in blood plasma proteins, especially albumin. Water is normally drawn into association with albumin in the circulatory system. When plasma albumin is very low

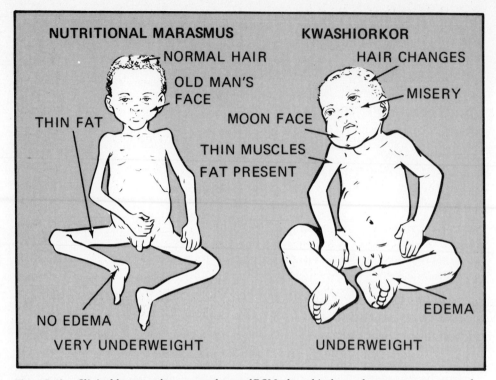

NUTRITIONAL MARASMUS   KWASHIORKOR

NORMAL HAIR   HAIR CHANGES

OLD MAN'S
FACE   MISERY

THIN FAT   MOON FACE

THIN MUSCLES

FAT PRESENT

NO EDEMA   EDEMA

VERY UNDERWEIGHT   UNDERWEIGHT

*Figure 5-12.   Clinical features of two severe forms of PCM—kwashiorkor and marasmus—contrasted
diagrammatically. Source: Jelliffe DB: Child Nutrition in Developing Countries—A
Handbook for Field Workers. Washington, D.C., U.S. Department of Health, Education,
and Welfare, Public Health Service Publication No. 1822, 1968.*

the water begins to seep out of the blood vessels into the tissues causing the edema. After
nutritional therapy has begun the edema disappears and the previously concealed, wasted
condition of the body is revealed.

Other symptoms include weight loss, stunted growth, retarded wound healing, anemia, decreased resistance to disease (especially due to decreased antibody formation), an
enlarged and fatty liver, vomiting, and diarrhea. Abnormal skin color changes occur along
with drying, peeling, and ulceration of the skin. Hair frequently becomes sparse and loses
pigmentation.

Improving the quality and quantity of a local food protein source is one major step in
alleviating PCM. Some successful attempts have been made to produce hybrid varieties of
grains such as wheat and corn which have improved amino acid patterns, and rice which
produces a higher yield. Cultivation of leguminous crops (peas, beans, lentils, and soybeans) in areas where protein deficiency occurs is encouraged because of their relatively
high protein content and favorable amino acid complementarity pattern with grains.[19]
Supplementation of plant protein with amino acid mixtures has been useful. Various organizations involved with the problems of hunger have sponsored research aimed at developing plant protein mixtures which are inexpensive, but contain a total amino acid
pattern of high biological value. One such mixture is called Incaparina. The acceptance of
mixtures of plant protein blends, or a blend of small amounts of animal protein with plant
proteins or any new foodstuff, depends largely upon socio-cultural factors as well as the
taste and food preferences of its intended consumers.

Key Points: Protein Deficiency

I.   Protein deficiency is a problem of international concern and occurs mostly in tropical and subtropical countries.

II   Terms associated with the study of protein deficiency are:

Kwashiorkor: a protein deficiency disease associated with inadequate protein intake with generally adequate caloric intake.

Marasmus: wasting condition associated with inadequate nutrient and caloric intake.

PCM: protein-calorie (or energy) malnutrition which includes Kwashiorkor and marasmus.

Nutritional edema: body tissues swelling with fluid as a result of a dramatic decrease in blood plasma protein, albumin.

III. Kwashiorkor most often occurs in the child who is weaned from the breast of his or her mother enabling the mother to nurse a newborn child.

A. Kwashiorkor is a disease resulting from emotional, psychological, economical, medical, and educational factors as well as nutritional factors.

B. Edema makes a child with kwashiorkor appear round and full concealing that child's wasted condition.

IV. Improvement of the food sources for, and the dietary intake of persons at nutritional risk, must take into account social, cultural, and religious factors as well as limitations set by individual customs and preferences.

Questions: Protein Deficiency

1. Protein deficiency is most common
    a. in the U.S.
    b. in the arctic regions
    c. in the tropical and subtropical countries

2. Protein deficiency in the U.S. is most often a result of _____ .

3. Identify the following descriptions according to the type of nutritional deficiency:
    a. A thin, emaciated baby with a protruding round belly has sunken cheeks and eyes, and a little old man appearance.
    b. A child about two years-old with a round, moon-shaped face has fluid-filled body tissues (edema), sparse and depigmented hair, many skin lesions, and frequent diarrhea.

4. Apathy and listlessness may be the body's attempt at _____ in PCM.

5. The separation of a child from what food source generally precipitates kwashiorkor?

6. It is not uncommon for a child who has been cured of kwashiorkor to return to the treatment clinic a second time with the same condition. What factors contribute to this occurrence?

7. Nutritional edema is the result of a protein intake deficiency and occurs when:
    a. white blood cell count drops
    b. red blood cell count drops
    c. blood plasma albumin levels drop

8. Nutritional edema is characterized by:
    a. swollen tissues and pitting of the skin when pressure is applied
    b. a thin emaciated body
    c. high blood plasma levels

9. Refer back to the many functions of proteins for review, then match the reasons for development of protein deficiency symptoms on the right to the symptoms listed on the left:

_____ 1. low resistance to infec-   a. decreased plasma protein production
           tion or disease   b. inadequate protein for growth and
_____ 2. fatty liver   maintenance of body tissues
_____ 3. retarded wound heal-   c. decreased antibody formation
           ing   d. decreased lipoprotein formation
_____ 4. depigmentation of   e. inadequate protein available for tissue
           skin and hair   growth or scar tissue formation
_____ 5. anemia   f. inadequate protein for pigment forma-
_____ 6. edema   tion
_____ 7. stunted growth and   g. inadequate protein for normal
           weight loss   amounts of hemoglobin production

10. Simple food supplementation programs are not enough to break the cycle of PCM occurrence because of extenuating economic, social, psychological influences, limited sanitation and nutrition knowledge, and limited health care facilities.
    a. True
    b. False

Answers: Protein Deficiency

1. c
2. neglectful care or ignorance of good nutrition principles
3. a. marasmus (total calorie deficiency)
   b. kwashiorkor (protein deficiency)
4. conserving energy
5. human breast milk
6. psychological/emotional disturbances in the mother-child relationship; inadequate nutrition knowledge and continued poor infant feeding practices
7. c
8. a
9. 1. c
   2. d
   3. e
   4. f
   5. g
   6. a
   7. b
10. a

INBORN ERRORS OF PROTEIN METABOLISM

A mutation in an individual's DNA can result in incorrectly formed or reduced production of enzyme proteins. The defective enzyme production results in some abnormality of metabolism—an inborn error of metabolism. The degree of malfunctioning metabolism which results depends in part on how the body accommodates and reacts to the products of the impaired metabolism, the quantity of such products, and the degree of structural change in the malformed enzyme. The expression of symptoms varies from slight to severe.

Phenylketonuria. Phenylketonuria (PKU) is the condition produced when an individual lacks the enzyme necessary to metabolize the essential amino acid phenylalanine to the nonessential amino acid tyrosine. Tyrosine is necessary for the formation of the pigment melanin and some hormones. Consequently, phenylalanine and the products of its abnormal metabolism accumulate in the blood and urine. Since phenylalanine is an essential amino acid, the child with PKU must have enough phenylalanine, tyrosine, and protein in his or her diet to allow for adequate protein synthesis. However, the diet has to be carefully controlled to eliminate excess phenylalanine.

Foods high in this amino acid, especially animal foods, must be deleted from the diet. Commercial formulas for the infant with PKU are available which are controlled in phenylalanine content. The phenylalanine blood level of the growing child must be regularly monitored and the diet adjusted as necessary. Food exchange lists based on the grouping of foods by similar phenylalanine content facilitate special diet planning for the individual with PKU.

Untreated phenylketonuria results in a build-up of phenylalanine and its metabolites and inadequate tyrosine to meet body needs. These conditions lead to slowed physical growth and the development of moderate to severe mental retardation. Children with this condition have light skin, blond hair, and blue eyes because phenylalanine cannot be converted to the compounds necessary for normal pigmentation. Such children are irritable, often hyperactive, and susceptible to convulsive seizures.[20]

An early diagnosis must be made in order to stop the negative progress of PKU. A simple chemical test of an infant's diaper wet with urine, or a blood serum test, can identify infants with PKU. PKU screening tests are required in most states.

Key Points: Inborn Errors of Protein Metabolism

I.   An inborn error of metabolism (abnormality of metabolism) is the result of a mutation in an individual's DNA which causes incorrectly formed or inadequately produced enzyme production.

II.   Phenylketonuria (PKU) occurs when an individual lacks the enzyme necessary to metabolize the essential amino acid phenylalanine.

$$\text{Phenylalanine} \not\to \text{Tyrosine}$$

III. Some phenylalanine is needed in the diet along with adequate amounts of tyrosine and protein to enable growth and new tissue formation.

IV.   Untreated phenylketonuria results in the build-up of phenylalanine and its metabolites and lack of adequate tyrosine for pigment formation and some hormone production, conditions responsible for the symptoms of PKU: hyperactivity, irritability, susceptibility to seizures, mental retardation, pale skin, blue eyes, and blond hair.

V.   The diet for the individual with PKU must be controlled to eliminate excess phenylalanine. Special infant formulas and food exchange lists are available for planning diets low in phenylalanine content.

Questions: Inborn Errors of Protein Metabolism

1.   Inborn errors of metabolism include disease conditions arising from a malformed or absent enzyme production.
      a.   True
      b.   False

2.   Phenylketonuria results from an inborn error of protein metabolism.
      a.   True
      b.   False

3.   The essential amino acid phenylalanine is normally metabolized to what nonessential amino acid?

4. Symptoms and/or characteristics of a child with untreated phenylketonuria are:
    a.   dark pigmentation
    b.   irritability
    c.   severe mental retardation
    d.   blond hair, blue eyes, very light skin
5. Though the incidence of PKU is very small, why do you suppose a test of an infant's diaper urine or blood serum test for PKU is required in most states?
6. Why must some phenylalanine be present in the PKU infant's or child's diet?

Answers: Inborn Errors of Protein Metabolism

1. a
2. a
3. tyrosine
4. b, c, d
5. The test is simple, inexpensive, highly accurate, and easily performed. It can also be utilized early enough to effectively treat an infant with a positive diagnosis and prevent the negative progress of the disease.
6. Phenylalanine is an essential amino acid. Some phenylalanine must be consumed to allow for growth and maintenance of body tissues.

VEGETARIANISM AND PROTEIN COMPLEMENTATION

Recently, many persons in the U.S. have chosen vegetarianism as an alternate to the more common meat-based diet. Reasons for choosing a vegetarian diet may be of traditional religious, cultural, social, or ethical origin. Some persons simply believe that a vegetarian diet is more healthful for them. Others see vegetarianism as a more economical diet choice. These persons are the so-called "new vegetarians."[21] Whatever their reasons for choosing a vegetarian diet all vegetarians share a common task—the need to make wise food choices in order to meet their nutritional needs from a more limited food selection.

Whenever a food group is omitted as a choice in diet planning, greater skill must be exercised in order to choose foods which meet individual nutrient requirements. For vegetarians this means more careful planning in protein food selections. Some vegetarians do include a few animal source protein foods such as milk, cheese, and eggs in their diets. The process of making protein food choices from selections available for this type of vegetarian is not as critical as it is for the vegetarian who excludes all animal source foods from his or her diet.

The four food groups are milk, meat, breads and cereals, fruits and vegetables. The vegetarian who omits all animal source foods is left with only half of the groups (breads and cereals; fruits and vegetables) from which to make all food selections. Other vegetarians who further exclude additional foods, or food groups, trim the choices from which they can make food selections to a relatively small number. Therefore, in order to plan diets using foods which adequately meet his or her nutritional needs, it is important for such a vegetarian to become knowledgeable about nutrition. Vegetarian diets can usually provide adequate nutrients to prevent deficiencies if sound nutrition principles are learned and practiced.[22]

The following are general classes of vegetarian diets:

1. Lacto-ovo-vegetarian diets (lacto=milk; ovo=egg) include animal source foods such as dairy products and eggs but exclude flesh foods.
2. Lactovegetarian diets (lacto=milk) include animal source foods such as milk and milk products but exclude flesh foods and eggs.
3. Vegan diets exclude all flesh and animal source foods such as meat, poultry, fish, eggs, and dairy products.

4.   Fruitarian diets include primarily fruits, with some honey, nuts, and oils.

Nutrient value of vegetarian diets. Since lacto-ovo-vegetarians include animal food sources which contain proteins of high biological value (complete proteins supplying all essential amino acids), their risk of protein deficiency is low. Vitamin B_{12} is available from milk and milk products. The use of whole grain cereals and breads which not only provide a good source of some protein, but iron and B-complex vitamins as well, is recommended. Because milk and milk products such as cheese and nuts (containing significant amounts of fats) are often used in relatively large quantities as protein sources, consumption of nonfat and low-fat milk may be indicated.[23] Whole milk, however, is recommended for children.

Individuals using vegan diets encounter a greater difficulty in obtaining adequate nutrient intake. The sheer bulk of food which must be consumed on vegan diets in order to meet calorie needs can be difficult for some persons to consume, especially children. Vitamin B_{12} is supplied only in foods from animal sources and a vitamin B_{12} deficiency may result from the use of a vegan diet. Storage levels of vitamin B_{12} in former meat eaters may be high in relation to daily needs for this vitamin and deficiency symptoms may not present themselves for a number of years.[24] The risk for vitamin B_{12} deficiency may be high for other persons, however, and a vitamin B_{12} supplement or the use of foods fortified with vitamin B_{12}, such as fortified soybean milk, is generally recommended.

When milk or milk products are omitted from vegetarian diets an inadequate intake of vitamin D, riboflavin, and calcium may occur.[25] Foods providing natural sources of vitamin D are limited although adequate exposure of the body to sunshine can cause significant formation of vitamin D in the skin. Dark green, leafy vegetables, legumes, whole grains, and limited amounts of nutritional yeast can provide significant sources of riboflavin in the vegan diet. Calcium absorption even from vegetables high in calcium content may be low. The use of fortified soy milk is generally recommended to provide a regular source of vitamins B_{12} and D, and calcium.

High amounts of phytic acid and fiber from cereal products consumed in a vegetarian diet interfere with iron and zinc absorption and, therefore, the potential risk of iron and/or zinc deficiency is greater for vegans.[26] Use of leavened bread is recommended because yeast lowers the phytate content of whole wheat flour used in breadmaking. Increased ascorbic acid (vitamin C) is recommended to enhance iron absorption along with the increased intake of iron-dense foods.[27]

Vegan and fruitarian diets are more restrictive in the foods they allow so their use presents greater difficulties in meeting all nutrient requirements. Deficiency symptoms may not appear until deficiency conditions are well advanced. *The younger the individual and the longer the time such a limited diet is used without recommended nutritional supplementation, the greater the risks for the development of nutrient deficiencies.*

Protein complementation. Protein complementation is the combining of protein foods with amino acid patterns that enhance the total protein value of each food. The amino acids in relatively large amounts (strengths) in one food are *eaten in the same meal* with a food low in those amino acids (weaknesses), but which contribute a good supply of amino acids either in low amounts or absent in the first food. In this way foods containing incomplete proteins can be made more complete by providing all essential amino acids, and a good spectrum of nonessential amino acids in sufficient amounts to meet body protein needs.

How can a person know which proteins to combine together to achieve enhanced protein complementation? At first this task would seem overwhelming because of the need to know the amino acid patterns of many different foods. Fortunately, there are some general rules-of-thumb which can help to simplify this process.

In general, enhanced protein combinations from non-meat sources which more adequately meet body protein needs can be obtained from combinations of grains (rice, wheat, corn, oats, barley, and rye) with milk or milk products; grains with legumes (peas, beans, lentils); seeds and nuts[28] with legumes.[29] There are many different ways of expressing the degree of improved amino acid complementation between food groups and Figure 5-13 is one.

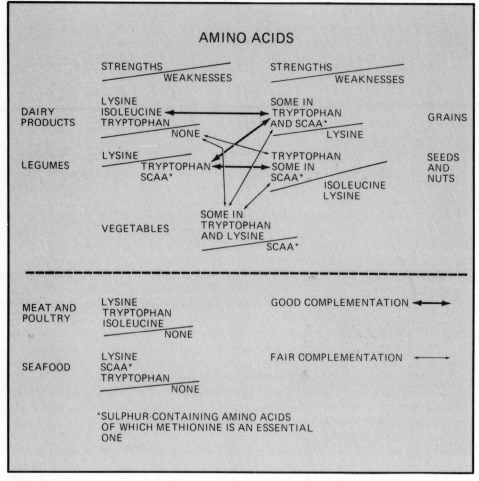

Figure 5-13. Relative *strengths and weaknesses of amino acids in food groups. Adapted from Lappé FM: Diet for a Small Planet, revised edition. New York, Ballantine Books, 1975.*

The supporting role vegetables can play in rounding out the protein complementation of different foods within a meal are shown in Figure 5-13. Meat, poultry, and seafood are included on this chart in order to demonstrate the ability of these high protein foods (even when used in relatively small amounts) to increase the total protein available from a meal of mixed foods or a prepared dish of mixed foods. Lappé has provided an in-depth study of protein complementation and gives practical guidelines, and many recipes for general consumer use, in food preparation using protein complementation principles.

Textured vegetable proteins are protein food products intended to replace and, in some cases, resemble meats. They are usually made from soybeans which are processed in different ways to produce bite-size particles or a stringy fiber-like product.[30] Some products are extenders to add to meat. They stretch the portions which can be obtained from the meat source while the meat improves the biological value of the soy protein. Others are formed to appear like and totally replace a meat such as a hamburger patty or bacon strip. Clamp gives a practical guide for the use of textured vegetable protein (TVP) products, soybeans, and other low-cost protein foods.[31]

The vegetarian needs to know how to use plant foods in order to make maximum use of the protein they contain. In view of the ever increasing world population, greater use of plant protein foods in order to meet our protein needs may need to be made by each of us.

Key Points: Vegetarianism and Protein Complementation

I.   Because vegetarians decrease the number of food groups from which they can make food selections, they must use greater skill in planning diets to meet individual nutrient requirements. Lacto-ovo-vegetarian and lactovegetarian diets provide food groups from which some animal source food selections can be made. These diets can supply high quality protein, adequate amounts of vitamins B_{12} and D, riboflavin, and calcium.

II.   Vegan and fruitarian diets are at risk of being deficient in vitamins D and B_{12}, riboflavin, calcium, iron, and zinc without nutritional supplementation of these nutrients.
   A.   Use of fortified soy milk is recommended in order to provide vitamins B_{12} and D, calcium, and protein.
   B.   Intake of citrus fruit is recommended several times daily to provide increased ascorbic acid intake which enhances iron absorption.
   C.   Selection of iron-dense foods is recommended along with a selection of whole wheat breads leavened with yeast because of its lowered phytate content.
   D.   Consumption of dark green, leafy vegetables, legumes, whole grains, and some nutritional yeast is recommended for sources of riboflavin in the diet.

III. Protein foods can be combined in ways which increase the total protein value of each food over that of each food eaten separately.
   A.   Foods with relatively large amounts of certain amino acids are matched with foods which have relatively low amounts of those same amino acids.
   B.   Enhanced matches can be made between food groups:
      1.   grains with milk or milk products
      2.   grains with legumes
      3.   seeds and nuts with legumes
   C.   Small amounts of fish, poultry, and meat can increase the total protein value of a mixed food dish.

IV.   Soybeans are made into textured vegetable protein (TVP) products which often resemble meats and are intended to replace a meat source in a meal. They are also made into extenders intended to be combined with a meat source. Extenders increase the number of servings which can be obtained from a meat source while retaining a total protein content of high biological value.

Questions: Vegetarianism and Protein Complementation

1.   One common problem shared by all vegetarians is:
   a.   that no vegetarian diets are healthful.
   b.   the limited availability of vegetable foods.
   c.   the need to make wise food choices in order to meet their nutritional needs from a more limited food selection.

2.   The fewer the food groups used in food selection the greater the (ease/difficulty) in obtaining all nutrient requirements from diet.

3.   Besides vegetables, fruit, cereals, and grains lacto-ovo-vegetarians also eat what animal source foods?

4. What diets include only vegetable and fruit food sources?
   a. lactovegetarian diets
   b. vegan diets
   c. fruitarian diets

5. Why do vegetarians have difficulty in obtaining adequate amounts of vitamin B_{12}?

6. Why are vegetarians especially encouraged to eat whole grain breads and cereals?

7. In addition to protein, legumes and cereals contain significant amounts of (carbohydrate/fat).

8. In addition to protein, whole milk, cheese, and nuts contain significant amounts of (carbohydrate/fat).

9. The risk of inadequate protein intake is greatest in the use of:
   a. lacto-ovo-vegetarian diets
   b. lactovegetarian diets
   c. vegan diets

10. Inadequate kcal intake is probable on vegan diets because consumption of _____ foods reduces appetite and often "fills up" a person before the total kcal intake requirement is met.

11. When milk or milk products are omitted from vegetarian diets inadequate intake of what three vitamins and mineral may occur?

12. What two substances from cereal products reduce iron and zinc absorption when these substances are present in relatively large amounts?

13. The intake of what vitamin increases iron absorption?
   a. vitamin D
   b. vitamin B_{12}
   c. vitamin C (ascorbic acid)

14. What fortified product is recommended for intake by vegans to provide a regular source of vitamins B_{12} and D, and calcium?

15. Why are vegan and fruitarian diets not recommended for children?

16. Protein complementation is:
   a. combining foods that taste good together
   b. combining foods with mutually supplemental amino acid patterns
   c. combining similar protein foods together

17. Why are small amounts of animal protein in a dish of mixed foods such as a casserole of noodles, chicken, and broccoli especially valuable?

18. Protein is best absorbed and utilized when complementary protein foods are eaten in the same meal.
   a. True
   b. False

19. Rate the following menus as examples of good or poor protein complementation and briefly explain the reason for your rating:
   a. Split pea soup
      Tossed green salad with vinegar and oil dressing
      Iced tea
   b. Macaroni and cheese
      Green beans with cashew nuts
      Jello
      Milk

c. Vegetable soup
   Hopping John
      (rice and black-eyed peas)
   Cornbread
   Lemonade

d. Cheese enchiladas
   Corn tortillas
   Refried beans
   Spicy rice
   Iced tea

20. What foods could be added to recipe "a" above to improve protein complementation?

21. The following are examples of the amino acid content of some incomplete proteins. Combine them into pairs which are good protein complements.

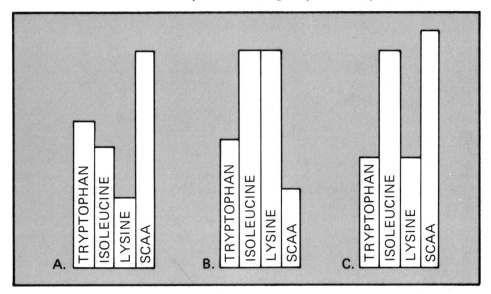

Figure 5-14.

Answers: Vegetarianism and Protein Complementation

1. c
2. difficulty
3. milk, milk products such as cheese, eggs
4. b
5. Vitamin B_{12} is found only in foods of animal origin.
6. Because whole grains offer more iron, B-complex vitamins, and protein than refined, white breads.
7. carbohydrate
8. fat
9. c
10. high-bulk
11. vitamins D and B_{12}, riboflavin, calcium
12. phytic acid and fiber
13. c
14. fortified soy milk
15. Because a child probably cannot consume the large quantity of high-bulk food

necessary to provide adequate kcal, calcium, vitamins and protein for activity, body metabolism, and growth. A child is much more likely to develop one or more nutrient deficiencies due to lower body reserves and a smaller intake of nutrients.

16. b
17. The meat makes more complete (complements) the protein from the grains (noodles) and vegetables (broccoli) and increases the total protein of this combination dish greater than if each food was eaten singly.
18. a
19. a. poor—no complement for the peas (legumes)
     b. good—macaroni (grains) plus cheese (dairy products) plus added nuts and vegetables for lesser but additional complementation.
     c. good—grains (rice and corn flour plus black-eyed peas—legumes) and lesser but additional vegetable complementation.
     d. good—cheese (dairy products) plus corn flour (grain) and beans (legumes) plus rice (grains).
20. Some examples:
     whole wheat breads or rolls; sesame and sunflower seeds in a salad; whole wheat toast with peanut butter; a glass of milk; meat chunks in the soup such as ham
21. A and B; B and C

REFERENCES

[1] This nitrogen must be obtained from dietary protein in order to make body protein. The human body cannot utilize "free" nitrogen as it occurs in the air. Approximately 1g of nitrogen within a food protein source represents 6.25g protein content.

[2] A **buffer** refers to having both acid and alkaline properties. A buffer can help keep a solution at a stable pH (level of acidity) by accepting or releasing hydrogen ions (H+). Refer to Chapter Thirteen for a more detailed description.

[3] The acidity of the stomach is about pH 1.5-2: very acidic.

[4] Denaturation of proteins also occurs during heating and cooking which makes the protein involved more "digestible." Denaturation of body proteins such as enzymes and hormones renders them inactive.

[5] **Gastric** refers to the stomach.

[6] Robinson CH: Fundamentals of Normal Nutrition, 3rd ed. New York, The Macmillan Company, 1978, p. 46

[7] Fontana VJ and Moreno-Pagan F: Allergy and diet. *In* Goodhart RS and Shils ME (eds): Modern Nutrition in Health and Disease, 6th ed. Philadelphia, Lea and Febiger, 1980, p. 1071

[8] **Catalyze** means to promote the occurrence and increase the rate of chemical reactions. Catalysts do not themselves participate in or become part of the products of a chemical reaction.

[9] Protein is most often a more costly source of energy than either carbohydrate or fat food sources. From an economical point of view, you should consume enough protein to meet body protein needs and look to carbohydrates and some fat for fulfilling remaining caloric needs.

[10] Munro HN and Crim MC: The proteins and amino acids. *In* Goodhart RS and Shils ME (eds): Modern Nutrition in Health and Disease, 6th ed. Philadelphia, Lea and Febiger, 1980, p. 90

[11] Kreutler PA: Nutrition in Perspective. Englewood Cliffs, NJ; Prentice-Hall, Inc., 1980, p. 146

[12] Whitney EN and Hamilton EMN: Understanding Nutrition. St. Paul, MN; West Publishing Company, 1977, p. 533

[13] The following article gives an interesting survey of the nutritional beliefs of many athletes, some of which are alarmingly ill-founded: Darden E: The nutrition of Olympic athletes. The Journal of Home Economics, 69, March 1977, pp. 40-43

[14] Transfer RNA is not a long strand but appears to be composed of small, separate units.

[15] **Homeostatic** refers to a state of equilibrium.

[16] Adrenocortical hormones are produced by the adrenal cortex, examples are the gluco-corticoids: corticosterone, hydrocortisone, and cortisone.

[17] McNutt KW and McNutt DR: Nutrition and Food Choices. Chicago, Science Research Associates, Inc., 1978, p. 413

[18] Williams SR: Nutrition and Diet Therapy. St. Louis, The C. V. Mosby Company, 1977, p. 341

[19] Robinson CH: Fundamentals of Normal Nutrition, 3rd ed. New York, The Macmillan Company, 1978, p. 457

[20] Kreutler PA: Nutrition in Perspective. Englewood Cliffs, NJ; Prentice-Hall, Inc., 1980, pp. 139-140

[21] Erhard D: The new vegetarians. Nutrition Today, 8, November-December 1973, pp. 4-12

[22] A helpful source of vegetarian diet information is the American Dietetic's Statement on vegetarianism:
Position paper on the vegetarian approach to eating. Journal of the American Dietetic Association, 77, July 1980, pp. 61-69

[23] Register UD and Sonnenberg LM: The vegetarian diet. Journal of the American Dietetic Association, 62, March 1973

[24] Nutrition and vegetarianism. Dairy Council Digest, 50, January-February 1979, p. 4

[25] Smith EB: A guide to good eating the vegetarian way. Journal of Nutrition Education, 7, July-September 1975, p. 109

[26] Swanson CA and King JC: Human zinc nutrition. Journal of Nutrition Education, 11, October-December 1979, p. 181

[27] Taber LAL and Cook RA: Dietary and anthropometric assessment of adult omnivores, fish-eaters, and lacto-ovo-vegetarians. Journal of the American Dietetic Association, 76, January 1980, p. 28

[28] The peanut is actually a legume. However, it has an amino acid pattern similar to nuts as well as a familiarity to most people as a nut, so it is treated as a nut.

[29] Lappé FM: Diet for a Small Planet, revised edition. New York, Ballantine Books, 1975, p. 153

[30] Lockmiller NR: What are textured protein products? Food Technology, 26, May 1972, pp. 55-57

[31] Clamp BA: Cooking with Low-Cost Proteins. New York, Arco Publishing Company, Inc., 1976

6
DIGESTION, ABSORPTION, AND METABOLISM: AN OVERVIEW

The processes involved in the digestion, absorption, and metabolism of macronutrients are given individually within each respective chapter on carbohydrates, lipids, protein, and water. However, there is a need to review the processes and correlations between them since they do not occur exclusively of one another but simultaneously and in association within the integrated whole of the body.

An emphasis is placed upon the simplification of learning through the use of notated visual aids and definitions of appropriate terminology. The use of diagrams which help the reader "see" the action described is a technique helpful towards attaining an understanding and retaining information. It also simplifies the reference work of the reader. Therefore, six large drawings are given to summarize digestive, absorptive, and metabolic processes:

1. an outline of organs involved,
2. a summary of the processes of digestion,
3. a summary of the processes involved in the digestion of the specific macronutrients,
4. a summary of the absorption of the macronutrients,
5. a summary of chemical processes involved in energy production, and
6. a summary of vitamin and mineral participation in processes of energy production.

Review of the more detailed descriptions can be made by rereading the appropriate section in each chapter on the macronutrient in question.

DIGESTION

Key Points: Definitions of Terms Associated with Digestive Processes

Acini—the secretory cells of glands such as the salivary glands, the pancreas, and the liver. They occur in aggregates resembling bunches of grapes. The secretions pour into collecting tubules which eventually lead to ducts.

Amylase—an enzyme which catalyzes the hydrolysis of starch to sugar. Salivary amylase (ptyalin) begins the enzymatic breakdown of starch in the mouth. However, salivary amylase is not very effective because of the short duration of time food is exposed to its action. Amylase is also contained in the pancreatic juice.

Bile—a secretion of the liver which is stored in the gallbladder. Bile contains bile salts, bile acids, bile pigments, cholesterol, and mucin. Bile emulsifies fat in the intestine and neutralizes intestinal acid contents. Emulsification is necessary for the digestion and absorption of fat.

Bolus—a portion of food which has been chewed and mixed with saliva.

Chief cells—the specialized cells of the tubular gastric glands which secrete pepsinogen, rennin, and some lipase.

Cholecystokinin—a hormone produced by cells of the intestinal wall when fat is present in the intestines. Cholecystokinin is secreted into the blood system and upon reaching the gallbladder stimulates that organ's contraction. Contraction of the gallbladder releases stored bile into the intestine.

Chyme—the term used for the semi-liquid substance produced by enzymatic and mechanical action upon ingested food. Chyme is released from the stomach into the duodenum.

Denaturation—the change in chemical and physical properties of protein molecules due to their exposure to such conditions as heat or acid. Denaturation results in the "uncoiling" of protein molecules and is usually irreversible. The uncoiled dietary protein is more digestible and the uncoiled body protein generally loses its ability to function properly.

Digestion—the mechanical and chemical breaking down of consumed food into its simpler substances in the gastrointestinal tract, which enables the nutrients in food to be absorbed and utilized by body cells.

Endocrine gland—a gland whose secretions go into the body, that is, directly into the bloodstream such as hormones of the pancreas (insulin), duodenal cells (cholecystokinin), mucosal cells of the stomach (gastrin), as well as hormones of the thyroid and pituitary glands.

Enterogastrone—the hormone produced by duodenal mucosa glands in response to the presence of dietary fat in the intestine (duodenum). Enterogastrone slows the motility of the stomach and the intestine which causes food to be held in the stomach longer; hence, the greater and longer-lasting feeling of satisfaction after eating a meal containing some dietary fat.

Enzymes—catalytic proteins which are complex compounds secreted by living cells. Enzymes cause or accelerate changes in other substances (substrates) without themselves being changed or becoming part of the products of the reaction. The suffix -ase means enzyme and follows the prefix denoting the substrate upon which an enzyme is specific for its action, such as lactase which causes the hydrolysis of lactose (sugar in milk). Enzymes are eventually used up so they must be continually synthesized within living cells.

Epiglottis—cartilage lid of the larynx which drops during swallowing and closes the entrance to the trachea preventing food and drink from entering the trachea (the windpipe).

Esophagus—the muscular tube extending from the pharynx to the stomach (the food pipe).

Exocrine gland—a gland whose secretions go outside the body by way of a duct, not into the bloodstream. Outside the body includes body cavities such as the mouth and intestinal lumen.

Gastric glands—tubular glands in the wall of the stomach which secrete enzymes, hydrochloric acid, and mucus into the stomach. Emotions greatly influence gastric gland secretion. Anger and hostility seem to increase their secretion while fear and depression seem to decrease their secretion.

Gastric juice—the collective secretions of the gastric (stomach) glands. It is composed of water, hydrochloric acid (HCl), and enzymes: pepsinogen (active form is pepsin), some lipase, and rennin (in infants). The stomach is protected from the strong HCl acid by the secretion of mucus from various specialized gastric cells. There is also an intrinsic factor (a special protein carrier) found in the stomach which enables the absorption of vitamin B_{12}.

Gastrin—a hormone secreted by certain mucosal cells of the stomach. Secretion of gastrin is stimulated by entrance of food into the stomach, especially by coffee, meat broths, and alcohol. Gastrin stimulates secretion by gastric glands.

Goblet cells—specialized cells of the stomach which secrete a thick protective mucus.

Heartburn—an uncomfortable burning sensation felt when some stomach contents containing HCl leak from the stomach into the esophagus when the cardiac sphincter (gastroesophageal constrictor muscle) fails to function properly.

Hormone—secretion of endocrine glands. Hormones elicit a specific response from certain organs. Hormones are considered regulators of body metabolism.

Intestinal juice *(succus entericus)*—the enzymatic secretions of the intestine: enterokinase (activates trypsinogen to trypsin), peptidases, a small amount of lipase, sucrase, maltase, and lactase. Mucus is also secreted by intestinal mucosal cells, especially in the duodenum.

Mastication—the chewing which breaks up food and mixes it with saliva.

Micelle—a complex of bile salts and lipid which is microscopic in size. Micelles enable the emulsification of fat within the watery contents of the intestine.

Mucus—the viscous secretion of epithelial cells containing mucin, a glycoprotein, salts and water. Mucus performs protective and lubricative functions.

Pancreatic juice—the thin, watery, alkaline juice secreted by the pancreas into the intestine which contains these enzymes: amylase (for starch), chymotrypsinogen and trypsinogen (inactive forms of proteases), peptidase (for peptides), and lipase (for fats). Pancreatic juice helps to neutralize the acid chyme as it enters the duodenum.

Parietal cells—the hydrochloric acid-producing cells of the gastric glands.

Peristalsis—the wave-like contraction and relaxation action of the esophagus and intestines which propels the contents of those organs forward along the alimentary canal.

Pylorus—the lower portion of the stomach leading into the duodenum and containing the pyloric sphincter.

Saliva—the secretion of the salivary gland which contains mucin, water, some salts, and the enzyme amylase which acts primarily upon cooked starch within the mouth. The thought, sight, or smell of food increases the flow of saliva as well as gastric juices.

Secretin—the hormone produced by cells in the wall of the duodenum when acidic chyme enters there. Secretin travels by way of the bloodstream to the pancreas and stimulates the flow of pancreatic juice into the intestine.

Sphincter—a ring-like muscle surrounding a natural body opening which is capable of contracting to close the opening or relaxing to open the opening.

Ulcer—erosion of a local area of some tissue surface where inflammation of tissue cells has led to cellular death and a sloughing off of these cells. Ulcers can proceed through cellular layers until bleeding and even perforation occurs.[1] Duodenal mucous gland secretions help protect the duodenum from the acidic chyme entering there. However, the capacity of mucous glands to secrete mucus, and gastric glands to secrete gastric juice, is under emotional influence and their increased or decreased secretory functions may be related to formation of peptic and duodenal ulcers.[2]

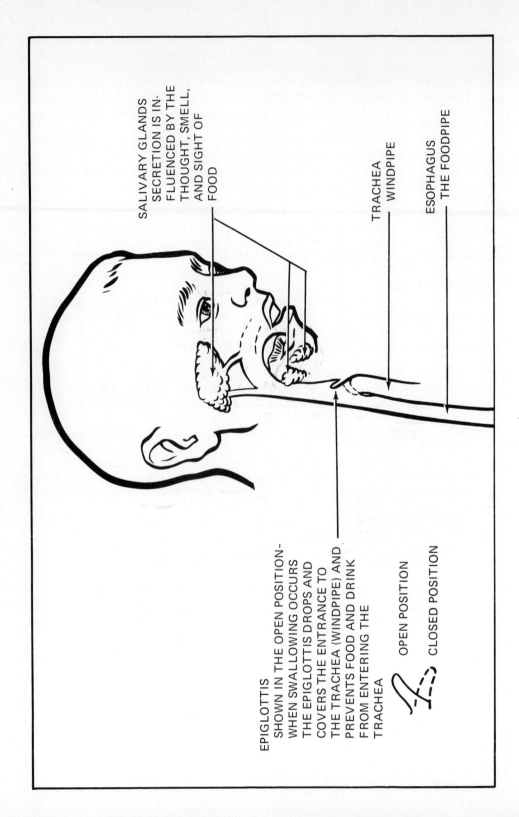

SALIVARY GLANDS
SECRETION IS IN-
FLUENCED BY THE
THOUGHT, SMELL,
AND SIGHT OF
FOOD

TRACHEA
WINDPIPE

ESOPHAGUS
THE FOODPIPE

EPIGLOTTIS
SHOWN IN THE OPEN POSITION—
WHEN SWALLOWING OCCURS
THE EPIGLOTTIS DROPS AND
COVERS THE ENTRANCE TO
THE TRACHEA (WINDPIPE) AND
PREVENTS FOOD AND DRINK
FROM ENTERING THE
TRACHEA

OPEN POSITION

CLOSED POSITION

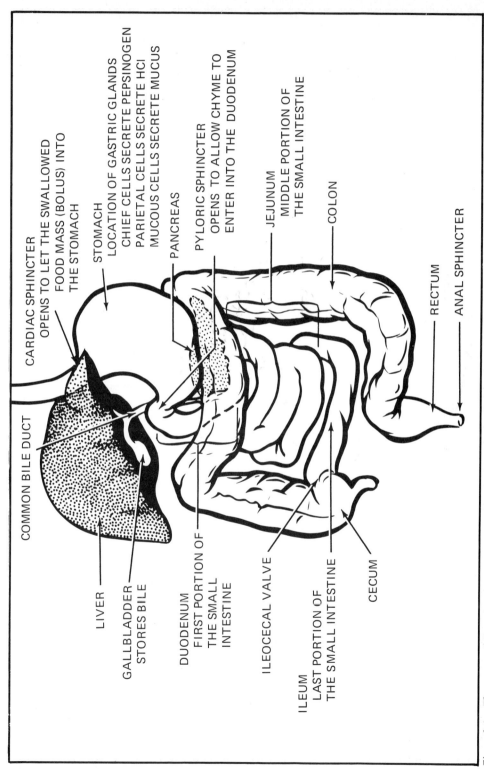

Figure 6-1. The organs of digestion.

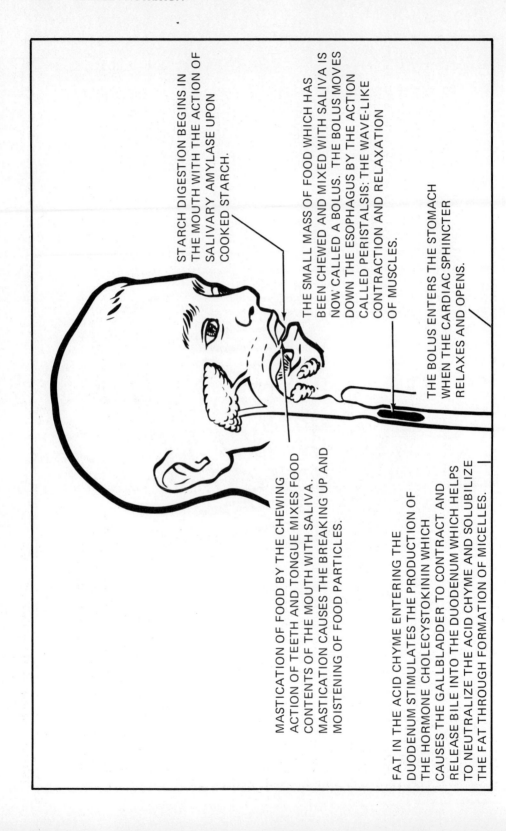

STARCH DIGESTION BEGINS IN THE MOUTH WITH THE ACTION OF SALIVARY AMYLASE UPON COOKED STARCH.

THE SMALL MASS OF FOOD WHICH HAS BEEN CHEWED AND MIXED WITH SALIVA IS NOW CALLED A BOLUS. THE BOLUS MOVES DOWN THE ESOPHAGUS BY THE ACTION CALLED PERISTALSIS: THE WAVE-LIKE CONTRACTION AND RELAXATION OF MUSCLES.

THE BOLUS ENTERS THE STOMACH WHEN THE CARDIAC SPHINCTER RELAXES AND OPENS.

MASTICATION OF FOOD BY THE CHEWING ACTION OF TEETH AND TONGUE MIXES FOOD CONTENTS OF THE MOUTH WITH SALIVA. MASTICATION CAUSES THE BREAKING UP AND MOISTENING OF FOOD PARTICLES.

FAT IN THE ACID CHYME ENTERING THE DUODENUM STIMULATES THE PRODUCTION OF THE HORMONE CHOLECYSTOKININ WHICH CAUSES THE GALLBLADDER TO CONTRACT AND RELEASE BILE INTO THE DUODENUM WHICH HELPS TO NEUTRALIZE THE ACID CHYME AND SOLUBILIZE THE FAT THROUGH FORMATION OF MICELLES.

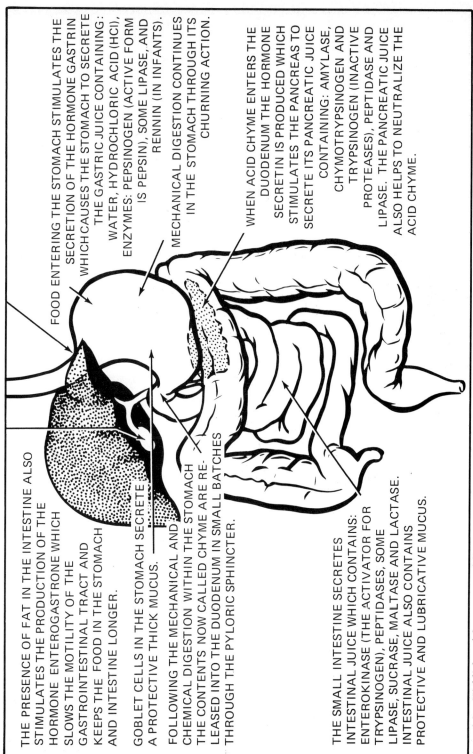

THE PRESENCE OF FAT IN THE INTESTINE ALSO STIMULATES THE PRODUCTION OF THE HORMONE ENTEROGASTRONE WHICH SLOWS THE MOTILITY OF THE GASTROINTESTINAL TRACT AND KEEPS THE FOOD IN THE STOMACH AND INTESTINE LONGER.

GOBLET CELLS IN THE STOMACH SECRETE A PROTECTIVE THICK MUCUS.

FOLLOWING THE MECHANICAL AND CHEMICAL DIGESTION WITHIN THE STOMACH THE CONTENTS NOW CALLED CHYME ARE RE-LEASED INTO THE DUODENUM IN SMALL BATCHES THROUGH THE PYLORIC SPHINCTER.

THE SMALL INTESTINE SECRETES INTESTINAL JUICE WHICH CONTAINS: ENTEROKINASE (THE ACTIVATOR FOR TRYPSINOGEN), PEPTIDASES, SOME LIPASE, SUCRASE, MALTASE AND LACTASE. INTESTINAL JUICE ALSO CONTAINS PROTECTIVE AND LUBRICATIVE MUCUS.

FOOD ENTERING THE STOMACH STIMULATES THE SECRETION OF THE HORMONE GASTRIN WHICH CAUSES THE STOMACH TO SECRETE THE GASTRIC JUICE CONTAINING : WATER, HYDROCHLORIC ACID (HCl), ENZYMES: PEPSINOGEN (ACTIVE FORM IS PEPSIN), SOME LIPASE, AND RENNIN (IN INFANTS).

MECHANICAL DIGESTION CONTINUES IN THE STOMACH THROUGH ITS CHURNING ACTION.

WHEN ACID CHYME ENTERS THE DUODENUM THE HORMONE SECRETIN IS PRODUCED WHICH STIMULATES THE PANCREAS TO SECRETE ITS PANCREATIC JUICE CONTAINING: AMYLASE, CHYMOTRYPSINOGEN AND TRYPSINOGEN (INACTIVE PROTEASES), PEPTIDASE AND LIPASE. THE PANCREATIC JUICE ALSO HELPS TO NEUTRALIZE THE ACID CHYME.

Figure 6-2.   Highlights of the processes of digestion.

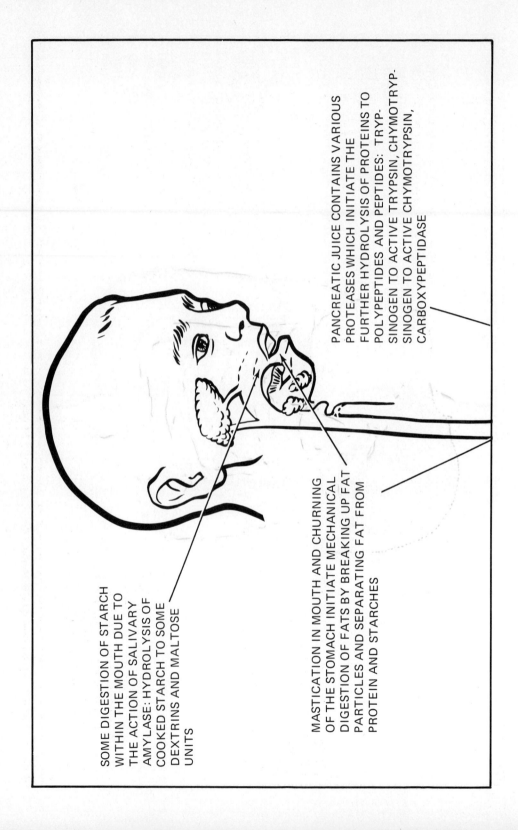

PANCREATIC JUICE CONTAINS VARIOUS PROTEASES WHICH INITIATE THE FURTHER HYDROLYSIS OF PROTEINS TO POLYPEPTIDES AND PEPTIDES: TRYP-SINOGEN TO ACTIVE TRYPSIN, CHYMOTRYP-SINOGEN TO ACTIVE CHYMOTRYPSIN, CARBOXYPEPTIDASE

SOME DIGESTION OF STARCH WITHIN THE MOUTH DUE TO THE ACTION OF SALIVARY AMYLASE: HYDROLYSIS OF COOKED STARCH TO SOME DEXTRINS AND MALTOSE UNITS

MASTICATION IN MOUTH AND CHURNING OF THE STOMACH INITIATE MECHANICAL DIGESTION OF FATS BY BREAKING UP FAT PARTICLES AND SEPARATING FAT FROM PROTEIN AND STARCHES

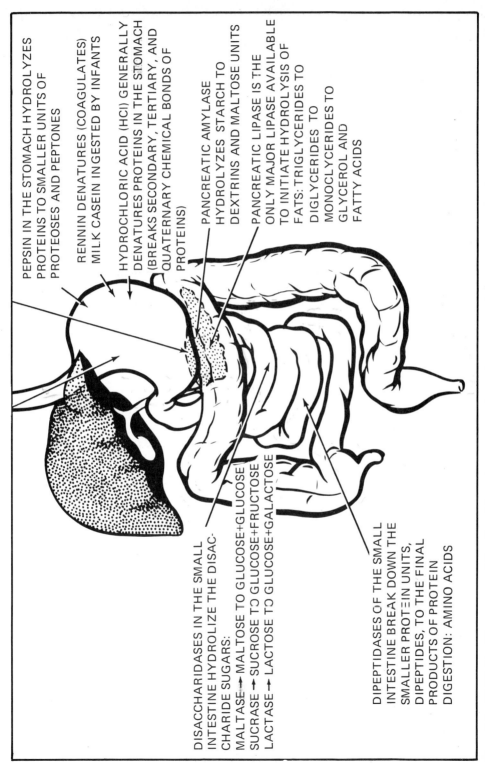

PEPSIN IN THE STOMACH HYDROLYZES
PROTEINS TO SMALLER UNITS OF
PROTEOSES AND PEPTONES

RENNIN DENATURES (COAGULATES)
MILK CASEIN INGESTED BY INFANTS

HYDROCHLORIC ACID (HCl) GENERALLY
DENATURES PROTEINS IN THE STOMACH
(BREAKS SECONDARY, TERTIARY, AND
QUATERNARY CHEMICAL BONDS OF
PROTEINS)

PANCREATIC AMYLASE
HYDROLYZES STARCH TO
DEXTRINS AND MALTOSE UNITS

PANCREATIC LIPASE IS THE
ONLY MAJOR LIPASE AVAILABLE
TO INITIATE HYDROLYSIS OF
FATS: TRIGLYCERIDES TO
DIGLYCERIDES TO
MONOGLYCERIDES TO
GLYCEROL AND
FATTY ACIDS

DISACCHARIDASES IN THE SMALL
INTESTINE HYDROLIZE THE DISAC-
CHARIDE SUGARS:
MALTASE → MALTOSE TO GLUCOSE+GLUCOSE
SUCRASE → SUCROSE TO GLUCOSE+FRUCTOSE
LACTASE → LACTOSE TO GLUCOSE+GALACTOSE

DIPEPTIDASES OF THE SMALL
INTESTINE BREAK DOWN THE
SMALLER PROTEIN UNITS,
DIPEPTIDES, TO THE FINAL
PRODUCTS OF PROTEIN
DIGESTION: AMINO ACIDS

Figure 6-3.   Highlights of the processes of digestion of the various macronutrients.

Questions: Digestion

1. Match the phrases on the right to the items on the left which they best describe.

   ____ 1. chyme
   ____ 2. bolus
   ____ 3. enterogastrone
   ____ 4. cholecystokinin
   ____ 5. chief cells
   ____ 6. acini cells

   a. stimulates the gallbladder to contract and release bile
   b. slows the motility of the stomach and intestines
   c. secretory cells of glands whose secretions are collected in tubules leading to a duct
   d. small mass of food which has been chewed and mixed with saliva
   e. the semi-liquid contents of the stomach which is emptied into the intestine
   f. secrete pepsinogen

2. Amylases can be found in:
   a. bile
   b. pancreatic juice
   c. saliva
   d. gastric juice

3. What are two functions of bile?

4. The breaking of quaternary, tertiary, and secondary bonds of proteins in the presence of HCl acid of the stomach, resulting in the uncoiling of protein molecules, is _____ .

5. Identify the correct answer in each sentence:
   a. The glands which secrete juices by way of ducts are (endocrine/exocrine) glands.
   b. The glands which secrete juices to the outside of the body are (endocrine/exocrine).
   c. The glands which secrete hormones directly into the bloodstream are (endocrine/exocrine).

6. Enzymes are:
   a. catalytic proteins
   b. not part of the chemical reaction or its products which they initiate
   c. used once and then degraded

7. Match the following phrases on the right to the item each best describes on the left.

   ____ 1. pyloric sphincter
   ____ 2. goblet cells
   ____ 3. peristalsis
   ____ 4. epiglottis
   ____ 5. esophagus
   ____ 6. secretin
   ____ 7. sphincter
   ____ 8. parietal cells

   a. stimulates flow of pancreatic juice
   b. wave-like contractions of the esophagus and intestines
   c. cartilage flap which closes the opening of the trachea during swallowing
   d. muscle regulating flow of chyme from stomach to duodenum
   e. secrete hydrochloric acid
   f. secrete thick mucus in stomach
   g. food tube
   h. a ring-like muscle controlling an opening of the body

8. Gastric gland secretion is stimulated by the hormone _____ .

9. Choose one correct answer for the following statements.
   a. Feelings of anger and hostility (increase/decrease) gastric gland secretions.
   b. Feelings of fear and depression generally (increase/decrease) gastric gland secretions.

10. Identify the major enzyme for protein in the gastric juice.

11. Vitamin B_{12} is freely absorbed from the intestine.
    a. True
    b. False

12. What uncomfortable sensation is produced when the cardiac sphincter muscle fails to sufficiently close after food enters the stomach and stomach motility increases?

13. Secretions of endocrine glands are called:
    a. enzymes
    b. hormones
    c. bile

14. Intestinal juice contains the major digestive lipase.
    a. True
    b. False

15. The hormone which activates trypsinogen to trypsin is:
    a. gastrin
    b. cholecystokinin
    c. enterokinase

16. The chewing of food is termed _____ .

17. A tiny bile salt/lipid complex which enables the emulsification of fat within the intestines is a _____ .

18. The substance which provides a protective coating in the stomach against the action of the strong hydrochloric acid is _____ .

19. The major lipase of the digestive system is found in the:
    a. intestinal juice
    b. gastric juice
    c. pancreatic juice

20. The pancreatic juice contains enzymes for the hydrolysis of starch, proteins, and fats.
    a. True
    b. False

21. The localized erosion of body tissue due to sloughed-off dead cells from an area of inflammation is termed an _____ .

22. Though the exact causes of peptic (stomach) or duodenal ulcers are not known the combination of increased _____ ; decreased _____ secretion appears implicated in ulcer formation.

Answers: Digestion

1. 1. e
   2. d
   3. b
   4. a
   5. f
   6. c
2. b and c

3. Emulsification of fats within the intestine; neutralization of acidic chyme in the intestine.
4. denaturation
5. a. exocrine
   b. exocrine
   c. endocrine
6. a and b
7. 1. d
   2. f
   3. b
   4. c
   5. g
   6. a
   7. h
   8. e
8. gastrin
9. a. increase
   b. decrease
10. pepsinogen (precursor) $\xrightarrow[\text{pepsin}]{\text{HCl}}$ pepsin
11. b
12. heartburn
13. b
14. b
15. c
16. mastication
17. micelle
18. mucus
19. c
20. a
21. ulcer
22. increased gastric juice (especially HCl) secretion; decreased mucous gland secretion.

ABSORPTION

Key Points: Definitions of Terms Associated with Absorptive Processes

Absorption—the taking into the body of nutrients ingested as food and drink. These nutrients cross cellular membranes of the gastrointestinal tract following the digestive processes by one of several means:

Passive diffusion—the crossing of water through pores in semi-permeable cellular membranes from an area of lesser solute concentration to an area of greater solute concentration. This water passes freely and is regulated by solute concentration and not by the cellular membrane. See Figure 13-5, Osmosis. Some electrolytes and certain other small molecules are also absorbed by this process from areas of their greater concentration to areas of their lesser concentration.

Facilitated diffusion (also termed carrier mediated diffusion or passive transport)—the crossing of molecules through semi-permeable cellular membranes from an area of greater concentration to an area of lesser concentration by means of a specific carrier molecule until molecular concentration is equalized on both sides of the membrane. By use of a specific carrier, some molecules are transported across the cellular membrane with the exclusion of others. No energy is required for facilitated diffusion.

Active transport—the crossing of molecules through semi-permeable membranes against a concentration gradient; in other words, movement continues even from a space of lesser concentration to one of greater concentration. Active transport also requires a specific carrier as in facilitated diffusion, but in addition requires an energy source.

Pinocytosis—the crossing of molecules through cellular membranes by the cell membrane actually wrapping around the particle to be absorbed, pulling the particle inward and releasing it into the cell. Pinocytosis results in the cell engulfing the particle it absorbs.

Artery—a vessel carrying blood away from the heart.

Binders—substances which combine with certain nutrients within the digestive tract that render the nutrient involved unabsorbable. Fiber can bind certain nutrients; oxalic and phytic acids found in some grains, and vegetables bind minerals such as iron and calcium.

Capillary—the smallest type of vessel within the circulatory system. Capillaries connect the arteries to the veins creating a closed circulatory system. Capillaries are narrow and thin-walled allowing for an easy exchange of substances between the fluids inside and outside the capillaries.

Carriers—substances which are specific agents for the carriage or transport of other substances.

Chylomicrons—the minute lipoprotein formed from the combining of a triglyceride, phospholipid, cholesterol, and protein. Chylomicrons enable the transport of digested fat within the blood system. They are formed within cells of the intestinal wall, absorbed into the lymph system, and later deposited in the blood. The blood appears milky after a fat-rich meal due to the presence of many chylomicrons. However, chylomicrons are soon broken down by the action of lipoprotein lipase, the clearing factor.

Enterohepatic circulation—the recirculation of bile salts from formation in the liver, to storage in the gallbladder, to emptying into the intestine where they emulsify and transport fat, to their separation from fat and reabsorption, and carriage back to the liver by the portal blood system. Upon return to the liver they re-enter the cycle again. Only a small amount is lost in the feces so this is a highly efficient and conservative system. New bile salts to replace that small amount which is lost are formed in the liver from cholesterol.

Hepatic vein—the vein which collects blood from capillaries of the liver and carries it to the heart.

Lacteal—the small vessel of the lymph system located within the villi of the intestine where certain nutrients, notably fat compounds, are collected.

Lipoprotein—a complex containing both lipid (fat) and protein. Lipoproteins make soluble the fat transported within the watery medium of the blood system.

Lymph—the interstitial fluid which closely resembles blood plasma and occurs outside the vascular system and around the outside of cells. It provides the medium for exchange of nutrients into and out of cells and is collected in a loosely organized system of vessels and ducts. Most substances absorbed originally into the lymph system eventually end up within the circulatory system. The thoracic duct empties collected lymph into the blood system at the vena cava which carries blood directly into the heart.

Mesentery—the thin membrane which lines the abdomen and holds the intestines to the abdominal wall. The mesentery contains blood vessels, lymph vessels, and nerves which connect to the intestines. The mesentery is wrapped around the intestines and gives the intestines support.

Microvilli—the minute projections from the surface of each villi which greatly add to the total area for absorption within the intestine. The large number of microvilli on each villi appear like microscopic bristles and form what is termed the "brush border."

Portal vein—the vein which collects blood from the capillaries of the intestines (mesenteric blood system) and carries the blood and many newly absorbed nutrients to the capillaries of the liver.

Thoracic duct—the collecting area for lymph fluid which is eventually emptied into the superior vena cava which carries blood directly into the heart. Thoracic refers to the chest which is the general location of this duct of the lymph system.

Vein—a blood vessel which carries blood toward the heart.

Villi—the very small projections on the internal surface of the intestines. These projections contain the capillaries and lacteals involved in the absorption of ingested nutrients. The villi also have other projections on their surfaces called microvilli which add to the surface area available for absorption (the microvilli form the brush border).

Questions: Absorption

1. The free crossing of water through a semi-permeable membrane from an area of lesser solute concentration to an area of greater solute concentration is:
    a. passive diffusion (osmosis)
    b. facilitated diffusion
    c. active transport

2. The carrier assisted diffusion of select molecules through a semi-permeable membrane which does not require an energy source is _____ . This type of diffusion occurs until the concentration of solute molecules is _____ on both sides of the semi-permeable membrane.

3. Some carriers will transport certain molecules through a semi-permeable membrane even from an area of lower concentration to an area of higher concentration (against a concentration gradient). This type of carrier transport requires energy and is termed _____ .

4. Some cells actually engulf a molecule by wrapping a part of the cell membrane around the molecule or particle and pulling it inward. This type of absorption is termed _____ .

5. Match the following phrases on the right to the items on the left which they best describe:

    _____ 1. lacteal
    _____ 2. capillary
    _____ 3. chylomicrons
    _____ 4. binders
    _____ 5. lymph
    _____ 6. lipoprotein
    _____ 7. carriers

    a. substances which form unabsorbable complexes within the digestive tract
    b. the smallest type of blood vessel which is narrow and thin-walled
    c. specific agents which "ferry" other substances
    d. lipoprotein complex formed within the cells of the intestinal wall following the absorption of fat
    e. smallest vessel of the lymph system which is located in the intestinal villi
    f. a water-soluble fat/protein complex in blood plasma
    g. interstitial fluid resembling blood plasma which provides the medium for exchange of nutrients into and out of cells

6. Bile salts are formed in the _____ ; are stored in the _____ ; emptied into the _____ ; reabsorbed from the intestine into the _____ ; and are carried back to the _____ with very little fecal loss for recycling.

7. The conservation system for the recycling of bile salts is called the _____ .

8. The thin membrane which contains blood vessels, lymph vessels, and nerves and both covers the intestines and holds the intestines to the abdominal wall is the _____ .

9. a. The vein carrying blood from the liver to the heart is the (hepatic vein/portal vein).
    b. The vein carrying blood from the intestines to the liver is the (hepatic vein/portal vein).

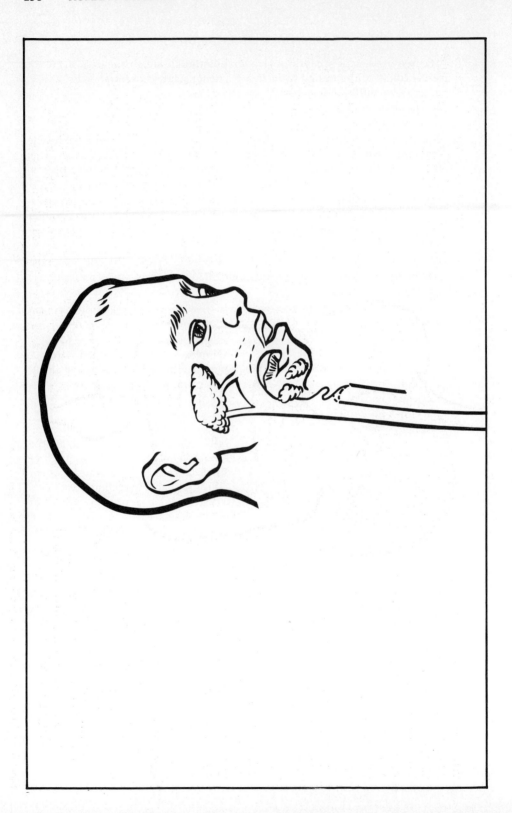

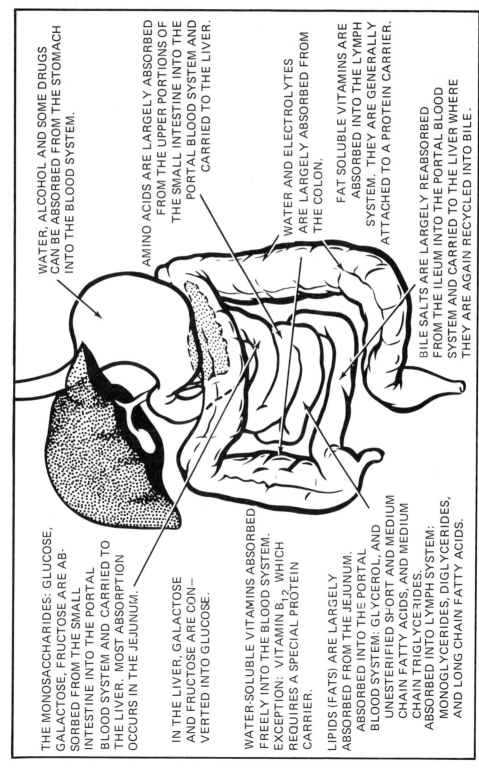

WATER, ALCOHOL AND SOME DRUGS CAN BE ABSORBED FROM THE STOMACH INTO THE BLOOD SYSTEM.

AMINO ACIDS ARE LARGELY ABSORBED FROM THE UPPER PORTIONS OF THE SMALL INTESTINE INTO THE PORTAL BLOOD SYSTEM AND CARRIED TO THE LIVER.

WATER AND ELECTROLYTES ARE LARGELY ABSORBED FROM THE COLON.

FAT SOLUBLE VITAMINS ARE ABSORBED INTO THE LYMPH SYSTEM. THEY ARE GENERALLY ATTACHED TO A PROTEIN CARRIER.

BILE SALTS ARE LARGELY REABSORBED FROM THE ILEUM INTO THE PORTAL BLOOD SYSTEM AND CARRIED TO THE LIVER WHERE THEY ARE AGAIN RECYCLED INTO BILE.

THE MONOSACCHARIDES: GLUCOSE, GALACTOSE, FRUCTOSE ARE ABSORBED FROM THE SMALL INTESTINE INTO THE PORTAL BLOOD SYSTEM AND CARRIED TO THE LIVER. MOST ABSORPTION OCCURS IN THE JEJUNUM.

IN THE LIVER, GALACTOSE AND FRUCTOSE ARE CONVERTED INTO GLUCOSE.

WATER-SOLUBLE VITAMINS ABSORBED FREELY INTO THE BLOOD SYSTEM. EXCEPTION: VITAMIN B_{12} WHICH REQUIRES A SPECIAL PROTEIN CARRIER.

LIPIDS (FATS) ARE LARGELY ABSORBED FROM THE JEJUNUM. ABSORBED INTO THE PORTAL BLOOD SYSTEM: GLYCEROL, AND UNESTERIFIED SHORT AND MEDIUM CHAIN FATTY ACIDS, AND MEDIUM CHAIN TRIGLYCERIDES. ABSORBED INTO LYMPH SYSTEM: MONOGLYCERIDES, DIGLYCERIDES, AND LONG CHAIN FATTY ACIDS.

Figure 6–4.   Highlights of the processes of absorption of the macronutrients.

10. The collecting area for lymph which is emptied into the superior vena cava is the
     a. common bile duct
     b. pancreatic duct
     c. thoracic duct

11. The thoracic duct is located in the following general area:
     a. upper abdominal region
     b. lower abdominal region
     c. upper chest region

12. The finger-like projections of the intestines containing capillaries and lacteals which greatly increase the surface absorption area of the intestines are the
     _____ .

13. Which minute intestinal projections form the "brush border?"

Answers: Absorption

1. a
2. facilitated diffusion (also termed carrier mediated diffusion or passive transport); equalized
3. active transport
4. pinocytosis
5. 1. e
    2. b
    3. d
    4. a
    5. g
    6. f
    7. c
6. liver; gallbladder; intestines; portal blood system; liver
7. enterohepatic circulation
8. mesentery
9. a. hepatic vein
    b. portal vein
10. c
11. c
12. villi
13. microvilli

METABOLISM

Key Points: Definitions of Terms Associated with Metabolic Processes

Acetyl CoA—also called *active acetate*. Acetyl CoA is the form in which two carbon fragments enter the citric acid cycle (also called the Krebs cycle after the man who was able to clarify the chemical reactions involved) which is the final pathway for all nutrients in energy metabolism. Acetyl CoA is formed from the combination of acetic acid (a two-carbon compound) and the chemical compound coenzyme A (which also contains one of the vitamins of the B-complex, pantothenic acid).

Anabolism—the term for building more complex substances from simpler ones such as new body tissue from nutrients ingested. This is an energy requiring process.

Basal metabolism—the energy expenditure by the body at rest and in a fasting state when nutrients are being metabolized but not absorbed.

Catabolism—the process of breaking down complex substances to simpler substances usually involving energy-producing oxidation reactions such as the breakdown of body fat to produce energy, carbon dioxide, and water.

Deamination—the removal of an amino group ($-NH_2$) from an amino acid. Deamination primarily occurs in the liver and kidneys and results in the formation of ammonia (NH_3) or the ammonium ion (NH_4^+) and a keto-acid.

Electron transport chain—also called *oxidative phosphorylation*. The transfer of hydrogen and electrons along with the energy of these high energy hydrogen bonds from NADH $+ H \rightarrow 0_2$ by way of intermediary compounds. Some heat is lost with each hydrogen transfer and each transfer causes some loss of energy of the bond until the final low energy H_2O (water) bond is formed. The energy lost from hydrogen transfer is captured in the phosphate bonds of ATP formed from ADP + P. Thus, the electron transport chain results in the formation of high energy bonds within compounds which can be stored and then broken when needed to release energy for energy-requiring work of the body. See Figure 6-5 for a more detailed explanation.

-emia—suffix referring to "in the blood," that is, uremia refers to accumulation of urea in the blood; glycemia refers to sugar in the blood; lipemia refers to fatty substances in the blood.

Glycolysis—the process of breaking down glucose. Specifically it refers to the anaerobic process of glucose catabolism from a molecule of glucose to two molecules of pyruvic acid (net production of two ATP plus 2 NADH + H), or two molecules of lactic acid (net production of two ATP). This glycolytic pathway is also called the Embden-Meyerhof pathway. Glycolysis takes place in the cell cytoplasm. See Figure 1-4 in Chaper One.

Gluconeogenesis—the formation of glucose from noncarbohydrate sources such as molecules of protein or fat. For example, refer to Figure 6-5 and follow the glycerol portion from fat back up the glycolytic pathway (seemingly, a reversal of glycolysis) to the formation of glucose (two three-carbon glycerol molecules can combine to form one six carbon glucose molecule). Also, deamination can allow some amino acids to enter the glycolytic pathway as pyruvic acid and proceed up to the formation of glucose.

Homeostasis—the state of equilibrium or stability of the processes of the body. This is a dynamic state where the body maintains uniformity while at the same time it experiences a constant exchange of body compounds.

Krebs cycle—also called the *tricarboxylic acid cycle or citric acid cycle*. This is the aerobic portion of energy production and occurs in the mitochondria of the cell. See Figure 1-4. It is the second phase of energy production from catabolism of a molecule of glucose and begins at pyruvic acid and continues clockwise around the cycle until water (H_2O) and carbon dioxide (CO_2) are formed and energy is produced and held within high energy bonds of

ATP molecules. See Figure 6-5. Two-carbon fragments obtained from fatty acids are converted to acetyl CoA and enter into the Krebs cycle. Following deamination, amino acid carbon skeletons can enter at several points in the Krebs cycle. *Consequently, the Krebs cycle is the final, common metabolic pathway for the various nutrients in energy production.* The Krebs cycle was named for Sir Hans Krebs who theorized and then confirmed this series of chemical processes for energy production.

Metabolism—Metabolism is the sum total of all the chemical changes which occur within living cells of the body including all the anabolic processes of new tissue development, as well as the catabolic processes of tissue breakdown and nutrient breakdown for the production of energy.

Oxidative phosphorylation—the electron transfer process which enables hydrogen from $NADH + H^+$ to combine with oxygen to form H_2O (water) with the capture of the high energy from the hydrogen bonds into phosphorus bonds as $ADP + P \rightarrow ATP$ through the passing of electrons by way of intermediary compounds. See Figure 6-5 for an explanation of electron transfer processes. Refer to the electron transport chain above.

Pyruvic acid—the three-carbon compound produced by catabolism of glucose within the glycolytic pathway which undergoes a chemical reaction to form acetyl CoA, the gateway substance into the Krebs cycle.

Urea—the non-toxic substance into which ammonia (NH_3) is formed within the liver. In this way ammonia can be carried within the blood to the kidneys for excretion within urine. Urea is the chief end-product of amino acid metabolism.

-uria—the suffix pertaining to the condition of the urine, that is, glycosuria represents sugar in the urine; lipuria represents fatty substances within the urine.

Energy metabolism. Energy production is a regulated, systematic process within the body. It is the result of chemical reactions occurring within all living cells. The energy formed is conservatively held within high energy phosphate bonds within certain molecular compounds, primarily adenosine triphosphate (ATP). These chemical bonds can be broken in time of need to release their captured energy to do work. Some heat loss occurs with the release of this energy. ATP is the primary source of energy for accomplishing all the work of the body.

The processes of energy production can be broken into two distinct phases, anaerobic[3] and aerobic.[4] The aerobic phase also contains a subphase, oxidative phosphorylation.

Anaerobic phase—glycolysis; the Embden-Meyerhof pathway; takes place within the cell's cytoplasm. This phase begins with a molecule of glucose and ends with the production of pyruvic acid or lactic acid.

Aerobic phase—TCA cycle; tricarboxylic acid cycle; Krebs cycle; takes place in the mitochondria of the cells. This phase begins with the change of pyruvic acid to the compound acetyl CoA and then continues in a cyclic pattern of chemical reactions which results in the formation of water, carbon dioxide, and compounds containing high energy hydrogen bonds.

Subphase—electron transport; oxidative phosphorylation. This part of the second phase begins with the compounds containing the high energy hydrogen bonds and includes the subsequent passage of these hydrogens and electrons to intermediary compounds. The passage of these hydrogens and their electrons produces small losses of heat, and the transfer of the energy within the bonds to newly formed phosphate bonds of ATP. ATP holds the energy until needed.

All phases of energy production depend upon enzymes to catalyze the individual chemical reactions involved (though these enzymes are not shown in Figure 6-5). Specific enzymes are needed for each chemical reaction as well as its reversal. *Hence, some steps are not reversible due to the absence of a catalyzing enzyme within the system such as for the conversion of acetyl CoA back to pyruvic acid.* There are actually three places within the glycolytic pathway which are not reversible. However, gluconeogenesis (the making of glucose from noncarbohydrate compounds such as amino acids) does occur through the bypassing of the non-reversal reactions with some new reactions.[5] *To simplify Figure 6-5, the glyolytic pathway from pyruvate back up to glucose is shown as reversible.*

The breakdown of carbohydrate to glucose units enables the entrance of carbohydrate into the energy production cycle. Fat breaks down to glycerol and fatty acids. Glycerol can go back into the glycolytic pathway to reform glucose or glycogen, or proceed down the pathway for energy production. Fatty acids release two-carbon fragments which are converted to acetyl CoA and enter the Krebs cycle for energy production. Amino acids can enter the Krebs cycle for energy production. Amino acids can enter the system at various points within the Krebs cycle. Some amino acids can also be converted to pyruvic acid which can proceed up toward formation of glucose and glycogen.[6] Most of the noncarbohydrate energy sources enter the Krebs cycle as acetyl CoA.

A brief analysis of the energy production pathways reveals some generalities.

1. All three macronutrients—carbohydrate, protein, and fat—can be used as energy sources.
2. An excess of dietary carbohydrate, protein, or fat can lead to fat formation (see junctions at glyceraldehyde-3-phosphate and acetyl CoA).
3. Amino acids can be used to make glucose (proceeding up the glycolytic pathway from pyruvic acid) while fatty acids cannot.
4. Only the glycerol portion of fat (about 10 percent of the triglyceride molecule) can be converted to glucose.

The Cori cycle. During heavy exercise when the need for energy production may exceed available oxygen for the complete combustion of glucose, energy production in the anaerobic phase continues. This energy production occurs from glucose through pyruvic acid to lactic acid (see Figure 6-5). The net amount of ATP produced during glycolysis is eight ATP. However, conversion of pyruvic acid to lactic acid requires $NADH + H^+$ to be oxidized to NAD^+ and the body loses the three potential ATP's from this $NADH + H^+$ ($NADH + H^+$ = three ATP). Since two molecules of pyruvic acid are produced from one molecule of glucose the reaction pyruvic acid → lactic acid occurs twice for every molecule of glucose and a total loss potential of six ATP is experienced. The eight ATP's produced during the phase of glycolysis to pyruvic acid are reduced by the six ATP lost through

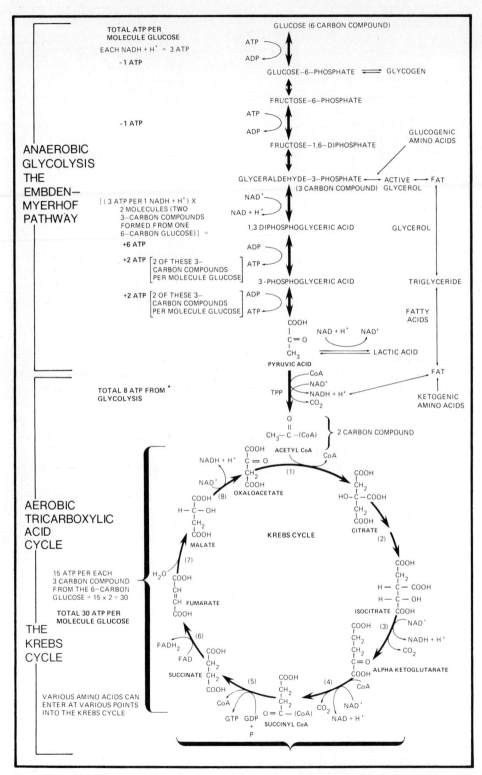

Figure 6-5:   Simplified highlights of energy production through glycolysis and the Krebs cycle.

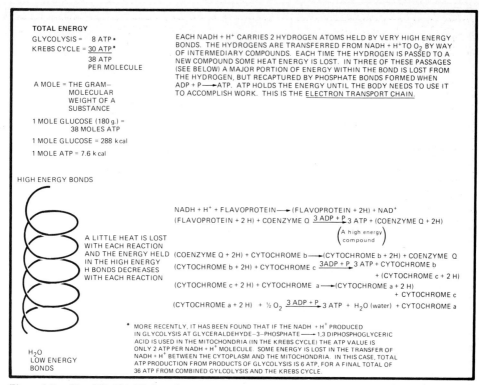

TOTAL ENERGY

GLYCOLYSIS = 8 ATP •

KREBS CYCLE = <u>30 ATP</u> *

38 ATP
PER MOLECULE

A MOLE = THE GRAM—
MOLECULAR
WEIGHT OF A
SUBSTANCE

1 MOLE GLUCOSE (180 g.) =
38 MOLES ATP

1 MOLE GLUCOSE = 288 k cal

1 MOLE ATP = 7.6 k cal

EACH NADH + H^+ CARRIES 2 HYDROGEN ATOMS HELD BY VERY HIGH ENERGY BONDS. THE HYDROGENS ARE TRANSFERRED FROM NADH + H^+ TO O_2 BY WAY OF INTERMEDIARY COMPOUNDS. EACH TIME THE HYDROGEN IS PASSED TO A NEW COMPOUND SOME HEAT ENERGY IS LOST. IN THREE OF THESE PASSAGES (SEE BELOW) A MAJOR PORTION OF ENERGY WITHIN THE BOND IS LOST FROM THE HYDROGEN, BUT RECAPTURED BY PHOSPHATE BONDS FORMED WHEN ADP + P ⟶ ATP. ATP HOLDS THE ENERGY UNTIL THE BODY NEEDS TO USE IT TO ACCOMPLISH WORK. THIS IS THE <u>ELECTRON TRANSPORT CHAIN.</u>

HIGH ENERGY BONDS

A LITTLE HEAT IS LOST
WITH EACH REACTION
AND THE ENERGY HELD
IN THE HIGH ENERGY
H BONDS DECREASES
WITH EACH REACTION

NADH + H^+ + FLAVOPROTEIN ⟶ (FLAVOPROTEIN + 2H) + NAD^+

(FLAVOPROTEIN + 2 H) + COENZYME Q $\underline{3\ ADP + P}$ 3 ATP + (COENZYME Q + 2H)

(A high energy compound)

(COENZYME Q + 2H) + CYTOCHROME b ⟶ (CYTOCHROME b + 2H) + COENZYME Q

(CYTOCHROME b + 2H) + CYTOCHROME c $\underline{3 ADP + P}$ 3 ATP + CYTOCHROME b
+ (CYTOCHROME c + 2 H)

(CYTOCHROME c + 2 H) + CYTOCHROME a ⟶ (CYTOCHROME a + 2 H)
+ CYTOCHROME c

(CYTOCHROME a + 2 H) + ½ O_2 $\underline{3\ ADP + P}$ 3 ATP + H_2O (water) + CYTOCHROME a

* MORE RECENTLY, IT HAS BEEN FOUND THAT IF THE NADH + H^+ PRODUCED IN GLYCOLYSIS AT GLYCERALDEHYDE–3–PHOSPHATE ⟶ 1,3 DIPHOSPHOGLYCERIC ACID IS USED IN THE MITOCHONDRIA (IN THE KREBS CYCLE) THE ATP VALUE IS ONLY 2 ATP PER NADH + H^+ MOLECULE. SOME ENERGY IS LOST IN THE TRANSFER OF NADH + H^+ BETWEEN THE CYTOPLASM AND THE MITOCHONDRIA. IN THIS CASE, TOTAL ATP PRODUCTION FROM PRODUCTS OF GLYCOLYSIS IS 6 ATP, FOR A FINAL TOTAL OF 36 ATP FROM COMBINED GLYCOLYSIS AND THE KREBS CYCLE.

H_2O
LOW ENERGY
BONDS

Figure 6-5. *Simplified highlights of energy production through glycolysis and the Krebs cycle (continued).*

conversion of pyruvic acid to lactic acid. The result is a net of only two ATP. Note, however, the importance of the production of NAD^+ from pyruvic acid → lactic acid which can be used at glyceraldehyde-3-phosphate → 1, 3 diphosphoglyceric acid to enable the anaerobic cycle to continue during times of intense physical exercise.

These ATP formed during anaerobic glycolysis can help produce enough energy to sustain an individual during heavy exercise. When the exercise ceases, the lactic acid accumulated in the muscle tissues is picked up by the blood and carried back to the liver where it is reconverted to pyruvic acid. The pyruvic acid then proceeds up the system to form glucose or down the system to produce energy as needed.

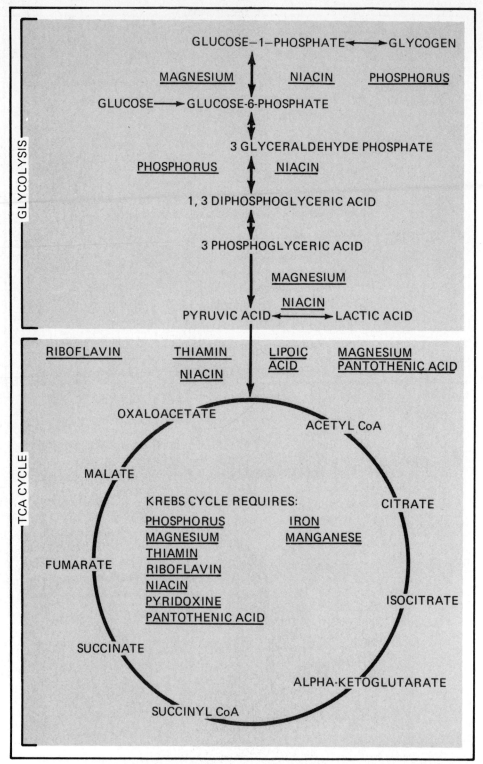

Figure 6-6. *Highlights of participation of some vitamins and minerals in the processes of energy production.*

Questions: Metabolism

1. What is the two-carbon compound which provides the entrance into the Krebs cycle for all nutrients?

2. What are other names for the Krebs cycle?
    a. TCA cycle
    b. citric acid cycle
    c. tricarboxylic acid

3. Coenzyme A contains which B-complex vitamin?

4. Match the phrases on the left to either of the terms on the right which they best represent:

    _____ 1. the making of protein   a. anabolism
              from amino acids   b. catabolism
    _____ 2. fat synthesis
    _____ 3. glycogen → glucose →
              H_2O + CO_2 + energy
    _____ 4. negative nitrogen balance (hint: refer to Chapter Five—Proteins)
    _____ 5. calorie intake below calorie expenditure resulting in weight loss
    _____ 6. healthy pregnancy of a young woman

5. The formation of glucose from deaminated amino acids is a process termed:
    a. glycolysis
    b. glycogenesis
    c. gluconeogenesis

6. Identify the proper term in each sentence:
    a. Glycolysis is an (aerobic/anaerobic) process.
    b. The Krebs cycle is an (aerobic/anaerobic) process.
    c. The electron transfer is an (aerobic/anaerobic) process.

7. Glycolysis takes place in the cell's _____ .

8. The Krebs cycle takes place in the cell's _____ .

9. An equal balance between body protein breakdown and body protein synthesis is representative of _____ .

10. The end-products from the reactions of the Krebs cycle are:
    a. water + energy
    b. water + carbon dioxide
    c. water + CO_2 + energy

11. All the processes of the living body including all the chemical changes which occur in living cells is known as:
    a. absorption
    b. digestion
    c. metabolism

12. What is the compound which contains high energy phosphate bonds that can be broken to release energy to accomplish body work?

13. The following reaction is an example of what type of chemical reaction?

$$R-CH-COOH \rightarrow R-\overset{\overset{\text{O}}{\|}}{C}-COOH + NH_3$$
$$|$$
$$NH_2$$

    an amino acid   keto-acid   ammonia

14. Energy produced from the transfer of hydrogen from NADH + H$^+$ to oxygen by way of various intermediary compounds is known as:
    a. glycolysis
    b. electron transport chain
    c. oxidative phosphorylation

15. What is the three-carbon compound formed at the end of glycolysis which undergoes a chemical reaction to form acetyl CoA, the gateway substance into the Krebs cycle.
    a. lactic acid
    b. pyruvic acid
    c. keto-acid

16. The toxic substance ammonia (NH_3) is converted to what nontoxic substance within the liver so it can be transported by the blood to the kidneys for excretion?

17. Match the phrases on the right to the items on the left which they best describe.
    _____ 1. glycemia   a. sugar in urine
    _____ 2. -emia   b. refers to the condition of the urine
    _____ 3. basal metabolism   c. refers to the condition of blood
    _____ 4. -uria   d. sugar in blood
    _____ 5. glycosuria   e. dynamic equilibrium
    _____ 6. homeostasis   f. energy expenditure by the body at rest and fasting

18. The amount of energy needed to carry on only the basic body functions necessary to the living body, excluding those needed for digestion, absorption, or physical exercise is termed _____ .

19. Why are some chemical reactions involved in energy production not reversible?

20. Why is it that fatty acids cannot be used to form glucose to replenish a low blood glucose supply?

21. One mole of glucose equals how many grams of glucose (see Figure 6-5)?

22. One mole of glucose produces 38 moles of ATP. One mole of any substance contains 6.02×10^{23} number of molecules. Therefore, how many molecules of ATP are produced by one mole of glucose?

23. One mole of ATP equals how many kcal? (See Figure 6-5.)
    a. 5
    b. 7.6
    c. 10

24. The downward spiral next to the electron transfer illustration in Figure 6-5 is meant to illustrate:
    a. the decrease in hydrogen energy bond value with each hydrogen and electron transfer
    b. the increasing energy value of the hydrogen bond with each hydrogen and electron transfer
    c. the continuous action of the electron transfer system

25. Water (H_2O) contains high energy bonds.
    a. True
    b. False

26. Some amino acids can form glucose.
    a. True
    b. False

27. The glycerol portion of a triglyceride (fat) can form glucose.
    a. True
    b. False

28. Which one of the following situations represents the body operating only at the basal metabolic rate?
    a. A young woman lying down, but awake, who is relaxed, has a normal body temperature, and is in a comfortable room temperature environment (about 72°F) 30 minutes after her last meal.
    b. The same woman in answer #a above but 10 to 12 hours after her last meal.
    c. The same woman in answer #a above but sound asleep one hour after her meal.

Answers: Metabolism

1. acetyl CoA (active acetate)
2. a, b, and c
3. pantothenic acid
4. 1. a
   2. a
   3. b
   4. b
   5. b
   6. a
5. c
6. a. anaerobic
   b. aerobic
   c. aerobic
7. cytoplasm
8. mitochondria
9. homeostasis
10. c
11. c
12. adenosine triphosphate (ATP)
13. deamination
14. b and c
15. b
16. urea
17. 1. d
    2. c
    3. f
    4. b
    5. a
    6. e
18. basal metabolism
19. A necessary catalyzing enzyme for that reaction is not present.
20. Fatty acids can be broken into two-carbon fragments which can be converted to acetyl CoA which then enters the Krebs cycle to produce energy. However, there is no enzyme available to convert acetyl CoA to pyruvic acid enabling it to proceed up the glycolytic pathway to form glucose.
21. 180g
22. 38 times (6.0235×10^{23}) = 22,889,300,000,000,000,000,000,000—this number is fantastically large and this many molecules of ATP are produced by 180g of glucose (about 6½ oz). This question was submitted just to illustrate the tremendous number of ATP's being produced constantly in the body and necessary to accomplish the work of the body.
23. b
24. a
25. b
26. a
27. a
28. b

REFERENCES

[1] Whitney EN and Hamilton EMN: Understanding Nutrition. St. Paul, MN; West Publishing Company, 1977, p. 162

[2] Mitchell HS et al: Nutrition in Health and Disease, 16th ed. Philadelphia, J. B. Lippincott Company, 1976, pp. 343-344

[3] **Anaerobic** means an absence of molecular oxygen.

[4] **Aerobic** means requiring molecular oxygen.

[5] Stryer L: Biochemistry. San Francisco, W. H. Freeman and Company, 1975, pp. 368-369

[6] The formation of glucose from noncarbohydrate sources such as amino acids is called *gluconeogenesis* (literally, the "making of new glucose").

7
INTRODUCTION TO VITAMINS

The term vitamin was composed from "vita" meaning necessary for life and "amine" because the researcher who coined the term found an amine (a nitrogen-containing compound) in the substance he was working with, thiamin.[1] Vitamine was the original spelling. The final "e" was dropped because few other vitamins contained an amine.

Vitamins are substances which are needed in very small amounts but, indeed, are necessary for life. They are organic compounds (remember, organic substances contain carbon). If you check the RDA table you will see that vitamins are recommended only in micrograms (millionths of a gram) or milligrams (thousandths of a gram). Their functions are much more varied than just the prevention of a deficiency disease.

Vitamins are necessary to life and essential in our diet because our bodies cannot manufacture them. Vitamins themselves are not a source of energy but are necessary for the occurrence of metabolic reactions which cause the release of energy from energy nutrients.

Synthetic vitamins are those produced in chemical laboratories and marketed in various preparations including tablets, capsules, and drops. Synthetic vitamins are used to enrich cereal products. Synthetic vitamins are equal in function and are not inferior to naturally occurring vitamins because their chemical configurations are identical.

Unfortunately, vitamins can be destroyed although they differ in the ease and conditions causing destruction. Some vitamins such as thiamin are easily destroyed by alkalis (baking soda). Others such as ascorbic acid are destroyed by oxidation.

Some vitamins exist in several related chemical forms, some of which may not be biologically active. Appropriate enzymes convert the inactive vitamin to the required active form. The inactive vitamin is known as a vitamin precursor or provitamin (pre and pro = before, so these terms designate "that which comes before the vitamin").

Antivitamins are vitamin antagonists. One way in which an antivitamin works is to take the required place of a vitamin similar in chemical structure in an enzyme. The vitamin is necessary for the proper functioning of the enzyme. However, with an antivitamin in the vitamin's place the enzyme is not active and cannot function properly. This situation occurs because the body cannot discriminate between a vitamin and its antivitamin. Another type of antivitamin can destroy or reduce the biological effectiveness of a vitamin. Refer to the section in Chapter 15 on the toxic substances in food for a description of thiaminase, a naturally occurring substance which destroys thiamin.

Most vitamins function as coenzymes, compounds necessary to activate enzymes. A coenzyme fits onto a specific site of a certain inactive protein called an apoenzyme. Coenzymes are sometimes referred to as prosthetic groups. *Together the coenzyme and apoenzyme form the active enzyme, technically called a holoenzyme.* When an antivitamin takes a coenzyme's place the resulting compound does not have the activity of an enzyme, and the metabolic function of the enzyme cannot be carried out. Undesirable intermediary products involved in the normal metabolic activity of the impaired enzyme build up and frequently become

153

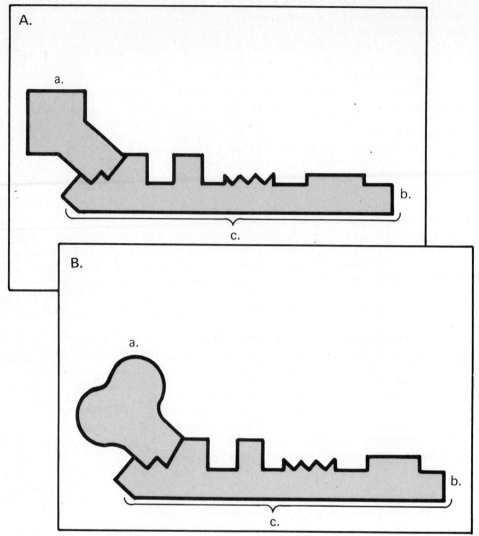

Figure 7-1.   *Example of a vitamin as a coenzyme and a vitamin antagonist.*
A. a. Vitamin as a coenzyme. b. Apoenzyme. c. Holoenzyme.
B. a. Vitamin antagonist. b. Apoenzyme. c. Holoenzyme.
This figure demonstrates how a vitamin can be replaced by a vitamin antagonist which
has a chemically similar shape. The antagonist "fits" into the place where the vitamin is
attached as a coenzyme portion of the holoenzyme. Part A is an active enzyme. Part B does
not have the proper enzyme activity.

responsible for the symptoms associated with a vitamin deficiency disease.

A vitamin deficiency can be caused by one of several conditions. *Most often it is the problem of frank inadequate intake.* It can also be the result of *malabsorption.* Vitamin intake may be adequate but conditions prevail which inhibit or retard absorption. The vitamin cobalamin (vitamin B_{12}) requires a specific protein produced by the gastric mucosa to act as a carrier in transporting the vitamin from the intestine to the bloodstream. If this protein is not produced then cobalamin cannot be absorbed and a deficiency disease, pernicious anemia, results.

Sometimes people tend to think that if a little of something is good then a lot is much better. In following this type of logic many persons consume megadose (very large) amounts of vitamins. In some cases a large vitamin intake conditions the body for an increased need for that vitamin. If the intake is suddenly curtailed an *induced deficiency* state can result.

Some disease conditions can increase the need for a vitamin above normal intake levels. Such conditions demand a higher requirement for a specific vitamin in order to prevent deficiency symptoms. Appreciable vitamin losses can occur under adverse conditions of food harvesting and storage. In addition, food processing methods and preparation methods can reduce the vitamin content of foods. See Table 7-1 for methods of food storage, processing, and preparation which help to conserve the vitamin content of foods.

The vitamins are generally divided into two classes: those that are water-soluble and those that are fat-soluble. The water-soluble vitamins are the B-complex vitamins and vitamin C. The fat-soluble vitamins are A, D, E, and K; vitamins which are distinctly different from one another.

The water-soluble vitamins are absorbed into the blood stream. Some are freely absorbed and others require an energy source and/or combination with another substance to facilitate absorption and transportation. Toxicity due to excesses of these vitamins is generally uncommon (but not unknown) because excess water-soluble vitamins are excreted in the urine. Only small amounts of water-soluble vitamins are stored in the body. Because there is minimal storage of water-soluble vitamins, they must be consumed regularly in the diet. Some of the water-soluble vitamins contain mineral elements in their chemical structure.

The fat-soluble vitamins are absorbed into the lymph system along with other fat compounds. Because contents of the lymph system are eventually dumped into the bloodstream, the fat-soluble vitamins must have appropriate lipoprotein carriers to make them soluble in the watery solution of blood. Fat-soluble vitamins are stored in the body when intake is in excess of need (this is reasonable since they are fatty substances, and fat in excess of need is stored in the body). Because they are stored, the deficiency symptoms associated with fat-soluble vitamins are relatively slow to develop. The body does not normally attempt to regulate the excess intake of fat-soluble vitamins by excreting them in the urine. Vitamins A, D, E, and K though different in chemical structure contain no other elements in their chemical structures than carbon, hydrogen, and oxygen.

Vitamin overdose. Partly because of the belief that more of a good thing is better and partly because people are always looking for easily obtainable and quick ways to gain better health, physical powers, mental alertness, and physical appearance, the consumption of vitamins in large doses continues.

The FDA conducted studies on excessive vitamin intake. It found that no additional benefits were derived for healthy persons from an intake in excess of recommended allowances but toxicity could occur from the overdose of some vitamins. Consequently, the FDA tried to restrict the sale of vitamin supplements containing over 150 percent of the U.S. RDA to a prescription basis only. The need for a prescription would have meant that an individual was consuming an increased vitamin intake on the advice of a physician. However, at the urging of opponents to this regulation the government overruled this regulation because it infringed on the rights of an individual to choose his own nutrient intake.[2]

The fact remains that excess vitamin intake has not been shown under research conditions to be beneficial for healthy persons and the threat of toxicity is probable from some vitamins taken in excess. The concept of needless excess vitamin intake is effectively presented in a film which correlates vitamin need to one lighted match necessary to light one candle. One lighted match accomplishes the job to a maximum. Ten lighted matches held together cannot light the candle any better than the one lit match.[3]

Indeed, many nutritionists feel that the excess intake of the water-soluble B-complex vitamins produces little benefit and perhaps increases hardship due to the excessive cost of some of the vitamin preparations. Most water-soluble vitamins taken in excess of need are readily excreted. Therefore, many nutritionists feel that the excessive intake of water-soluble vitamins, at best, produces only a high-cost urine! Excessive intakes of fat-soluble vitamins, however, can be toxic.[4]

Table 7-1.   Tips on maximizing vitamin retention in fruits and vegetables.

---

1. Use fresh fruits and vegetables as quickly after harvesting as possible. To the home gardener this means from garden to the table within a short time. To the food shopper this means within a few days of purchasing.
2. More vitamins are preserved when cooked whole and unpared than when pared, cut, and cooked, that is, vitamin content of a potato baked in the skin is higher than for a half cup of mashed potatoes which were pared, cut, boiled, and whipped.
3. Lengthy cooking times increase vitamin loss.
4. Cooking in large amounts of water increases vitamin loss through leaching.
5. Adding alkalis (baking soda) to cooking water destroys certain vitamins.
6. Use of a vegetable peeler reduces food loss and, therefore, vitamin loss as compared to use of a knife for paring. Peeling by any method exposes greater surface area of a food to oxygen which increases vitamin loss due to oxidation.
7. Use of cooking methods which shorten cooking time and use small amounts of water reduce vitamin loss in foods, such as stir-frying. However, very high heat such as required in pressure cooking increases some vitamin destruction.
8. The darker outside leaves of some leafy vegetables are higher in carotene (vitamin A) content. Discard bruised or dried outside leaves; add leaves which are edible but not attractive in cooked dishes; use cosmetically attractive inner leaves for salads.
9. Slice or otherwise cut fruits and vegetables just before their use in order to prevent extensive vitamin destruction due to oxidation. The smaller the cut pieces the greater the oxidation potential.
10. Store canned fruits and vegetables in a cool, dry storage area. Glass jars should also be stored in a dark place.
11. Vegetables which are cooked until they are heated through but remain crisp have milder flavor, better color, and retain more nutrients than vegetables cooked until soft.

Key Points: Introduction to Vitamins

I. Vitamins are necessary to life. They perform specific metabolic functions. Vitamins are essential in our diets though only in very small amounts because our bodies cannot manufacture them.

II. Many vitamins perform as coenzymes which are compounds necessary to activate enzymes. Some substances called antivitamins can take the place of a vitamin in its coenzyme position and cause the inactivation of the enzyme.

III. Vitamin deficiencies can be the result of inadequate intake, malabsorption, induction from previous excessive intake, and certain disease conditions and body states.

IV. Vitamins are generally divided into two classes:
Water-soluble—the B-complex vitamins and ascorbic acid (vitamin C)
Fat-soluble—vitamins A, D, E, and K
   A. Water-soluble vitamins are not stored in appreciable amounts; are less likely to become toxic at moderate levels above recommended intakes; must be con-

sumed regularly to avoid deficiency symptoms; are absorbed into the portal blood system; and some require a carrier for absorption and transport.

   B. Fat-soluble vitamins (especially A, D, and E) are stored in appreciable amounts; can become toxic because of accumulation in body tissues; are slower in exhibiting deficiency symptoms; are absorbed into the lymph system; require lipoprotein carriers.

V. There is no evidence of additional benefits derived for healthy persons from excessive vitamin intake and the risk of toxicity from an overdose of some vitamins is increased.

VI. Though not a direct source of energy, vitamins are needed as coenzymes in the chemical reactions necessary for energy production from other nutrients.

VII. The chemical structures of the various vitamins differ greatly. Fat-soluble vitamins contain only C, H, and O. Water-soluble vitamins contain additional elements.

Questions: Introduction to Vitamins

1. The term vitamin was chosen in part because it means:
    a. necessary to food
    b. necessary to diet
    c. necessary to life

2. Vitamins are needed in very (small/large) amounts

3. Why are vitamins essential in our diet?

4. Synthetic vitamins are nutritionally equivalent to naturally occurring vitamins.
    a. True
    b. False

5. Vitamins are not a source of energy but are necessary for the metabolic processes involved in _____ .

6. What kind of vitamins are used to enrich cereal products?
    a. naturally occurring vitamins
    b. synthetic vitamins
    c. provitamins

7. A precursor or provitamin is an (active/inactive) form of a vitamin.

8. Most vitamins function as _____ .

9. Antivitamins (vitamin antagonists) are:
    a. frequently similar in chemical structure to a vitamin.
    b. capable of destroying or reducing the biological effectiveness of a vitamin.
    c. essential to the human diet.

10. When an antivitamin is present the body (can/cannot) discriminate between it and its associated vitamin.

11. Coenzymes are compounds which are necessary to activate enzymes.
    a. True
    b. False

12. The inactive protein portion of an enzyme is called:
    a. a coenzyme
    b. a prosthetic group
    c. an apoenzyme

13. Without the proper coenzyme attached an enzyme is (active/inactive).

14. Identify three reasons why a person may develop a vitamin deficiency.

15. Vitamin losses from fruits and vegetables can occur as a result of poor conditions of harvesting and storage.
    a. True
    b. False

16. Why is vitamin loss greater when potatoes are mashed or whipped than when baked in the skin?

17. Rate the following food preparation methods from most to least likely to cause large losses of vitamins.
    a. cooking fruits and vegetables whole and unpared
    b. dicing fruits and vegetables into small pieces
    c. cutting fruits and vegetables into medium-size, chunky pieces

18. It is preferable to use (small/large) amounts of water when cooking vegetables in order to conserve vitamins.

19. The practice of adding baking soda to simmering legumes (beans and peas) assists in softening their cellulose content but increases _____ .

20. Which vegetable preparation method tends to conserve the most vitamins?
    a. boiling
    b. simmering
    c. stir-frying

21. Vegetables cooked until soft have (greater/lesser) vitamin loss than vegetables cooked until heated through but still remain crisp.

22. Which leaves of a green leafy vegetable contain the greatest vitamin A content?

23. Vitamin loss is increased for many foods during the storage period by light (through glass containers), increased temperatures, and moistness. Therefore, what is a description of the best storage facility for foodstuffs?

24. Excessive vitamin intake has:
    a. not been demonstrated as beneficial in humans
    b. been shown to cause toxicity by some vitamins
    c. been shown to cause increased excretion of the water-soluble vitamins

25. Classify the following terms as either descriptive of water-soluble or fat-soluble vitamins.
    a. water-soluble
    b. fat-soluble

    _____ 1. absorbed into the blood system
    _____ 2. are stored in appreciable amounts in the body
    _____ 3. are absorbed into the lymph system
    _____ 4. require a lipoprotein carrier in the bloodstream
    _____ 5. are excreted in the urine
    _____ 6. must be regularly consumed in the diet because storage in the body is minimal

    _____ 7. deficiencies are slow to develop
    _____ 8. B-complex and vitamin C
    _____ 9. vitamins A, D, E, and K
    _____ 10. sometimes contain mineral elements in their chemical structure
    _____ 11. are chemically composed only of carbon, hydrogen, and oxygen

Answers: Introduction to Vitamins

1. c
2. small
3. They are essential because our body cannot manufacture them even though our bodies need them.
4. a
5. energy production
6. b
7. inactive
8. coenzymes
9. a, b
10. cannot
11. a
12. c
13. inactive
14. inadequate intake of vitamins; malabsorption of the vitamin; induced deficiency by abruptly ceasing an excessive intake of a particular vitamin at a level to which the body has become accustomed; disease conditions which increase the requirement for a vitamin above normal intake.
15. a
16. A greater area of the potato has been exposed to moist heat, vitamins have been leached by the boiling water, and a greater surface area has been exposed to oxygen.
17. b, then c, then a
18. small
19. vitamin destruction
20. c
21. greater
22. the darker colored, outer leaves
23. a cool, dark, dry storage place
24. a, b, c
25.

1.	a	7.	b
2.	b	8.	a
3.	b	9.	b
4.	b	10.	a
5.	a	11.	b
6.	a		

ENRICHMENT OF FOODS

Enrichment of foods began with the addition of iodine (a mineral) to salt and later vitamin D to milk. During the early 1940's a more formal enrichment program was begun. At present, enrichment standards for cereals and grains are set for three vitamins and one mineral: thiamin, riboflavin, niacin, and iron. Certain other nutrients such as vitamins A and D and calcium may be optionally fortified in a food within limitations.

There are actually three general categories for the addition of nutrients to food: enrichment, fortification, and restoration. *Enrichment* involves, as mentioned above, the addition of thiamin, riboflavin, niacin, and iron to cereals and grains at levels established by law which are intended to compensate for losses of these nutrients during processing. Actually, iron and riboflavin are added in amounts greater than found in whole grains. Enrichment is not mandatory. However, if enrichment is done it must be done according to enrichment standards. Also, if a food product states on the label that it is enriched it must have nutrients added according to enrichment standards for that food. In other words, the nutrients may not be added in arbitrary quantity.

Fortification is the addition of nutrients to foods which do not normally contain significant amounts of the nutrients chosen for fortification. However, the food chosen for fortification needs to be appropriate for the addition of a specific nutrient such as milk fortified with vitamin D. Vitamin D is necessary for the efficient utilization of calcium. Milk is an excellent source of calcium; therefore, milk is a good carrier food for the nutrient vitamin D.

Restoration is a term which means the addition of nutrients to processed foods to a level approximating those before the food went into processing. Most nutrient additions are for the enrichment or fortification, and many foods are both enriched and fortified.

The Food and Drug Administration (FDA) is the official regulator of enrichment and fortification because of its authority to set food standards and regulate food additives.[5] If enrichment or fortification is done, then the standards set by the FDA must be used.

An example of the FDA's part in setting these standards is exemplified by the past controversy over superenrichment with iron. The FDA, at the urging of the American Bakers Association, proposed to increase the level for iron enrichment to nearly three times the level which had been used. Several respected professional medical and nutrition associations favored the increase to help reduce the occurrence of iron deficiency anemia.[6]

Persons opposed to this new regulation were concerned about problems of toxicity which might arise as a result of high iron intake for some individuals; the actual benefits of such an increase because of the low absorption rate of iron, especially from cereal and grain sources; and the possible masking of a pathological condition because of apparent high iron serum levels in the blood of persons consuming regular high levels of iron. Some opponents felt there was little evidence to support the increased level chosen as a known level for improvement of iron stores in the body.[7] Subsequently, the opponents successfully made their case and the FDA dropped the increase in iron for enriched and fortified food products in 1978.[8]

The FDA keeps several guidelines in mind when establishing levels of standards for the addition of various nutrients to certain foods, according to policies stated by the Food and Nutrition Board.[9] Some of the factors taken into account are the loss of nutrients from some foods in processing, the possibility of misleading consumers about the total nutritive value a fortified food will add to diet, the appropriateness of a food as a carrier for an added nutrient, the target population for whom the nutrient is intended, the interaction of the added nutrient and the other ingredients of the food carrier, and the physiological availability of the added nutrient from a particular food.

Enrichment of breads, cereals, and grains was justified on the basis that the foodstuffs in this category were relatively inexpensive staples and, therefore, likely to be eaten regularly by the population most in need of the fortified nutrients.

Enrichment and fortification of foods with vitamins (and some minerals) has decreased the incidence of various deficiency diseases: iodine to prevent goiter, iron to control iron deficiency anemia, niacin to prevent pellagra, and vitamin D to prevent rickets.

Enrichment and fortification are certainly to be considered valid approaches to meeting the nutrient needs of specific populations for whom certain nutrient availability and intake are low. However, enrichment and fortification programs should not be considered substitutes for a varied and balanced diet. Enrichment and fortification do not insure adequate, well-rounded nutrient intake by persons to maintain good health.[10] *There is still a need to encourage wise diet planning through selection and consumption of a wide variety of foods which will meet the nutritional requirements of healthy individuals.*

Key Points: Enrichment of Foods

I.   Enrichment is the addition of thiamin, riboflavin, niacin, and iron to grains/breads to levels established by law and at least to levels normally found in natural sources before processing.

II. Fortification is the addition of nutrients to foods which are not normally natural sources for those nutrients. The chosen food must be an appropriate carrier for the added nutrient.

III. The FDA sets standards for and regulates the addition of nutrients to food: enrichment and fortification.

IV. Some of the guidelines used by FDA to establish levels of standards for nutrient addition to foods are:
   A.   loss of nutrients during processing,
   B.   possible misrepresentation of the nutritional value of enriched and fortified foods,
   C.   appropriateness of a food as a carrier for a nutrient, including the consideration of interaction with the various nutrients within that food, and the physiological availability of the added nutrient from that food,
   D.   target population for whom the nutrient is intended.

V.   Enrichment and fortification of foods with various vitamins and minerals has eliminated certain nutrient deficiency diseases.

VI. Addition of nutrients to a food is no substitute for obtaining necessary nutrients from a varied diet.

Questions: Enrichment of Foods

1.   a.   What was the first nutrient intentionally added to a foodstuff to prevent a deficiency disease?
     b.   What was the food carrier?
     c.   What was the deficiency disease?

2.   What four nutrients are added in "enriched" cereal and grain foods?

3.   Any of the four nutrients added to enriched foods may be added in amounts set by the food processor.
     a.   True
     b.   False

4.   The addition of nutrients to a food in amounts not naturally found in that food is
     _____ .
     a.   enrichment
     b.   fortification
     c.   restoration

5.   The addition of nutrients to cereals and grains in amounts at least as great and slightly greater than found in whole grains is _____ .
     a.   enrichment
     b.   fortification
     c.   restoration

6.   The addition of nutrients to a food in approximate amounts found in that food before processing is meant by the term:
     a.   enrichment

b. fortification

c. restoration

7. Enrichment and fortification of "fabricated" foods can make those foods nutritionally equivalent to the natural, common foods they are intended to replace.
   a. True
   b. False

8. What agency is responsible for setting enrichment and fortification standards?

9. Why were increased amounts of iron once proposed for the standard regulating iron enrichment? Why was the proposal not adopted?

10. The absorption rate for iron from cereal foods is (high/low).

11. Review the guidelines FDA follows when establishing standards for food enrichment and fortification. On the basis of general nutrition knowledge and these guidelines, identify from the following the appropriate conditions for fortification or enrichment.
    a. addition of protein to candy sold in the U.S.
    b. addition of a nutrient whose intake is frequently found to be low by individuals in numerous sections of the country to a reasonably priced, regularly consumed, and compatible food
    c. addition of vitamin B_{12} to a food to prevent pernicious anemia
    d. addition of iron to baby cereals to prevent iron-deficiency anemia and to supplement low levels of iron found in breast milk and cow's milk, the food staples of infants
    e. addition of vitamin D to cola drinks

12. Enrichment and fortification programs should not take the place of a varied, well-balanced diet as a primary source for necessary nutrients for healthy persons.
    a. True
    b. False

13. Enrichment and fortification programs are effective in reducing incidence of some deficiency diseases.
    a. True
    b. False

Answers: Enrichment of Foods

1. a. iodine
   b. salt
   c. goiter
2. thiamin, riboflavin, niacin, iron
3. b
4. b
5. a
6. c
7. b; enrichment or fortification with certain nutrients does not compensate for other macronutrient or micronutrient constituents of the natural, common food.
8. FDA
9. to prevent the seemingly widespread occurrence of iron-deficiency anemia; possible toxicity from too high an intake of iron by some persons, questionable measurable benefits of such an intake, possible masking of a serious disease because of apparently high iron serum levels in the blood of persons with a regular high iron intake

10. low
11. b, d
12. a
13. a

Table 7-2.   Comparison of enriched and unenriched white bread and whole wheat bread.

	Iron content mg	Thiamin content mg	Riboflavin content mg	Niacin content mg
1. White unenriched bread, 1 slice (23g)	0.2	.02	.02	0.2
2. White enriched bread, 1 slice (23g)	0.6	.06	.05	0.6
3. Whole wheat bread, 1 slice (23g)	0.5	.06	.02	0.6

From: Bowes and Church's Food Values of Portions Commonly Used, 13th edition. Revised by Pennington JAT and Church HN, Philadelphia, J.B. Lippincott Company, 1980

REFERENCES

[1] The original spelling of thiamin was thiamine. The final "e" is dropped in more recent texts. Either spelling is still acceptable.

[2] White HS: Consumer's right to choose (letter). Journal of Nutrition Education, 10, October-December 1978, pp. 150-51

[3] Educational film "Vitamins from Foods," National Dairy Council

[4] A good review on megavitamin intake, especially for the general consumer is: Mayer J: Megavitamin madness: How much is too much? Family Health, 12, February 1980, pp. 48-49

[5] Hopkins H: Speaking out on fortifying foods. FDA Consumer, 12, December 1978-January 1979, pp. 18-20

[6] Hamilton EMN and Whitney EN: Nutrition: Concepts and Controversies. St. Paul, MN; West Publishing Company, 1979, pp. 292-294

[7] Elwood PC: The enrichment debate. Nutrition Today, 12, July-August 1977, pp. 18-24

[8] Anatomy of a decision. Nutrition Today, 13, January-February 1978, pp. 6-10 and 28-29

[9] General policies in regard to improvement of nutritive quality of foods. Food and Nutrition Board, National Academy of Sciences-National Research Council, Washington, D.C., 1973

[10] Mertz W: Fortification of foods with vitamins and minerals. Annals of the New York Academy of Sciences, 300, November 3, 1977, pp. 151-60

8
THE WATER-SOLUBLE VITAMINS

VITAMIN C (ASCORBIC ACID)

The well-documented discovery by Dr. James Lind of a cure for scurvy, the consumption of lime or orange juice, is familiar to most people. It is unfortunate that 50 years passed from the time Lind made his discovery in 1747 until the British Navy required rations of these citrus fruits on British sailing vessels. In the meantime many British sailors on ships sailing long exploration voyages succumbed to this painful disease.

Ascorbic acid is similar in chemical structure to glucose. Man is one of the few animal species lacking the necessary enzyme to convert glucose to ascorbic acid. It is felt that this enzyme lack is due to an inherited metabolic error—a genetic mutation.

The vitamin C recommendation in the revised 1980 RDA was raised from 45 mg for adult women and men to 60 mg for both population groups. The raise was made to increase body "pools" of ascorbic acid and to enhance greater absorption and utilization of iron.[1] The best food sources for vitamin C are citrus fruits. Other fruits and vegetables supply most of the remaining vitamin C in our diets. Milk, meats, eggs, grains, and cereals are poor sources of vitamin C. Vitamin C is easily destroyed by heat, oxidation, and alkali (such as baking soda), and is leached into cooking water as well. Vitamin conservation methods during cooking and food preparation are given in Table 7-1 (see Chapter Seven) and should be followed to preserve appreciable amounts of vitamin C in foods.

Conditions which have been shown to increase ascorbic acid requirements are:

1. stress—emotional or environmental
2. use of certain drugs such as oral contraceptive agents*
3. tissue healing of wounds
4. fever and infection
5. growth—such as that found during childhood or pregnancy
6. smoking*

The vitamin C deficiency disease is scurvy. Vitamin C is a primary substance necessary for proper collagen formation. Collagen is a protein which performs in the body as an intercellular "cementing" substance (sometimes referred to as "ground substance") upon which the body builds strong supportive tissue. Collagen is necessary for the formation and maintenance of bone matrix (the groundwork protein into which mineral salts are deposited), cartilage, dentin (the inner substance of teeth), and connective tissue. Most of the symptoms of scurvy are due to a breakdown of collagen formation and maintenance:

*Vitamin C plasma levels are lowered under conditions of cigarette smoking and oral contraceptive use. However, the significance of this lowering effect on ascorbic acid requirements has not yet been established.

fragile vascular capillaries which rupture easily causing hemorrhages (bleeding) in the skin, painful bleeding in the bones and joints, susceptibility to bone fractures, poor wound healing (because of inadequate ground substance for scar tissue formation), and bleeding and receding "spongy" gums with loosened teeth.

Scurvy is seldom seen in the United States though some vitamin C deficiency (without the development of scurvy symptoms) has been noted for certain population groups whose intake of vitamin C-rich fruits and vegetables is low, such as adolescent and older males. A nursing baby receives some ascorbic acid in human milk. Most commercial formulas are fortified with ascorbic acid. The bottle-fed infant not receiving a vitamin C fortified formula requires supplementation with citrus juice (or supplemental preparation if allergy develops to the juice) to prevent symptoms of deficiency. Most infants need a vitamin C food source or supplement by six months of age.

Anemia is also a condition found in adult scurvy. Ascorbic acid is instrumental in reducing ingested iron to the ferrous iron (Fe^{++}) state necessary for absorption. Ascorbic acid also helps to mobilize stored body iron. Folacin (a B-complex vitamin necessary to prevent megaloblastic anemia) requires ascorbic acid for conversion to its active form. Iron and folacin levels adequate for the prevention of anemia are, therefore, maintained in part by the presence of vitamin C.

Megadose intakes of vitamin C. So much controversy has arisen about the value of consuming megadose (very large) amounts of vitamin C that a discussion of this topic is warranted here. Recent reviews of creditable clinical trials using large doses of vitamin C disclosed that the use of vitamin C megadoses only reduced the incidence of colds by about one percent and the length of colds by one-tenth of a day.[2] The researchers concluded that such minor benefits are not worth the potential risks of such large doses of vitamin C.

What are some of the risks of excessive vitamin C intake? Some conditions associated with megadose vitamin C intakes are:

1. receiving false positive test results for glycosuria (glucose in the urine) as occurs with diabetic individuals,
2. interference with tests used to determine whether occult blood is in stools (could cause a failure to diagnose a serious intestinal disorder),
3. diarrhea,
4. possible increase in the formation of uric acid and oxalate stones (kidney stones),
5. interference with the anticoagulant action of drugs intended to reduce blood clotting,
6. possible cause of infertility and abortion and malformation of a fetus, and
7. impaired bacteria-killing ability of white blood cells.

The RDA given for ascorbic acid takes into consideration different breakdown rates for that vitamin in different individuals, efficiency of absorption, development of an adequate body pool, differences due to sex and age, and intake needs to prevent scurvy. The 60 mg allowance is felt to be generously ample for most healthy American adults. Higher dosages should be taken only under the advice of a physician. A moderate increase in ascorbic acid intake through the increased intake of natural food sources containing ascorbic acid may not be harmful and may be beneficial during times of illness or stress.

In conclusion, a summary of the findings of two competent, independent researchers is appropriate:[3] It would be a mistake for the layman to consume megadoses of ascorbic acid because of the risks associated with such an intake in order to obtain the minor, and even questionable, benefits of reducing the occurrence and severity of cold symptoms.

B-COMPLEX VITAMINS

Thiamin. Thiamin is a vitamin essential to carbohydrate metabolism. Thiamin pyrophosphate (TPP) is the active vitamin and it is TPP that is one of the crucial cofactors necessary for the formation of acetyl CoA from pyruvic acid. Acetyl CoA is the gateway substance into the Kreb's cycle for energy production from glucose. (Refer to Chapter Six for a more detailed description of the Kreb's cycle.)

Thiamin cannot be stored in the body in appreciable amounts. Excesses are generally excreted in the urine. Consequently, a dietary deficiency of thiamin will cause a rapid depletion of thiamin reserves.

Thiamin allowances are generally based upon caloric need because of thiamin's role in energy metabolism. However, a minimal intake of 1 mg of thiamin per day is recommended for adults to maintain body stores when caloric intake is restricted.[4] This allowance also takes into consideration the amount needed to prevent clinical symptoms, amount usually excreted, and certain enzyme activity dependent upon thiamin.

Adult RDAs vary from 1 to 1.5 mg/day computed on a 0.5 mg/1,000 kcal basis. Although thiamin is contained in many different foods it is not generally found in concentrated amounts. Pork, oysters, organ meats, and some legumes are fairly high in thiamin content. Milk and enriched breads and grains supply significant amounts of thiamin because of the quantity of these foods consumed. Thiamin is destroyed by moist heat. A considerable loss of thiamin occurs when the liquids in which vegetables are cooked are discarded. Pork drippings also contain discarded thiamin. Consumption of polished rice and the practice of washing rice greatly reduces the thiamin available from rice—factors of importance in countries where rice is a staple in the diet.

Beriberi, a deficiency disease, is due to a lack of thiamin. Symptoms of beriberi include a heaviness and weakness of legs along with pain in calf muscles due to cramping, and a burning and numbness in the feet. Also present are nausea, lack of appetite, irregular heart beat, general nervous irritability, and emotional instability. Most of these symptoms are due to tissue starvation and toxicity from metabolic intermediate products which are not broken down because energy metabolism is slowed or altered. "Wet" beriberi indicates the presence of edema; "dry" beriberi indicates emaciation and neural disorders.

Alcoholics who replace food with alcohol in their diet, and who might have some liver damage, frequently suffer thiamin deficiency. Thiamin deficiency in alcoholics may contribute to their characteristic development of mental confusion, loss of memory, and brain damage.

Riboflavin. Riboflavin is a component of a yellow-green fluorescent pigment in milk (flavin denotes "fluorescence"). Riboflavin is not readily soluble so its loss in cooking water is less than for thiamin. Riboflavin is also fairly stable to heat and acid. However, riboflavin is destroyed by alkali (such as baking soda) and ultraviolet light rays.

Riboflavin is part of two coenzymes necessary to activate certain hydrogen transfer reactions of the Krebs cycle (flavin mononucleotide, FMN, and flavin adenine dinucleotide, FAD) and to carry out electron transfer reactions (oxidative enzyme systems) necessary for the production of energy. Riboflavin is also a component of enzymes necessary for the metabolism of fatty acids and amino acids.

Riboflavin allowances remain about the same whether computed on energy intake, protein allowance, or metabolic body size. The 1980 revised RDA's range from 1.2 to 1.7 mg/day for adults based on 0.6 mg/1,000 kcal intake. The higher ranges are for men who generally have greater size, protein, and energy intakes than women. Requirements are increased during periods of growth. Use of oral contraceptives may increase requirements for riboflavin.

Milk and milk products supply nearly half of the average person's riboflavin requirement. The remainder is supplied by meat, poultry, fish, eggs, green leafy vegetables, and enriched or whole grain cereals.

Symptoms of riboflavin deficiency result in tissue erosion and aggravation of tissue injury. Because of the use and activity of mouth and nasal areas, fissures develop at the mouth and nasal angles which do not heal easily *(cheilosis)*. Other skin changes such as a greasy dermatitis develop, the tongue becomes swollen and deeply reddened *(glossitis)*, and eyes become teary while the cornea is invaded by blood vessels.

Niacin. Niacin is necessary as a component of coenzymes needed to activate reactions involved in carbohydrate, protein, and fat energy metabolism (nicotinamide adenine dinucleotide, NAD, and nicotinamide adenine dinucleotide phosphate, NADP). Since riboflavin is also involved as a coenzyme in these energy-production reactions, a deficiency of niacin produces symptoms similar to those of a deficiency of riboflavin. Niacin deficiency is frequently found in association with riboflavin and thiamin deficiencies. In addition, niacin is a component of the coenzyme necessary for the synthesis of fatty acids.

Niacin is resistant to destruction by heat, light, oxygen, acid, and alkali. However, because niacin is very soluble in water, losses which occur during cooking are due mainly to losses in discarded liquids.

Two forms of equal biologic activity constitute this vitamin: niacin (nicotinic acid) and nicotinamide. *The essential amino acid tryptophan is a precursor of niacin.* Thiamin, riboflavin, and vitamin B_6 are necessary to convert tryptophan to niacin. The 1980 revised RDAs give the niacin recommendations in niacin equivalents. One niacin equivalent (NE) equals 1 mg niacin or 60 mg of dietary tryptophan. The adult RDAs range between 13 and 19 niacin equivalents based on 6.6 niacin equivalents per 1,000 kcal. A minimum intake of 13 niacin equivalents is recommended even for caloric intakes of less than 2,000 kcal.

Diets based on corn without the benefit of additional milk or meat result in a deficiency of niacin because corn protein is very low in tryptophan. The favored foods of the south—sweet potatoes, cornbread, cabbage, rice, greens, grits, gravy, syrup, biscuits, and coffee—are low in protein and tryptophan. Enrichment of grains and cereals with niacin has eliminated pellagra, the niacin deficiency disease, from the poorer population of the south.

The deficiency disease due to a lack of niacin is pellagra. The symptoms of pellagra are in large part due to the decreased energy production consequent of niacin deficiency. There is general fatigue, weakness, loss of appetite, headache, nausea, vomiting, and diarrhea. The tongue, lips, and mouth become red and sore. A dermatitis develops which is greatly aggravated by exposure to sunlight. There is in more advanced stages an observed dementia involving hallucinations and delusions similar to insanity. These symptoms include the four "D's" of untreated pellagra: dermatitis, diarrhea, dementia, and death.

Administration of niacin to a niacin-deficient person with symptoms of dementia will alleviate the neurological symptoms. However, consumption of megadoses of niacin will not necessarily alleviate conditions of schizophrenia and depression not related to a niacin deficiency. Megavitamin therapy has been tried with schizophrenic individuals without documented success. The American Psychiatric Association has stated that positive results of megavitamin therapy have not been confirmed and has condemned the publicity methods of megavitamin proponents.[5]

Vitamin B_6. Pyridoxine, pyridoxal, and pyridoxamine are three equally effective forms of the vitamin substance labeled vitamin B_6. *The active form of vitamin B_6 is the coenzyme pyridoxal phosphate involved principally in amino acid metabolism.* Some of the enzymes requiring vitamin B_6 are necessary for transamination, deamination, decarboxylation, transulfuration, and tryptophan conversion to niacin.

Pyridoxine is also necessary for proper action of the enzyme which breaks down glycogen to glucose, and for a reaction involved in the formation of hemoglobin. This vitamin is also necessary to many other enzyme-activated reactions. It is not surprising that a deficiency of this vitamin, with its many functions, produces generalized symptoms of ill health: mental depression, nausea, vomiting, and sometimes a greasy dermatitis.

Vitamin B_6 recommendations are in milligrams and range between 2 and 2.2 mg/day for adults. Vitamin B_6 intake requirements are related to protein intake. High protein diets increase the requirement for vitamin B_6. Pregnancy and lactation also increase intake needs. The use of oral contraceptives may increase the vitamin B_6 requirement as does isonicotinic acid hydrazide (INH) used in the treatment of tuberculosis.

Detailed lists of foods containing vitamin B_6 are not generally available. Food sources which provide significant amounts of vitamin B_6 are fish, poultry, meats, avocados, bananas, peanuts, walnuts, and legumes.[6]

Vitamin B_6 deficiency is difficult to isolate because the effective forms of the vitamin are found in a wide variety of foods. However, deficiency states have been induced in humans for study trials and inadvertently in infants fed a commercial formula in which the vitamin was destroyed during heat processing. Deficiency symptoms include irritability, nervousness, depression, convulsions, difficulty in walking, weight loss, dermatitis, decreased conversion of typtophan to niacin, and anemia. The occurrence of vitamin B_6 deficiency in alcoholics is relatively high.

Toxicity due to an increased oral intake of vitamin B_6 is unlikely. Extremely high intakes may cause sleepiness. Storage of vitamin B_6 in human tissues is extremely small.

Vitamin B_{12}. Cobalamin is the accepted generic term for vitamin B_{12}. Cyanocobalamin is the most stable form of this vitamin which is nutritionally active when ingested or given by injection to man. Cyanocobalamin is therefore the commercially produced form.

Vitamin B_{12} is a chemically large and complex compound. This vitamin requires a special intrinsic factor, a glycoprotein, produced by glands in certain parts of the stomach for its absorption. This *intrinsic factor* combines with free vitamin B_{12} in the stomach. Vitamin B_{12} is normally ingested in a protein complex form, the *extrinsic factor*. The hydrochloric acid and enzymes present in gastric juice release the vitamin from its protein association. The vitamin B_{12}/intrinsic factor complex travels to the ileum where it is attached for a short period of time in the presence of calcium to ileal mucosal cells. It is finally absorbed into the portal blood system. Once in the blood vitamin B_{12} is attached to special protein carriers.

Vitamin B_{12} recommended intake is measured in micrograms. The revised 1980 RDA for vitamin B_{12} is 3 μg for both adult males and females. Requirement is increased during pregnancy and lactation. This vitamin is stored in the body but in very small amounts. Vitamin B_{12} deficiency symptoms take several years to become apparent, and the deficiency is more often the result of a lack of intrinsic factor production (a genetic disorder). However, deficiency can also be due to the inadequate production of gastric hydrochloric acid as sometimes occurs in old age.

Vitamin B_{12} is produced by certain bacteria in the intestines of animals. This occurs in the colon of man, but vitamin B_{12} cannot be absorbed from the colon.[7] Vitamin B_{12} is only found in plant food sources when they have been contaminated by the vitamin-producing microorganisms. The best food sources are meat, meat products, eggs, and milk and milk products. Because dietary sources of vitamin B_{12} are all of animal origin vegetarians are at risk of developing a dietary deficiency of vitamin B_{12}.

The deficiency disease for vitamin B_{12} is pernicious anemia, a fatal disease without appropriate treatment. Vitamin B_{12} is most successfully administered to persons with pernicious anemia by injection for direct absorption into the bloodstream. This procedure enables by-passing the gastrointestinal system and the need for the intrinsic factor. Vitamin B_{12} is also necessary for the normal maintenance of the protective covering of nerve fibers, the myelin sheath. Nerve damage is associated with extended vitamin B_{12} deficiency.

Folacin. Folacin is also referred to as folic acid, pteroylglutamic acid or folate. It was once termed the citrovorum factor (CF). The term folacin is derived from the Latin *folium* meaning leaf because of its presence in green, leafy vegetables.

Folacin is absorbed in the small intestine but its absorption rate differs for its various chemical forms. Folacin is attached to a protein carrier for both transportation and storage.

Folacin is necessary as a coenzyme in reactions involving the transfer of single carbon units as found in the chemical reactions of amino acid metabolism and DNA synthesis.

Some folacin is produced by bacteria within the intestines but how much of this is available for absorption and utilization is unknown. The current RDA for folacin in male and female adults is 400 μg. This recommendation is doubled in pregnancy and increased to 500 μg during lactation.

Foods generally high in folacin are liver, organ meats, yeast, fresh green vegetables, some fresh fruits, and legumes. Folacin is destroyed by oxidation and long cooking processes.[8]

A deficiency of folic acid produces a megaloblastic (or macrocytic) anemia. The red blood cells are large, nucleated, and reduced in number. There is also a reduction in white blood cells. Deficiency is generally due to a dietary lack because folacin (in its free form) is freely absorbed. However, deficiency may also result during conditions of increased need such as pregnancy, use of contraceptive pills, certain disease conditions, and malabsorption syndromes. Deficiency may produce glossitis (reddened, swollen tongue) and diarrhea.

Folacin has the ability to mask the condition of pernicious anemia by correcting red blood cell size and maturation at least temporarily. Because of the seriousness of pernicious anemia and possible misdiagnosis of this condition, as well as the fact that folacin does not prevent the nerve damage which occurs with vitamin B_{12} deficiency and pernicious anemia, intake of large supplements of folacin is discouraged except under the advice of a physician.

Pantothenic Acid. The term pantothenic acid was derived from the Greek word *pantos* meaning "from everywhere" or "in all places." This describes the food sources of pantothenic acid: many and varied, as well as the location of the vitamin in the body: in all cells and tissues.

Pantothenic acid is a constituent of Coenzyme A, the cofactor necessary for reactions involving the release of energy from carbohydrates, gluconeogenesis (the making of glucose from noncarbohydrate sources), the synthesis of fatty acids, steroid hormones, porphyrins (constituents of hemoglobin), and acetylcholine (a substance necessary for normal nerve transmission). Because of the many metabolic reactions in which Coenzyme A is involved, deficiency symptoms for pantothenic acid are generalized: retarded growth, gastrointestinal disorders, neuromuscular disorders, respiratory infections, and mental depression.

The 1980 revised RDA gives a safe and adequate dietary intake range for pantothenic acid between 4 to 7 mg/day for adults. Some pantothenic acid is produced by intestinal microorganisms but the extent of the contribution from this source is not known.

Some of the best food sources for pantothenic acid are organ meats, egg yolk, whole grains, and legumes. Additional, appreciable amounts are found in milk, fruits, and vegetables.

Biotin. Biotin is a relatively simple chemical compound necessary as a coenzyme in reactions involved in the metabolism of fat and carbohydrate. *Biotin is important to carboxylation reactions* (the adding of or transferring of carbon dioxide from one compound to another). Carboxylation reactions are necessary for the synthesis of fatty acids and some amino acids. The 1980 revised RDA set the estimated safe and adequate dietary intake of biotin between 100 to 200 μg for adults.

Good dietary sources of biotin are organ meats, egg yolks, legumes, tomatoes, and nuts. Biotin is also produced by intestinal microorganisms. This biotin seems to be well-utilized by man. Raw egg white contains a glycoprotein, avidin, which binds biotin and makes it unavailable for absorption from the intestines. Avidin in cooked egg white does not bind biotin. Biotin deficiency symptoms which have been induced in man are a scaly dermatitis, weakness, muscular pain, pallor, nausea, and loss of appetite.

VITAMIN-LIKE FACTORS

Choline. Choline, a chemical substance found in all body cells, is synthesized by the body.

Choline is part of the phospholipid lecithin and is termed a lipotropic agent because of its apparent influence on the mobilization of fat from the liver by promoting the formation of lipoproteins (transport forms of fatty substances). A deficiency of choline can lead to the development of a fatty liver.

Choline is a component of acetylcholine which is necessary for normal nerve transmission. Choline is able to donate methyl groups necessary for various chemical reactions.[9] There is no RDA or recommended intake range for choline since it is probably synthesized by the body in sufficient amounts to meet body needs.

Inositol. This substance is sometimes called muscle sugar because it has a structure related to glucose and is a component of muscle phospholipids. It was once thought to be a vitamin but it is now known to be produced in sufficient quantity by the body to meet body needs. Inositol is found in fruits, vegetables, whole grains, meats, and milk. Inositol may possess some lipotropic properties.

Lipoic acid. Lipoic acid was so-named because it is a fat-soluble acid (lipo = fat). The primary importance of lipoic acid is as a coenzyme in the reaction converting pyruvic acid to acetyl CoA (active acetate). It is also necessary for another chemical reaction of the Krebs cycle. These reactions are vital to carbohydrate metabolism and the production of energy. Refer to Figures 6-5 and 6-6. Lipoic acid is synthesized by the body.

Table 8-1.   Some of the best dietary sources for the various water-soluble vitamins.

Ascorbic Acid	Thiamin	Riboflavin	Niacin
Citrus fruits	Pork	Organ meats	Liver
Brussels sprouts	Oysters	Milk	Tuna fish
Strawberries	Organ meats	Milk products	Peanuts
Greens	Legumes	Oysters	Peanut butter
Cantaloupe	Oranges	Muscle meats	Peas
	Enriched	Enriched	Pork
	breads	breads and	Chicken
	and	cereals	Enriched breads
	cereals		and cereals

Vitamin B_6	Vitamin B_{12}	Folacin	Pantothenic Acid
Fish	Liver	Liver	Organ meats
Poultry	Meat	Organ meats	Fresh vegetables
Meats	Shellfish	Yeast	Whole grains
Avocados	Eggs	Fresh green	Yeast
Bananas	Milk	vegetables	Egg yolk
Peanuts		Fresh fruits	
Walnuts		Legumes	
Legumes			

Biotin

Organ meats
Egg yolks
Legumes
Tomatoes
Nuts

Key Points: The Water-Soluble Vitamins

I. Excesses of the water-soluble vitamins above body needs are generally excreted from the body. However, some toxic and undesirable conditions can occur from megadose intakes of some water-soluble vitamins.

II. Water-soluble vitamins are generally not stored in appreciable amounts in body tissues. Therefore, daily intake of these vitamins is recommended to maintain optimum body levels and proper body functioning.

III. Ascorbic acid is necessary for proper collagen formation and maintenance. Collagen is the foundation substance necessary for building strong, supportive body tissues. Conditions of emotional stress, the intake of certain drugs, growth, and body tissue repair during healing can increase ascorbic acid requirements. Ascorbic acid greatly enhances the absorption of dietary iron.

IV. Most of the B-complex vitamins function as coenzymes necessary in various enzyme systems involved in the oxidation of carbohydrate, fat, and protein for energy production.

V. Though each of the B-complex vitamins performs specific metabolic functions, the functions of the B-complex vitamins are interrelated. Consequently, a deficiency of any one seldom produces isolated deficiency symptoms though certain symptoms may be more apparent than others. A lack of one of the B-complex vitamins also affects the degree to which the other B-complex vitamins are utilized. Therefore, therapeutic supplements generally are given which contain all the B-complex vitamins.

VI. Folacin and vitamin B_{12} are necessary for proper formation of red blood cells. Folacin can be obtained from plant and animal food sources. Vitamin B_{12} is available only from animal food sources and may need to be supplemented in the diets of vegetarians who exclude all animal and animal source foods from their diets.

VII. Vitamin B_6 is a coenzyme necessary for chemical reactions involved in amino acid (protein) metabolism. Vitamin B_6 is also necessary for conversion of glycogen to glucose and the formation of hemoglobin.

VIII. Some vitamin-like factors include choline, inositol, and lipoic acid. These factors perform specific metabolic functions but are not true vitamins because they are synthesized by the body in amounts necessary to meet body needs.

Questions: The Water-Soluble Vitamins

1. A cure for scurvy was discovered more than two centuries ago.
   a. True
   b. False

2. The symptoms of scurvy are all primarily the result of a breakdown in the formation and maintenance of the ground substance _____ .

3. Match the phrases on the right to the items on the left which they best describe.

   _____ 1. pernicious anemia
   _____ 2. cheilosis
   _____ 3. bone matrix
   _____ 4. tryptophan
   _____ 5. glossitis
   _____ 6. beriberi
   _____ 7. pellagra

   a. the groundwork protein into which mineral salts are deposited
   b. the deficiency disease produced by a lack of adequate thiamin
   c. swollen and reddened tongue characteristic of the deficiency of some B-complex vitamins
   d. cracks and fissures at the angles of the

       mouth and nose due to riboflavin de-
       ficiency

e. a precursor for niacin

f.   the deficiency disease produced by a
    lack of adequate niacin

g. a deficiency disease in which a dietary
    deficiency or inability to absorb vitamin
    B_{12} results

4.   List at least three symptoms of scurvy.

5.   Which population groups most often have low serum levels of ascorbic acid?
     Why?

6.   All infants need a vitamin C dietary supplement (such as citrus juice) by what
     age?

    a. three months

    b. six months

    c. 12 months

7.   Thiamin in the form of TPP is especially necessary for:

    a. protein synthesis

    b. fat synthesis

    c. energy production

8.   To what causes are the symptoms of beriberi most often due?

9.   The thiamin allowance is generally based upon caloric need and intake. What is
     the minimum daily recommended intake for thiamin when caloric intake is lim-
     ited?

    a. 0.5 mg

    b. 1 mg

    c. 2 mg

10.   Thiamin is easily destroyed by:

    a. light

    b. cold

    c. moist heat

11.   A food source particularly rich in thiamin is:

    a. pork

    b. potato

    c. pineapple

12.   Why are enriched grains a good source of thiamin though their thiamin content is
     not high?

13.   Why is the addition of a pinch of baking soda to some green vegetables during the
     cooking process to preserve the bright green color not a good practice?

14.   Why should milk be contained in dark glass bottles or opaque plastic containers?

15.   Diets based on what grain product are typically deficient in niacin?

16.   Why are diets that are sufficient in protein usually sufficient in niacin?

17.   Niacin deficiency is frequently found in association with deficiencies of what
     other vitamins?

    a. thiamin

    b. ascorbic acid

    c. riboflavin

18.   What are the four "D's" of pellagra?

19.   Administration of megadoses of niacin will alleviate the schizophrenic and de-

pressed conditions of only niacin-deficient individuals.
a. True
b. False

20. Vitamin B_6 is especially vital to:
a. protein metabolism
b. carbohydrate metabolism
c. fat metabolism

21. Vitamin B_6 requirements are increased:
a. with increased energy intake
b. with increased protein intake
c. during pregnancy and lactation

22. There are two factors important to the availability of vitamin B_{12} in the prevention of pernicious anemia. Vitamin B_{12} is the _____ factor; a specific gastric glycoprotein is the _____ factor.

23. Vitamin B_{12} is absorbed into the portal blood system. Does it travel freely in the blood or require a protein carrier?

24. The daily requirement for vitamin B_{12} for an adult is:
a. 3 mg
b. 3 μg
c. 3 g

25. A deficiency of vitamin B_{12} produces:
a. pernicious anemia
b. cheilosis
c. nerve damage

26. Why are strict vegetarians at risk of developing a deficiency of vitamin B_{12}?

27. What kind of anemia is produced by a deficiency of folacin?
a. pernicious anemia
b. microcytic anemia
c. megaloblastic anemia

28. Which conditions may result in folic acid deficiency?
a. a strict vegetarian diet
b. use of contraceptive pills and/or pregnancy
c. malabsorption syndromes

29. Why are intakes of large supplemental amounts of folacin not recommended?

30. The adult recommended folacin intake is doubled during pregnancy.
a. True
b. False

31. Pantothenic acid is available from limited food sources.
a. True
b. False

32. Pantothenic acid is necessary as a constituent of _____ .

33. Coenzyme A is necessary for:
a. carbodydrate metabolism
b. the synthesis of fatty acids
c. gluconeogenesis

34. The 1980 revised RDA gives a safe and adequate dietary intake range for pantothenic acid as:
a. 2-3 mg/day
b. 4-7 μg/day
c. 4-7 mg/day

35. Match the phrases on the right to the items on the left which they best describe.

    _____ 1. avidin
    _____ 2. inositol
    _____ 3. biotin
    _____ 4. choline
    _____ 5. acetylcholine
    _____ 6. lipotropic
    _____ 7. lipoic acid

    a. important to carboxylation reactions (transfer of CO_2)
    b. the "raw egg white injury factor" which binds biotin
    c. constituent of lecithin
    d. term which means "affinity for fat"
    e. muscle sugar
    f. coenzyme in the reaction converting pyruvic acid to acetyl CoA
    g. substance of which choline is a constituent and which is necessary for normal nerve transmission

36. Refer to Table 8-1 which gives some of the best sources for the various B-complex vitamins.
    a. Can you make a generalization about the best food groups from which to obtain the B-complex vitamins?
    b. What advice could you give to a friend who wants to know how to obtain adequate amounts of the B-complex vitamins in his or her diet?
    c. Which is the only vitamin for which meat is not listed as a good food source?

Answers: The Water-Soluble Vitamins

1. a
2. collagen
3. 1. g
    2. d
    3. a
    4. e
    5. c
    6. b
    7. f
4. Any of the following: hemorrhages in the skin due to ruptured vascular capillaries; painful, bleeding bones and joints; susceptibility to bone fractures; poor wound healing; bleeding and receding "spongy" gums with loosened teeth.
5. Adolescent boys and older men; their intake of fresh fruits and vegetables is low.
6. b
7. c
8. Tissue starvation and the build-up of undesirable metabolic intermediate products due to the interruption of energy metabolism.
9. b
10. c
11. a
12. because they are consumed in significant amounts
13. Baking soda is an alkali and destroys some vitamin activity such as that for thiamin and riboflavin.
14. because ultraviolet light destroys riboflavin and milk is a good source of riboflavin
15. corn
16. because they contain the amino acid tryptophan which can be converted to niacin
17. a and c
18. dermatitis, diarrhea, dementia, death
19. a

20. a
21. b, c
22. extrinsic; intrinsic
23. It requires a protein carrier.
24. b
25. a, c
26. Because vitamin B_{12} is only available from animal food sources.
27. c
28. b, c
29. Excess folacin can mask the presence of pernicious anemia and cause a misdiagnosis of this serious disease. Misdiagnosis can also allow possible nerve damage to occur as a result of vitamin B_{12} deficiency.
30. a
31. b
32. Coenzyme A
33. a, b, c
34. c
35. 1. b
    2. e
    3. a
    4. c
    5. g
    6. d
    7. f
36. a. No; all four food groups are represented as sources of the composite B-complex vitamins.
    b. Eat a variety of foods from the four food groups every day.
    c. ascorbic acid

REFERENCES

[1] Recommended Dietary Allowances, Ninth Revision Edition. Food and Nutrition Board, National Academy of Sciences-National Research Council, Washington, D.C.; 1980, p. 76

[2] Chalmers TC: Effects of ascorbic acid on the common cold. American Journal of Medicine, 58, 1975, p. 523

[3] Levy JV and Bach-y-Rita P: Vitamins—Their Use and Abuse. New York, Liveright, 1976, pp. 29-30

[4] Recommended Dietary Allowances, Ninth Revised Edition. Food and Nutrition Board, National Academy of Sciences-National Research Council, Washington, D.C.; 1980, p. 83

[5] Darby WJ, McNutt KW, and Todhunter EN: Niacin. In Present Knowledge in Nutrition, 4th ed. New York and Washington, D.C.; The Nutrition Foundation, Inc., 1976, pp. 170-171

[6] One list of moderate length giving the vitamin B_6 content in micrograms of selected foods can be found in: Sauberlich HE and Canham JE: Vitamin B_6. In Goodhart RS and Shils ME (eds): Modern Nutrition in Health and Disease, 6th ed. Philadelphia, Lea and Febiger, 1980, pp. 217-18

[7] Herbert V: Vitamin B_{12}. In Present Knowledge in Nutrition, 4th ed. New York and Washington, D.C.; The Nutrition Foundation, Inc., 1976, p. 193

[8] Hebert V, Colman N and Jacob E: Folic Acid and Vitamin B_{12}. In Goodhart RS and Shils ME (eds): In Modern Nutrition in Health and Disease. Philadelphia, Lea and Febiger, 1980, p. 247

[9] A methyl group is chemically known as an alkyl radical: —CH_3.

9
THE FAT-SOLUBLE VITAMINS

The fat-soluble vitamins are A, D, E, and K. Because they are soluble in fat they share some common characteristics with lipids in body absorption and metabolism.

1. Factors which decrease absorption of fat also decrease absorption of fat-soluble vitamins. Refer to Table 4-1 for a summary of factors affecting the absorption of fat.
2. All the fat-soluble vitamins are composed entirely of the elements carbon, hydrogen, and oxygen.
3. Fat-soluble vitamins are absorbed into the lymph system from the intestines along with other fatty substances.
4. Fat-soluble vitamins can be stored in the body and an excess intake can lead to toxicity in some cases.
5. Because fat-soluble vitamins can be stored in the body, deficiency symptoms are slower to develop than those for water-soluble vitamins.
6. Ingested mineral oil is not absorbed but passes through the intestines and is excreted in the feces. Fat-soluble vitamins are soluble in mineral oil. Consequently, the ingestion of mineral oil renders fat-soluble vitamins unavailable for absorption.

VITAMIN A

Active forms of vitamin A are retinol, retinaldehyde, and retinoic acid. Vitamin A is generally transported and stored in the body in the form of retinyl esters. Vitamin A also occurs in a precursor form (provitamin A) that must be converted in the body to biologically active forms of vitamin A. Vitamin A is easily oxidized though it is relatively stable to heat, acid, and alkali. Vitamin E seems to play a role in the protection of vitamin A from destruction by oxidation.

The greatest stores of vitamin A in the human body are found in the liver. In time of need the retinyl esters are converted to retinol and attached to a specific protein carrier for transport to body tissues. Protein deficiency will cause a decrease in the production of the specific protein carrier. This results in the decreased transport of vitamin A and a decreased availability of vitamin A to body tissues.

Functions of Vitamin A

1. *Vitamin A is necessary for proper adaptation to changes in light by the eye.* Rhodopsin, a light sensitive pigment, composed of opsin (a protein) and retinaldehyde (a vitamin A compound), is the substance necessary for normal vision in dim light. Rhodopsin is located in the light receptors in the retina[1] of the eye termed rods. When light strikes the rods the rhodopsin splits into its opsin and retinaldehyde components.

177

In the dark, these components are recombined in order to be ready to split again when initiated by light. A little vitamin A is lost each time splitting occurs. Consequently the blood must carry a constant supply of vitamin A to the rods. A deficiency of vitamin A retards this splitting/recombining process and leads to a condition termed *night blindness*. This type of night blindness can be corrected by administering a proper amount of vitamin A.

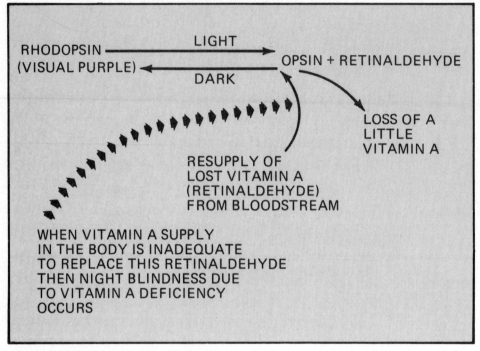

Figure 9-1.   Role of vitamin A in normal vision.

2. *Vitamin A is necessary for the maintenance of healthy, functional epithelial tissue (skin and mucous membranes) which help protect against invading disease-producing bacteria.* In the absence of adequate vitamin A the epithelial tissues fill with keratin (a protein normally found in nails and hair). This process is called keratinization. The keratin causes the cells to become dry and hard, resulting in loss of proper cell function. These cells eventually die. When these dead cells accumulate on epithelial surfaces they can be invaded by infection-producing bacteria.

The reactions of epithelial tissue to vitamin A deficiency are:

A. The conjunctiva (a thin, transparent membrane covering the eye) becomes dry and dull. This is termed *xerosis.*

B. The cornea of the eye (the thick, translucent membrane covering the front of the eye) becomes dry and thick leading to loss of sight. This condition is non-reversible and is termed *xerophthalmia.* The tear ducts dry and no longer function to lubricate or cleanse the eye and infections easily occur.

C. The skin becomes dry and scaly and keratinized epithelial cells plug oil glands. This leads to the formation of hard pimple-like formations around hair follicles—a condition termed follicular hyperkeratosis.

D. Mucus production is severely limited and mucous membranes of the gastrointestinal tract, respiratory tract, genital and urinary tracts are adversely affected. Resistance to infection in these areas is low.

3.   *Vitamin A is necessary for growth.* A deficiency of vitamin A results in retarded growth perhaps because it is necessary for normal RNA metabolism and protein synthesis[2], or because it causes a loss of appetite. Bone growth is also slowed.

Preformed vitamin A (retinol) is found in animal foods, and provitamin A (carotene) is found in yellow and yellow-orange plant pigments. A large portion of the carotenes in deep yellow to yellow-orange fruits and vegetables such as apricots, carrots, and sweet potatoes can be converted to vitamin A by man as well as other animals. Carotenes are also present in deep green vegetables. Of the carotenes, β-carotene provides the most vitamin A for man. The biological activity of β-carotene is about half that of an equal amount of retinol.

The revised 1980 RDA gives the RDA for vitamin A in retinol equivalents:[3]

1 retinol equivalent = 1 μg retinol

= 6 μg β-carotene

= 12 μg other provitamin A

= 3.33 IU vitamin activity from retinol

= 10 IU vitamin A activity from β-carotene

Refer to Appendix B for information on how to calculate the retinol equivalents for vitamin A from retinol, β-carotene, and other provitamin A sources. The RDAs for adults range from 800 to 1000 retinol equivalents with increases for pregnancy and lactation.

Food sources of vitamin A are organ meats, cream, butter, and egg yolk. Margarine is fortified with vitamin A. Provitamin A food sources include deep green and yellow vegetables and fruits. Refer to Table 2-6 for examples of good sources of vitamin A.

Vitamin A deficiency is the major cause of blindness in developing countries[4] and is second only to protein-calorie malnutrition in prevalence of nutritional deficiency disease world-wide.

Because vitamin A can be stored in appreciable amounts in the body toxicity can occur from megadoses of this vitamin. Many of the symptoms of hypervitaminosis A are similar to vitamin A deficiency: bone and joint pain, abnormal bone growth and fragility; dry, scaly skin, loss of appetite, and gastrointestinal disorders. Hypervitaminosis A can also cause headache, sleeplessness, abnormal or loss of menstruation, and enlargement of the liver and spleen. Polar bear liver contains toxic amounts of vitamin A and has caused intoxication in some Arctic explorers who consumed this liver.

VITAMIN D

Vitamin D consists of a group of steroid compounds which possess antirachitic properties, that is, prevent rickets. Ergocalciferol (D_2) and cholecalciferol (D_3) are two nutritionally important chemical forms of vitamin D which are formed from vitamin D precursors.

However, cholecalciferol can be formed on the skin in the presence of sunlight from a precursor and then absorbed. In this way vitamin D has hormone-like properties.

Vitamin D is vital to normal calcium and phosphorus metabolism Vitamin D enhances the absorption of calcium from the intestine and is thought to also improve the absorption of phosphorus. Vitamin D enables the normal mineralization of bones and cartilage. This function prevents the development of rickets in young children and osteomalacia in adults. It may also contribute to the prevention of osteoporosis in the elderly though there are other factors which also affect the development or prevention of osteoporosis.[5] Vitamin D also aids in maintaining critical calcium serum levels for proper neuromuscular functioning.

Pharmacological doses (drug amounts) of vitamin D are given in the treatment of rickets. Rickets most likely results from a dietary lack of vitamin D concurrent with inadequate exposure to sunshine.

The 1980 revised RDA gives the recommendation for vitamin D in micrograms of cholecalciferol. Formerly it was given in International Units (IU). Ten micrograms (µg) of cholecalciferol equals 400 IU of vitamin D. The allowance of 10 µg cholecalciferol is recommended for infants, children, and adolescents. Adults have a recommendation of 5µg which is doubled during pregnancy and lactation. The requirement for the normal adult can usually be met by adequate exposure to sunlight. However, this exposure can be limited by certain climatic conditions or air pollution thus necessitating the use of dietary sources.[6]

Preformed vitamin D food sources are limited to yeast, fish liver oils, egg yolk, and liver. The most common sources of vitamin D are exposure to sunlight and vitamin D fortified foods such as milk and butter. The appropriateness of milk as a carrier for added vitamin D is discussed in Chapter Seven, Introduction to Vitamins (Enrichment).

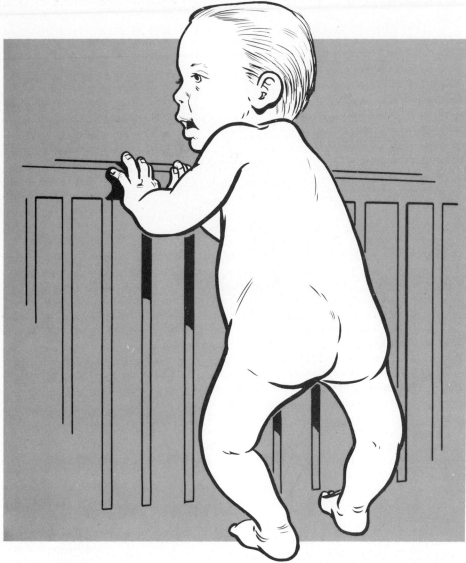

Figure 9-2.   Infant with bowed legs characteristic of rickets.

A prolonged deficiency of vitamin D most commonly leads to the development of rickets in children and osteomalacia in adults. Rickets is characterized by stunted growth, enlarged ankles and wrists, bowed legs, a hollow chest and projected sternum, and often a narrow pelvis and undesirable spinal curvatures. These symptoms are due to inadequate absorption and utilization of calcium and phosphorus resulting in faulty mineralization of bones and even teeth. Osteomalacia is the adult form of rickets which leads to a reduction in the mineral content of bones and results in softened, fragile bones.

A vitamin D supplement is generally recommended for breast-fed infants because the vitamin D content of human milk is low.[7] A supplement is also recommended for strict vegans who eliminate animal source foods from their diet.

Toxicity can occur from an excessive intake of vitamin D because it is stored in adipose tissues and the liver. Toxicity involves damage through calcification of soft tissues such as renal (kidney) tubules, the heart, and blood vessels which is not always reversible. Other toxicity symptoms include nausea, vomiting, and diarrhea. Excessive vitamin D intake can also lead to an increased formation of kidney stones.

VITAMIN E

Tocopherol is the name used to describe vitamin E. There are numerous tocopherol compounds. However, the α-tocopherol (alpha-tocopherol) is the one most commonly designated as active vitamin E.

The functions of vitamin E in man have been the subject of popular press and controversy. It has been purported to be effective in treating muscular dystrophy, cancer, sterility, and increasing sexual prowess. Unfortunately, actual results from scientific tests have not been able to demonstrate the ability of vitamin E to function in man to prevent or enhance any of the above listed conditions. *The only demonstrated function of vitamin E is that of an antioxidant which protects polyunsaturated fats and vitamin A from oxidation (and, therefore, destruction) in the body.*

The premature infant has a low plasma concentration of vitamin E and may be susceptible to red blood cell hemolysis. Amounts of vitamin E and polyunsaturated fats in infant formulas therefore need to be carefully monitored.[8] The vitamin E content in breast milk is adequate for normal nursing infants.

The vitamin E content in American diets varies greatly according to the type of fat consumed. Vitamin E need is increased with greater ingestion of polyunsaturated fatty acids (PUFA). However, oils high in PUFA are the vegetable oils which are also rich in vitamin E. Because of the absence of reported and confirmed vitamin E deficiencies it appears that the typical American diet is adequate in vitamin E.

The 1980 revised RDA for vitamin E expresses this vitamin's requirement in mg instead of International Units. However, the recommended intakes do not differ substantially from previous recommendations.[9] The RDA for adults varies from 8 to 10 mg α-tocopherol equivalents (α-T.E.). Though some legumes, grains, liver, and eggs supply fair to small amounts of vitamin E, the best sources are oils of vegetable origin.

Toxicity from an excessive intake of vitamin E is rare and has not been reported in consistent findings. However, since vitamin E is fat-soluble and can be stored in the body to some degree caution should be exercised in ingesting excessively large doses to avoid potential toxicity.

VITAMIN K

Vitamin K is represented by several compounds in the chemical group termed quinones. Menaquinone is the form synthesized by intestinal bacteria in man, phylloquinone is the form found in green plants, and menadione is the synthetic form of the vitamin.

The only known function of vitamin K is its necessity for prothrombin formation as well as some other blood-clotting factors in the liver. A deficiency of vitamin K results in defective blood coagulation.

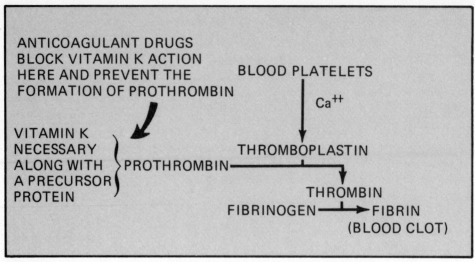

Figure 9-3.   Role of vitamin K in reactions leading to the normal clotting of blood.

Vitamin K is measured in micrograms and the recommended safe and adequate intake for adults is 70 to 140 µg/day. Vitamin K is also synthesized by bacteria in the lower intestinal tract although maximum absorption occurs from the upper intestine.

A dietary deficiency of vitamin K is not likely as it occurs in many green, leafy vegetables. Fruits, cereals, dairy products, and meats supply small amounts. Dietary sources are also supplemented by the vitamin K formed in the intestines by microorganisms normally living there. These bacteria are missing in the sterile intestines of the newborn infant, however, and hemorrhage in newborn infants can occur. This hemorrhage condition is corrected by therapeutic administration of vitamin K. Medical supervision is required for use of supplemental vitamin K because excesses can be toxic causing hemolytic anemia and liver damage.

Dicumarol and warfarin are anticoagulant drugs which prevent blood coagulation because they are antagonistic to the action of vitamin K, therefore preventing the formation of prothrombin. These drugs are used to treat conditions such as coronary thrombosis or thrombophlebitis (blood clots in vessel walls).

Key Points: The Fat-Soluble Vitamins

  I.   The fat-soluble vitamins A, D, E, and K are affected generally by the same factors which influence the absorption and metabolism of lipids in the body.

       A.   Though different in chemical structure, each of the fat-soluble vitamins is composed only of the elements carbon, oxygen, and hydrogen.

       B.   Fat-soluble vitamins can be stored to varying degrees in the body. Consequently, deficiency symptoms are slower to develop in the face of inadequate intake than deficiency symptoms from inadequate intake of water-soluble vitamins; and elevated levels of fat-soluble vitamins in various tissues can be toxic to the body.

  II.   Vitamin A is necessary for normal vision in dim light, maintenance of healthy skin and mucous membranes, and normal body growth. Preformed vitamin A is obtained from animal foods and provitamin A from carotene found in plant pigments. The RDAs for vitamin A are given in retinol equivalents (R.E.). Vitamin A deficiency is the major cause of blindness in developing countries and deficiency symptoms are accentuated in protein deficiency states.

III.   Vitamin D can be formed in the skin when exposed to sunlight, a hormone-like property. Vitamin D is necessary for normal calcium and phosphorus metabolism. Vitamin D promotes the normal mineralization of bones and cartilage preventing the disease rickets in children and osteomalacia in adults. The RDAs for vitamin D are measured in micrograms. Milk fortified with vitamin D is a reliable dietary source for this vitamin.

IV.   Vitamin E activity is most often attributed to the α-tocopherol compound. At present, the only *demonstrated* function of vitamin E is as an antioxidant valuable for its protective action against destruction by oxidation of polyunsaturated fats and vitamin A. The best sources of vitamin E are also those which contain large amounts of polyunsaturated fatty acids: vegetable oils. The RDAs for vitamin E are expressed in terms of α-tocopherol equivalents (α-T.E.).

V.   Vitamin K activity is attributed to several compounds in the chemical group termed quinones. The only known function of vitamin K is its necessity for prothrombin formation as well as other factors required for proper blood clotting. The recommended safe and adequate intakes are measured in micrograms and range between 70 to 140 μg/day for adults. Absorption of vitamin K produced by intestinal bacteria is significant.

Questions: Fat-Soluble Vitamins

1.   The presence of bile in the intestine is necessary for the adequate absorption of the fat-soluble vitamins.
    a.   True
    b.   False

2.   Regular ingestion of mineral oil is recommended as a laxative.
    a.   True
    b.   False

3.   Fat-soluble vitamins are absorbed into the (portal blood system/lymph system).

4.   The RDAs for vitamin A are based on:
    a.   retinol equivalents
    b.   retinaldehyde equivalents
    c.   retinoic acid equivalents

5.   A deficiency of what macronutrient can produce a drop in serum vitamin A levels?
    a.   fat
    b.   carbohydrate
    c.   protein

6.   What food sources contain preformed vitamin A?

7.   Why is non-fat milk fortified with vitamin A?

8.   The biological activity of β-carotene is half that of retinol.
    a.   True
    b.   False

9.   Rhodopsin is formed by the combination of _____ (a protein) and _____ (a vitamin A compound).

10.   Why must some vitamin A be continually supplied to the rods in the retina of the eye?

11.   Why has vitamin A been called the anti-infection vitamin?

12. Vitamin A deficiency results in retarded growth though the exact role vitamin A plays in promotion of growth is as yet unknown.
    a. True
    b. False

13. Vitamin A deficiency is a major cause of blindness in undeveloped countries.
    a. True
    b. False

14. Match the phrases on the right to the items on the left which they best describe:

    _____ 1. xerophthalmia
    _____ 2. rhodopsin
    _____ 3. keratin
    _____ 4. night blindness
    _____ 5. follicular hyperkerato-
              sis
    _____ 6. xerosis

    a. thickening and drying of the conjunctiva of the eye
    b. irreversible thickening and drying of the cornea of the eye which leads to blindness
    c. pimple-like bumps on dry, scaly skin due to vitamin A deficiency
    d. visual purple
    e. inability to visually adjust to variances in light conditions often due to vitamin A deficiency
    f. the protein which causes epithelial cells to become hard and dry in vitamin A deficiency

15. Carotene, provitamin A, is contained in significant amounts in:
    a. corn, green beans
    b. spinach, collard greens
    c. apricots, pumpkin

16. Vitamin A consumption in capsule form is dangerous because amounts ingested can be many times the RDA for vitamin A and can lead to hypervitaminosis of vitamin A and _____ .

17. Antirachitic means to:
    a. prevent night blindness
    b. prevent rickets
    c. prevent blood clotting

18. Vitamin D is unique in that it possesses _____ activity.

19. Naturally preformed vitamin D is found in many varied food sources.
    a. True
    b. False

20. Vitamin D in the form of cholecalciferol is formed on the skin by the exposure to:
    a. heat
    b. cold
    c. sunlight

21. Vitamin D functions to:
    a. enhance calcium and even phosphorus absorption
    b. enhance mineralization of bones and cartilage
    c. lower serum calcium levels

22. What two factors probably act together in the formation of vitamin D deficiency?

23. 400 IU of vitamin D equal how many micrograms of cholecalciferol?
    a. 5

    b. 10

    c. 15

24. Why is the RDA for vitamin D higher in infancy, childhood, and adolescence than in adulthood? Why do adults have an established RDA for vitamin D?

25. How can the vitamin D allowance usually be met by healthy adults?

26. What atmospheric condition associated with modern times can reduce the effectiveness of sunshine to produce vitamin D conversion on or in the skin?

27. Excess vitamin D:
    a. is stored in adipose tissue and the liver.
    b. can cause calcification of soft tissue such as blood vessels and renal tubules.
    c. is excreted in the urine.

28. The active form of vitamin E is called:
    a. ergocalciferol
    b. menadione
    c. alpha-tocopherol

29. The only demonstrated function of vitamin E in man is that of:
    a. increasing sexual prowess
    b. increasing fertility
    c. an antioxidant

30. The vitamin E content in breast milk is adequate for healthy nursing infants.
    a. True
    b. False

31. The RDA for vitamin E is measured in _____ .

32. Supplemental vitamin E is not necessary even with a high intake of polyunsaturated fats.
    a. True
    b. False

33. Vitamin K is represented by compounds of what chemical group?
    a. tocopherols
    b. calciferols
    c. quinones

34. There is no RDA for vitamin K because an unmeasurable amount is produced by intestinal microorganisms and significantly absorbed by the body.
    a. True
    b. False

35. The only known function of vitamin K is its:
    a. necessity for formation of blood clotting factors
    b. antioxidant property
    c. antirachitic property

36. Why are newborn infants sometimes subject to hemorrhagic disease?

37. Excessive administration of menadione (synthetic vitamin K) is toxic.
    a. True
    b. False

38. Substances which are antagonistic to the action of vitamin K are termed:
    a. antirachitic agents
    b. anticoagulants
    c. antisterility agents

Answers: Fat-Soluble Vitamins

1. a
2. b
3. lymph system
4. a
5. c
6. animal source foods: whole milk, organ meats, eggs, cream
7. because fat-soluble vitamin A is removed with the fat in processing non-fat milk
8. a
9. opsin; retinaldehyde
10. Because some retinaldehyde is lost after each splitting/recombining reaction of rhodopsin and this is a continuous action necessary for vision in dim light.
11. Because it is necessary for forming and maintaining healthy epithelial tissues with normal mucus secretion which are resistant to invasion by infection-producing bacteria.
12. a
13. a
14. 1. b
    2. d
    3. f
    4. e
    5. c
    6. a
15. b, c
16. toxicity
17. b
18. hormone-like
19. b
20. c
21. a, b
22. a dietary lack of vitamin D and inadequate exposure to sunshine
23. b
24. Because of the increased need for vitamin D during periods of bone growth; adults have a requirement in order to maintain bone mineralization and structure and to reduce resorption of bone.
25. by adequate exposure to sunshine
26. air pollution (smog)
27. a, b
28. c
29. c
30. a
31. α-T.E.—alpha-tocopherol equivalents
32. a
33. c
34. a
35. a
36. The intestines are sterile and vitamin K-producing bacteria are not yet present.
37. a
38. b

REFERENCES

[1] The retina is the internal back surface of the eye. The optic nerve is sensitive to the energy changes produced by the splitting/recombining processes involving rhodopsin. The optic nerve transmits these energy changes as a kind of electrical "code" to the brain which deciphers the "code" in visual terms.

[2] Smith JE and Goodman DS: Vitamin A metabolism and transport. *In* Present Knowledge in Nutrition, 4th ed. New York and Washington, D.C.; The Nutrition Foundation, Inc., 1976, p. 70

[3] Recommended Dietary Allowances, Ninth Revised Edition. Food and Nutrition Board, National Academy of Sciences-National Research Council, Washington, D.C.; 1980, p. 57

[4] McNutt KW and McNutt DR: Nutrition and Food Choices. Chicago, Science Research Associates, Inc., 1978, p. 427

[5] Refer to Chapter Eleven—The Macrominerals (Calcium)—for further explanation and differentiation of rickets, osteomalacia, and osteoporosis.

[6] Recommended Dietary Allowances, Ninth Revised Edition. Food and Nutrition Board, National Academy of Sciences-National Research Council, Washington, D.C.; 1980, p. 61

[7] Recent research suggests the possible presence of a water-soluble form of vitamin D in breast milk which may significantly increase the total vitamin D content of human milk.

[8] Hemolysis (rupturing of red blood cells) occurs because red blood cell membranes contain a high percentage of polyunsaturated fats. These membranes are subjected to potential destruction by oxidation when exposed to oxygen in the lungs.

[9] Munro H: The ninth edition of recommended dietary allowances. Food and Nutrition News, 51, February 1980, p. 2

10
AN INTRODUCTION TO MINERALS

Macrominerals (listed in decreasing order of predominance in the body):
Calcium (Ca), Phosphorus (P), Potassium (K), Sulfur (S), Sodium (Na), Chlorine (Cl), and Magnesium (Mg).

Microminerals (present in the body in amounts less than .005 percent of body weight):
Iron (Fe), Zinc (Zn), Manganese (Mn), Fluorine (F), Copper (Cu), Cobalt (Co), Iodine (I), Selenium (Se), Molybdenum (Mo), Chromium (Cr).

Some researchers prefer to subgroup the microminerals in such a way as to emphasize their known essentiality:

Microminerals for which there is no question about their importance to health: Iron (Fe), Iodine (I), and Fluorine (F). Microminerals for which essentiality is accepted and whose functions are fairly well understood: Zinc (Zn), Manganese (Mn), Copper (Cu), Cobalt (Co), Selenium (Se), Molybdenum (Mo), and Chromium (Cr).

Microminerals which appear to be essential but whose functions are not well defined: Nickel (Ni), Vanadium (V), Tin (Sn), and Silicon (Si).

Microminerals are sometimes referred to as "trace elements." The trace elements are present in the body in quantities less than 0.005 percent of the body weight and are required in the diet in amounts no greater than a few milligrams daily. The macro- and microminerals listed above are essential to human nutrition. There are other minerals present in the body which are not known to be essential and some of these are contaminants. *Minerals are essential when they cause improvement in health and growth.*

Table 10-1. **Selected Mineral Content of Some Foods: Constituents of 100g of edible portion (approximately 3½ ounces).***

	Calcium mg.	Phosphorus mg.	Minerals Iron mg.	Sodium mg.	Potassium mg.
Dairy Products:					
Buttermilk	121	95	trace	130	140
Milk, whole cow	118	93	trace	50	144
Milk, non-fat cow	121	95	trace	52	145
Cream, light	102	80	trace	43	122
Cream, sour +	120	85	—	45	75
Whey, dried	646	589	1.4	—	—
Fats:					
Mayonnaise	18	28	.5	597	34
Fruits:					
Apples, raw	6	10	.3	1	110
Bananas	8	26	.7	1	370

Table 10-1.   Selected Mineral Content of Some Foods: Constituents of 100g of edible portion (approximately 3½ ounces)* (continued).

	Calcium mg.	Phosphorus mg.	Minerals Iron mg.	Sodium mg.	Potassium mg.
Peaches, raw	9	19	.5	1	202
Raisins, dry	62	101	3.5	27	763
Fruit Juices:					
Orange	11	17	.2	1	200
Prune	14	20	4.1	2	235
Tomato	7	18	.9	200	227
Grains and Flours:					
Flour, enriched wheat, all-purpose	16	87	2.9	1	86
Wheat, germ	47	1084	8.9	2	947
Wheat, whole meal	41	372	3.3	3	370
Beef:					
Hamburger, cooked	11	194	3.2	47	450
Liver, raw	8	352	6.5	136	281
Tongue, raw	8	182	2.1	73	197
Sugars and Sweets:					
Hard candy	21	7	1.9	32	4
Sugar, cane or beet	—	—	.1	1	3
Miscellaneous:					
Cola beverages	—	—	—	—	—

**Adapted from:* Composition of Foods. Agriculture Handbook No. 8, Agricultural Research Service, United States Department of Agriculture, 1975

+*Value from:* Bowes and Church: Food Values of Portions Commonly Used. Philadelphia, J. B. Lippincott Company, 1970

FUNCTIONS OF MINERALS

General functions of minerals are:

1. Involvement in the structure of all body cells.
2. Components of some enzymes, vitamins, and other vital body compounds.
3. Regulation of osmotic pressure and water balance.
4. Regulation of the permeability of cell membranes.
5. Regulation of acid-base balance.
6. Regulation of responses of nerves to stimuli.
7. Regulation of muscle contractions.

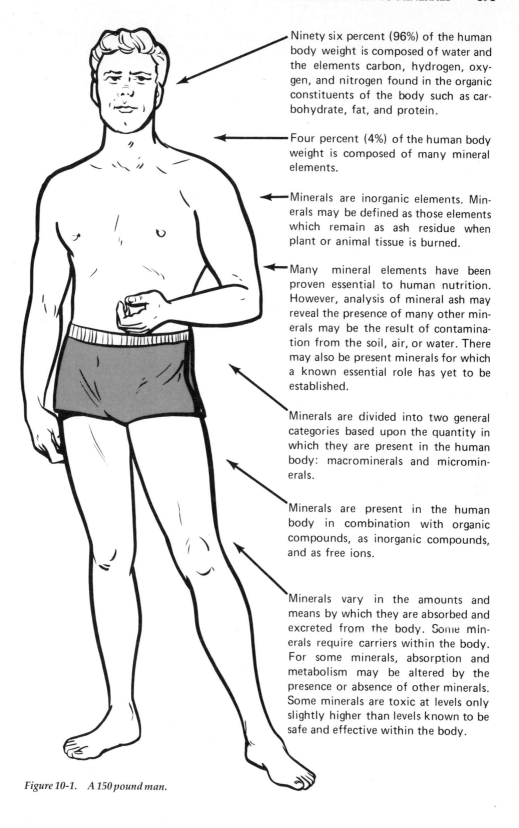

Ninety six percent (96%) of the human body weight is composed of water and the elements carbon, hydrogen, oxygen, and nitrogen found in the organic constituents of the body such as carbohydrate, fat, and protein.

Four percent (4%) of the human body weight is composed of many mineral elements.

Minerals are inorganic elements. Minerals may be defined as those elements which remain as ash residue when plant or animal tissue is burned.

Many mineral elements have been proven essential to human nutrition. However, analysis of mineral ash may reveal the presence of many other minerals may be the result of contamination from the soil, air, or water. There may also be present minerals for which a known essential role has yet to be established.

Minerals are divided into two general categories based upon the quantity in which they are present in the human body: macrominerals and microminerals.

Minerals are present in the human body in combination with organic compounds, as inorganic compounds, and as free ions.

Minerals vary in the amounts and means by which they are absorbed and excreted from the body. Some minerals require carriers within the body. For some minerals, absorption and metabolism may be altered by the presence or absence of other minerals. Some minerals are toxic at levels only slightly higher than levels known to be safe and effective within the body.

Figure 10-1.   A 150 pound man.

Some specific functions of minerals and the minerals participating in those functions:

1.   Involvement in the structure of hard tissue, bones, and teeth: Ca, P, Mg, Cu, F

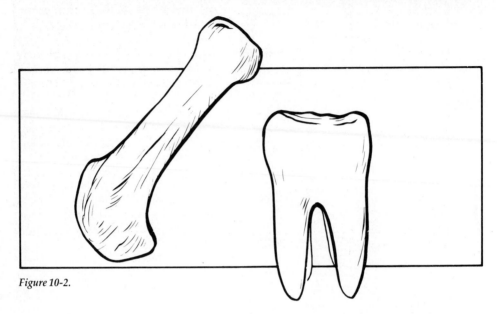

Figure 10-2.

2.   Are part of some enzymes and vitamins or activate enzymatic reactions: Ca, P, Mg, Na, S, Fe, Cu, Mn, Co, Zn, Mo, Se

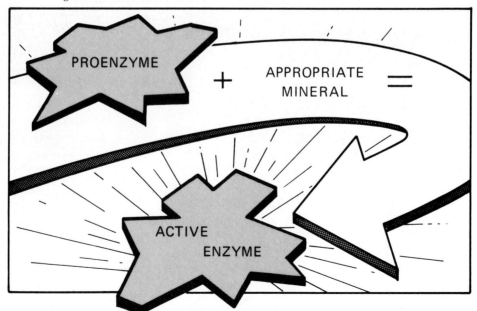

Figure 10-3.

3. Regulation of osmotic pressure and water balance: Na, K, Cl

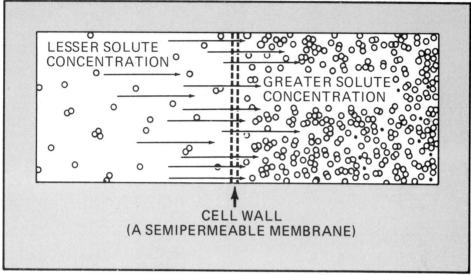

Figure 10-4. Illustration of osmotic pressure and water balance.

4. Regulation of the permeability of cell membranes: Ca, Na, Cr, P

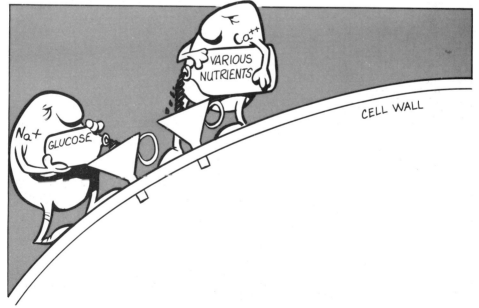

Figure 10-5.

5.   Regulation of acid-base balance: P, Na, K, Cl

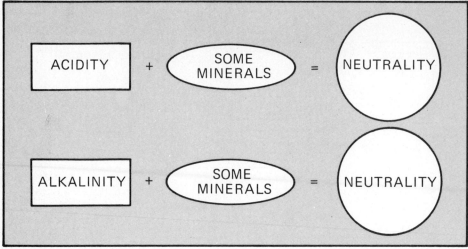

Figure 10-6.

6.   Regulation of responses of nerves to stimuli: Ca, Mg, Na, K

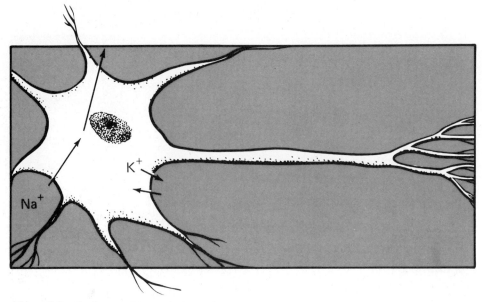

Figure 10-7.   During nerve transmission, sodium (Na) and potassium (K) exchange places: sodium enters the cell and potassium exits the cell. They return to their respective areas of concentration after the nerve impulse passes.

7.   Regulation of muscle contractions: Ca, Mg, Na, K

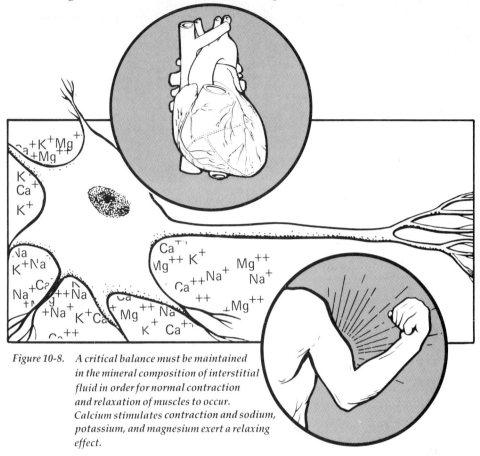

Figure 10-8.   *A critical balance must be maintained in the mineral composition of interstitial fluid in order for normal contraction and relaxation of muscles to occur. Calcium stimulates contraction and sodium, potassium, and magnesium exert a relaxing effect.*

8.   Essential components of other body compounds such as hormones (I) and hemoglobin (Fe).

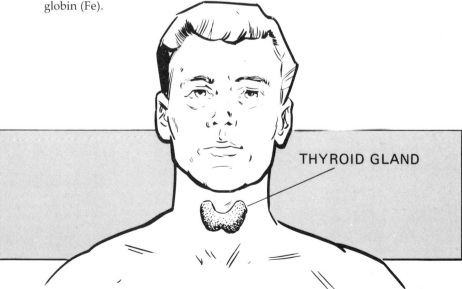

Figure 10-9.   *The thyroid gland secretes thyroxine, a hormone which contains iodine.*

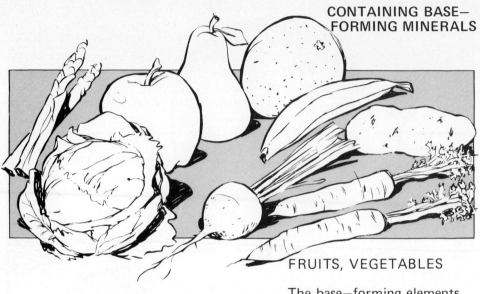

CONTAINING BASE—
FORMING MINERALS

FRUITS, VEGETABLES

The base—forming elements
Sodium (Na)   Magnesium (Mg)
Potassium (K) Iron (Fe)
Calcium (Ca)

CONTAINING ACID—
FORMING MINERALS

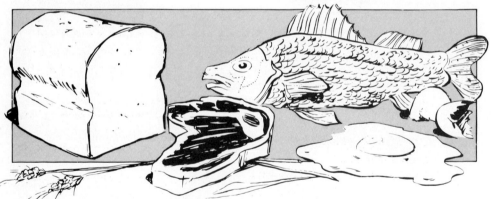

CEREAL PRODUCTS, PROTEIN FOODS

The acid—forming elements
Sulfur (S)
Phosphorus (P)
Chlorine (Cl)

Figure 10-10.   Foods grouped according to their predominant base-forming or acid-forming mineral content.

Key Points: An Introduction to Minerals

I. Minerals are inorganic elements that are present in the body in various forms: as constituents of organic compounds, inorganic compounds, and as free ions.

II. Approximately four percent of human body weight is composed of various mineral elements, some of which have no known essential role in human nutrition. Those essential minerals present in amounts greater than .005 percent of body weight are termed essential macrominerals; those minerals present in amounts less than .005 percent of body weight are termed microminerals or trace elements.

III. Some mineral elements perform only one known essential function while others perform various essential and often unrelated functions.

IV. Minerals are generally present in food in water-soluble forms. Consequently, many of the same food preparation methods suggested for maximum conservation of water-soluble vitamins are recommended to conserve the mineral content of foods.

V. Amounts and methods of absorption and excretion vary for the different minerals. Absorption and metabolism of many minerals are influenced by the presence or absence of other minerals. Some minerals are toxic when present in the body in even small amounts above nutritionally safe and effective amounts.

VI. Discovery of the essentiality of trace minerals is due especially to improved technology in assay and determination equipment and research methods. Research on the need for other minerals continues. Consequently, the microminerals reinforce the need for a balanced and varied diet in order to insure the consumption of known and potentially essential nutrients.

Questions: An Introduction to Minerals

1. Minerals are (organic/inorganic) compounds.
2. Compute the approximate weight of the minerals which would be present in a man weighing 150 pounds.
3. Ash residue is what remains after a plant or animal has been completely _____ . Therefore, minerals are (combustible/noncombustible).
4. Are all minerals present in the human body known to have an essential role?
5. Are all minerals essential in human nutrition known and their specific functions established?
6. If it is possible that all minerals essential in human nutrition are not known and their specific functions are not established, defend the statement that it may not be wise for a person to eat only synthetic or processed foods.
7. Webster's Dictionary defines macro as "involving large quantities." Keeping this definition in mind define "macromineral."
8. Webster's Dictionary defines micro as "involving minute quantities." Therefore, what would constitute a "micromineral?"
9. Enzymes, hormones, and vitamins are organic compounds. Is it possible for these compounds to contain minerals?
10. Essential trace elements are all those elements found in the body in quantities less than 0.005 percent of the body weight.
    a. True
    b. False
11. Approximately two percent of body weight is calcium and approximately one percent of body weight is phosphorus. What is the calcium to phosphorus ratio in the body?
12. A man weighs 150 pounds. Approximately .23 percent of body weight is sulphur; .005 percent body weight is iron; and .00005 percent is iodine. What is the weight of sulphur, iodine, and iron in this man?
13. The two minerals found in the greatest quantity in the human body are _____ and _____ . This is due to their presence in _____ and _____ , the hard tissues of the body.

14. Some elements are expressed in their ionized form as: Na^+, K^+, Ca^{++}, Mg^{++}, Cl^-, HCO_3^-, $HPO_4^=$, $SO_4^=$. What conclusions can you draw about the unique characteristics of an ion?

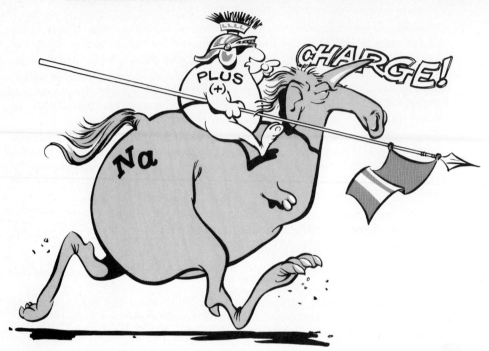

Figure 10-11. *Minerals often occur in the body as ions which carry an electrical charge. Cations have a positive charge and anions have a negative charge.*

15. It is important to be familiar with the symbols representing the mineral elements as these symbols are frequently used in literature dealing with nutrition in order to save writing space. Match the following symbols with the appropriate element:

_____ 1.	Calcium	a.	Mg
_____ 2.	Phosphorus	b.	S
_____ 3.	Sulfur	c.	Ca
_____ 4.	Sodium	d.	K
_____ 5.	Chlorine	e.	Na
_____ 6.	Magnesium	f.	Cl
_____ 7.	Iron	g.	P
_____ 8.	Zinc	h.	Cu
_____ 9.	Copper	i.	Fe
_____ 10.	Chromium	j.	F
_____ 11.	Manganese	k.	Mn
		l.	Co
		m.	Cr
		n.	Mo
		o.	Se
		p.	I
		q.	Zn

16. When are minerals determined to be essential in human nutrition?

17. Place the following elements under their appropriate classification:

    Micronutrients   Macronutrients   Elements

Cu	S	Na	Zn
Cl	I	K	P
Mg	Cr	Ca	Fe
Se	Mo	Mn	F

18. Refer to Table 10-1 for the mineral content of selected foods. What advantage can you give for encouraging a child to choose fruit juices instead of cola drinks?

19. Which is the most mineral-rich form of grain listed? Using the values listed for all-purpose flour and whole wheat meal, what advantage can you find for consuming whole wheat bread?

20. What is an obvious advantage for encouraging a child to choose a fruit snack such as raisins as a sweet treat versus hard candy or other sugar treats?

21. Compare the mineral contents of the meats listed in Table 10-1, the Table of Food Composition.
    a. Which meat is highest in iron?
    b. Which meat is highest in phosphorus?
    c. Could one make the assumption that meats seem, generally, to be a good source of minerals?

22. Minerals are located _____ in the body.
    a. only in soft tissues
    b. only in hard tissues
    c. in the structure of all cells

23. If minerals become more concentrated in fluid on one side of a semipermeable membrane, water will flow to the space of _____ .

24. Osmosis is the diffusion of water through a semipermeable membrane, passing from the side of lower solute concentration to that of the higher solute concentration. Minerals are solutes in body fluids. Consequently, minerals aid in the regulation of _____ .

25. Minerals help to regulate the acid-base balance of the body. Therefore, minerals help to maintain the body fluid's _____ .
    a. acidity
    b. alkalinity
    c. neutrality

26. Some minerals such as calcium and sodium have an ability to regulate the cellular absorption of some other nutrients. Therefore, these minerals function as _____ .

27. Several minerals must be present and in balance in the extracellular fluid for normal transmission of nerve impulses. These minerals are regulators of the responses of nerves to stimuli and are needed in their _____ form.
    a. insoluble salt
    b. ionized

28. Tetany is a body state marked by severe, intermittent spastic contractions of the muscles and by muscular pain. Rigor is characterized by the muscle fibers being in a state of constant contraction. An excess or decrease in the normal balance of some minerals can produce forms of tetany and rigor. Therefore, the function of some minerals is the _____ .

29. Refer to the functions of minerals and the groups of minerals performing those functions.

a. Which are the minerals that perform as regulators of responses of nerves to stimuli?

b. Are these the same minerals involved in the regulation of muscle contractions?

30. The general classes of foods containing a preponderance of base-forming minerals are _____ .

21. The general classes of foods containing a preponderance of acid-forming minerals are _____ .

32. Some citrus fruits such as oranges have organic acids which give them a sour, acidic taste. Are these fruits acid-forming or base-forming foods?

33. Therefore, the factors that must determine the acid-forming or base-forming properties of a food are the properties of the _____ .

34. Match the following elements to the food groups according to their acid- or base-forming properties:

_____ 1. Sulfur   a. fruits and vegetables (base-forming)
_____ 2. Calcium   b. cereal products and protein foods
_____ 3. Phosphorus   (acid-forming)
_____ 4. Potassium
_____ 5. Iron
_____ 6. Chlorine

35. Most of the minerals in foods occur as mineral salts, most of which are water-soluble. Therefore, can minerals be lost in the cooking water of foods? If so, list some ways to reduce this type of mineral loss. (Hint: refer to Chapter Seven, Table 7-1, for some tips applicable to mineral conservation.)

36. The range between safe and toxic levels of some minerals within the body may be quite narrow.
a. True
b. False

Answers: An Introduction to Minerals

1. inorganic
2. $150 \times 0.04 = 6$ pounds
3. burned; noncombustible
4. no
5. probably not
6. Synthetic or processed foods are enriched and/or fortified with nutrients known to be essential in human nutrition and which are found naturally in the "natural" food source which the new food is intended to replace. However, trace minerals which may be essential in human nutrition, although their essentiality has not yet been established, may be lost in the refining/processing of foods. These are not added to synthetic foodstuffs. It seems best to eat a wide variety of all common foods in order to obtain all nutrients of known essentiality, and possibly others not yet established as essential in human nutrition including various minerals.

7. Those minerals present in relatively large quantities in the body; all the macro-minerals are known to be essential in human nutrition.
8. Those minerals present in the body in very small amounts.
9. Yes, minerals are part of various organic compounds in the body.
10. b: Not all elements found in the body in less than 0.005 percent of the body weight are known to be essential in human nutrition.

11. 2:1

12. sulphur (.0023 × 150)=.345 pounds; iron (.00005 × 150)=.0075 pounds; iodine (.0000005 × 150)=.000075 pounds

13. calcium and phosphorus; bones and teeth

10. It is an atom or a group of atoms that carries an electrical charge.

15.
   1. c
   2. g
   3. b
   4. e
   5. f
   6. a
   7. i
   8. q
   9. h
   10. m
   11. k

16. when they cause improvement in health and growth

17.

Micronutrients			Macronutrients		
Cu	Mo	Zn	Cl	Na	S
Se	Mn	Fe	Mg	K	Ca
I	F	Cr	P		

18. In addition to carbohydrates, the child will consume both micro- and macro-minerals missing in cola drinks.

19. wheat germ; consumption of greater quantities of both micro- and macrominerals

20. Raisins offer a large percentage of mineral content versus minimal mineral value from hard candy or sugar.

21. a. liver
    b. liver
    c. yes

22. c

23. greater mineral (solute) concentration

24. osmotic pressure and water balance

25. c

26. regulators of the permeability of cell membranes

27. b

28. regulation of muscle contractions

29. a. Ca^{++}, Mg^{++}, Na^+, K^+
    b. yes

30. vegetables and fruits

31. cereal products and protein foods such as meat, fish, and eggs

32. base-forming

33. minerals which the foods contain

34.
   1. b
   2. a
   3. b
   4. a
   5. a
   6. b

35. Yes. Reduce the amount of water used in cooking; cook for short periods of time in moist heat; use steam cooking methods to reduce leaching by water; use such

methods as stir-frying which are short cooking time—small amount of water methods; use water from cooking in soups, gravies, and other dishes so the minerals dissolved in it will be consumed rather than poured down the drain.

36.   a

11
THE MACROMINERALS

CALCIUM

Calcium is present in the largest amount of all the minerals in the human body. The bones and teeth contain the greatest percentage of this mineral, 99 percent in the form of various calcium salts. The remaining one percent of calcium occurs in body fluids, soft tissue, and membrane structures.

Absorption of calcium. Normally, approximately 30 to 40 percent of dietary calcium is absorbed.[1] Calcium is absorbed by an active transport, energy-requiring mechanism. Some calcium ions are also absorbed by passive diffusion.[2] *Body need is the major factor governing the amount of calcium that will be absorbed.* Calcium absorption is increased during periods of growth and also during pregnancy and lactation. However, there are other important factors which influence the level of absorption of this mineral:

1. Presence of adequate vitamin D because vitamin D enhances calcium absorption.
2. Presence of an acid environment because acidity enhances calcium absorption.
3. Intake of calcium and phosphorus in an approximate ratio of 1:1 because calcium absorption is optimal when the calcium:phosphorus intake is in this proportion. This ratio is an inverse relationship: as calcium intake increases, phosphorus absorption decreases; as phosphorus intake increases, calcium absorption decreases.
4. Presence of certain amino acids because some amino acids enhance calcium absorption.
5. Presence of lactose (milk sugar) because lactose enhances the intestinal absorption of calcium.

Calcium salts are more soluble in an acid solution. Most absorption occurs from the duodenum, the section of the small intestine closest to the stomach, because the chyme is still relatively high in gastric acid (HCl) in this region.

There are several factors which hinder the absorption of calcium:

1. Vitamin D deficiency.
2. Excessive intake of dietary fats. The fatty acids and glycerides combine with calcium to form insoluble soaps through a process called saponification. These soaps are then excreted with the feces instead of being absorbed.
3. Excessive increase in phosphorus intake. An increase in phosphorus intake alters the desirable calcium:phosphorus ratio.
4. An alkaline environment. Calcium is insoluble in an alkaline medium.
5. Presence of binding agents such as oxalic and phytic acids. These acids combine with calcium to form insoluble calcium complexes.

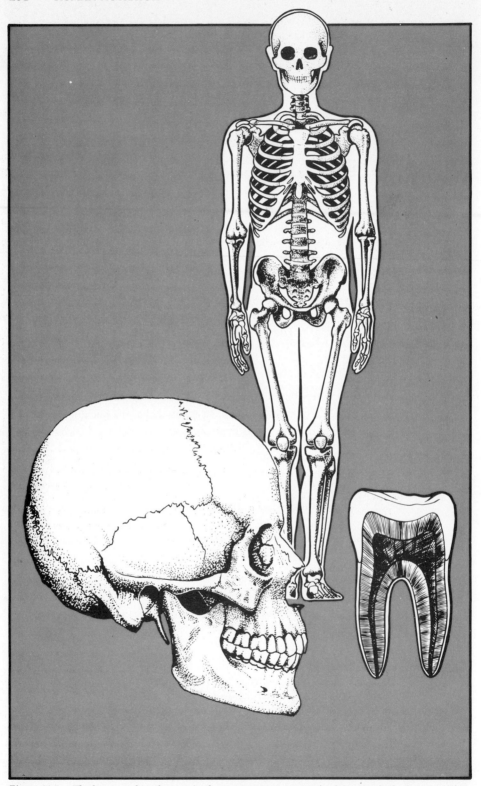

Figure 11-1. *The bones and teeth contain the greatest percentage of calcium in the body.*

6. Increased gastrointestinal motility. The rapid passage of food through the intestinal tract decreases the time in which absorption may take place and reduces contact with absorptive surfaces of the intestines.

7. Increased stress. Stress seems to reduce calcium utilization.

8. Immobilization. Lack of physical exercise and decreased uprightness of the body seem to increase calcium resorption from bone and, therefore, decrease calcium absorption and utilization.

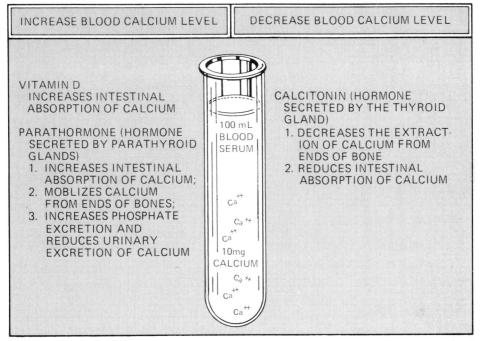

INCREASE BLOOD CALCIUM LEVEL

DECREASE BLOOD CALCIUM LEVEL

VITAMIN D
  INCREASES INTESTINAL
  ABSORPTION OF CALCIUM

PARATHORMONE (HORMONE
  SECRETED BY PARATHYROID
  GLANDS)
  1. INCREASES INTESTINAL
     ABSORPTION OF CALCIUM;
  2. MOBLIZES CALCIUM
     FROM ENDS OF BONES;
  3. INCREASES PHOSPHATE
     EXCRETION AND
     REDUCES URINARY
     EXCRETION OF CALCIUM

100 mL
BLOOD
SERUM

10mg
CALCIUM

CALCITONIN (HORMONE
  SECRETED BY THE THYROID
  GLAND)
  1. DECREASES THE EXTRACT-
     ION OF CALCIUM FROM
     ENDS OF BONE
  2. REDUCES INTESTINAL
     ABSORPTION OF CALCIUM

Figure 11-2. *The balance of calcium and phosphorus in the blood and the balance of calcium between the bone compartments and the circulating serum calcium (remarkably maintained at a constant average of 10 mg per 100 mL of blood serum) is regulated through interactions of calcium, phosphorus, vitamin D, and the hormones parathormone and calcitonin. Blood serum calcium level is **not** affected by calcium intake.*

Functions of calcium. Calcium is necessary:

1. For the formation of bones and teeth which provide the structural framework of the body as well as calcium reserves for maintaining proper serum calcium levels.

2. For the permeability of cells to various substances.

3. For the regulation of muscular contraction and relaxation.

4. For catalyzing some of the reactions involved in blood clotting.

5. As an activator for some enzymes.

6. For the normal transmission of nerve impulses.

Ionized calcium plays an important role in the clotting of blood. The calcium stimulates the release of thromboplastin from the blood platelets. The thromboplastin in the presence of calcium then catalyzes the conversion of prothrombin to thrombin, an enzyme. Thrombin, also in the presence of calcium, catalyzes the formation of fibrin (the blood clot) from fibrinogen.

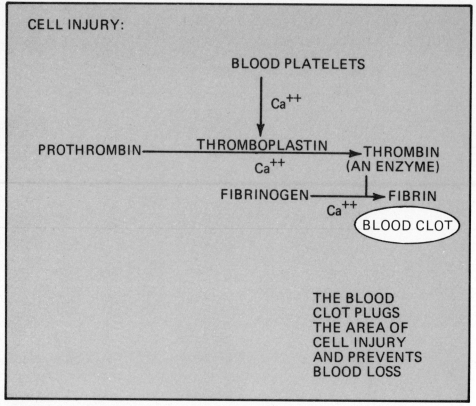

CELL INJURY:

BLOOD PLATELETS

Ca^{++}

PROTHROMBIN —————— THROMBOPLASTIN ————→ THROMBIN
Ca^{++} (AN ENZYME)

FIBRINOGEN ————→ FIBRIN
Ca^{++}

BLOOD CLOT

THE BLOOD
CLOT PLUGS
THE AREA OF
CELL INJURY
AND PREVENTS
BLOOD LOSS

Figure 11-3. Series of reactions leading to blood clot formation.

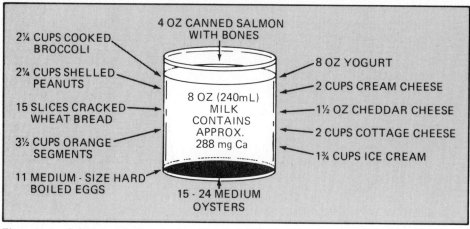

4 OZ CANNED SALMON
WITH BONES

2¼ CUPS COOKED BROCCOLI

2¼ CUPS SHELLED PEANUTS

15 SLICES CRACKED WHEAT BREAD

3½ CUPS ORANGE SEGMENTS

11 MEDIUM - SIZE HARD BOILED EGGS

8 OZ (240mL)
MILK
CONTAINS
APPROX.
288 mg Ca

8 OZ YOGURT

2 CUPS CREAM CHEESE

1½ OZ CHEDDAR CHEESE

2 CUPS COTTAGE CHEESE

1¾ CUPS ICE CREAM

15 - 24 MEDIUM OYSTERS

Figure 11-4. Calcium equivalents for 8 oz (1 cup) of milk. The 1980 revised RDAs recommend a daily intake of 800 mg calcium by the healthy adult.

Suboptimal intakes of calcium may result in retarded calcification of bones and teeth in the young. Acute deficiency of calcium is not usually seen without a concurrent lack of both phosphorus and vitamin D. Such deficiency leads to stunted growth and rickets, as evidenced by bowing of the legs, enlargement of the ankles and wrists, and a hollow chest.

Adults, too, can suffer adverse physiological consequences from an extended unavailability of calcium. The gradual drainage from the bones to replace calcium ions that are lost daily from the body leads to thin, fragile bones which break easily and which heal with difficulty. Osteomalacia (an adult form of rickets) is the softening of bones due to the reduction in the mineral content of the bone (not a reduction in bone size). Osteomalacia, like rickets, is probably more a result of vitamin D deficiency than calcium deficiency.

Osteoporosis is the actual diminishing of total bone content in the skeleton. Osteoporosis usually presents itself during advanced age and most frequently in women. Although the cause of osteoporosis is not known, a low calcium intake over a period of years may be implicated.[3] Presently there is no conclusive evidence to implicate calcium deficiency as the primary cause of osteoporosis in humans.[4]

It appears that a high protein intake for an extended period of time causes an increase in calcium excretion. If osteoporosis is proven to be caused by calcium deficiency, then increased protein intake may influence the development of osteoporosis. The increased calcium excretion associated with high protein intakes may be due to the phosphorus content of protein which in turn, alters the dietary calcium to phosphorus ratio. A high protein intake also increases the formation of acidic metabolic by-products. This higher acid load enhances the dissolution of bone.[5]

PHOSPHORUS

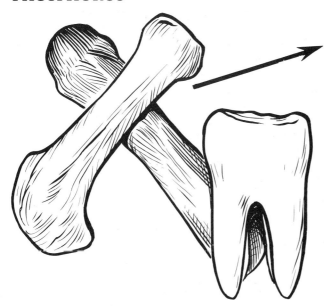

PHOSPHORUS IS AN IMPORTANT CONSTITUENT OF BONES AND TEETH. **IN BONES, THE RATIO OF CALCIUM TO PHOSPHORUS IS 2:1.** APPROXIMATELY 80% OF BODY PHOSPHORUS CONTRIBUTES TO MINERALIZATION OF BONES AND TEETH. ALONG WITH CALCIUM, PHOSPHORUS IS IN A DYNAMIC STATE OF DEPOSITION AND REABSORPTION IN BONES.

Figure 11-5.

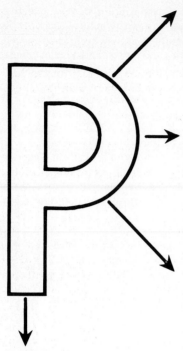

PHOSPHORUS REGULATES THE RELEASE OF ENERGY THROUGH PHOSPHORUS-CONTAINING SUBSTANCES SUCH AS **ADP-ATP** AND PHOSPHORYLATED VITAMINS. MONOSACCHARIDES ARE ALSO PHOSPHORYLATED DURING ENERGY METABOLISM.

PHOSPHORUS FACILITATES ABSORPTION AND TRANSPORTATION OF VARIOUS NUTRIENTS THROUGH THE PROCESS OF PHOSPHORYLATION. PHOSPHOLIPIDS IN THE CELL MEMBRANE REGULATE THE TRANSPORT OF VARIOUS SUBSTANCES INTO AND OUT OF CELLS. LIPOPROTEINS CONTAINING PHOSPHORUS FACILITATE THE TRANSPORTATION OF FATTY SUBSTANCES IN THE WATERY MEDIUM OF BLOOD.

PHOSPHORUS IS PART OF ESSENTIAL BODY COMPOUNDS SUCH AS THE ACTIVE FORMS OF VITAMINS, **TPP** (THIAMIN), AND THE NUCLEIC ACIDS, **DNA** AND **RNA**.

PHOSPHORUS IS PART OF COMPOUNDS WHICH SERVE AS NECESSARY BUFFERS TO CONTROL THE ACID–BASE BALANCE OF BLOOD.

Figure 11-6.

Table 11-1.   Phosphorus content of some representative foods.

Food	P (mg/100g or 3½ oz)
Cheddar cheese	478
Peanuts	415
Chicken, light meat	265
Cod, broiled	260
Bread, whole wheat	234 (or 52 mg/slice)
Beef, lean ground	233
Pork, loin, lean and fat, cooked	229
Eggs, hard cooked	200 (2 medium)
Bread, white, enriched	99 (or 22 mg/slice)
Milk, whole	93 (277 mg/cup)
Peas, cooked	89
Oatmeal	69 (158 mg/cup, cooked)
Rice, cooked	28 (42 mg/cup, cooked)

A diet that furnishes sufficient protein and calcium will also furnish sufficient phosphorus.

Carbonated soda drinks such as colas, root beers, and ginger ale offer large amounts of phosphorus: average around 70 mg/12 oz beverage.

Adapted from: Bowes and Church's Food Values of Portions Commonly Used, 13th edition. Revised by Pennington JAT and Church HN, Philadelphia, J. B. Lippincott Company, 1980

Phosphorus is more efficiently absorbed than calcium: approximately 70 percent of phosphorus is absorbed versus 30 to 40 percent of calcium. However, the absorption of phosphorus is closely related to that of calcium and the factors that influence the absorption of calcium also affect phosphorus.

The consumption of antacids, especially those containing aluminum hydroxide, closely following food ingestion, that is at mealtimes, can greatly reduce the availability of phosphorus for absorption. Aluminum hydroxide binds phosphorus into an insoluble compound which renders phosphorus unavailable for absorption.

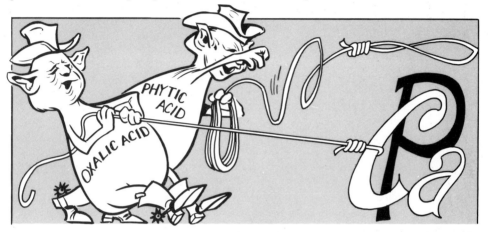

Figure 11-7.   Oxalic and phytic acids "tie up" calcium and phosphorus rendering them unavailable for absorption. Oxalic acid is predominant in foods such as spinach, beet tops, rhubarb, collards, and chocolate. Phytic acid is predominant in whole grains and some legumes such as soybeans.

Key Points: Calcium and Phosphorus

   I.   Calcium is the mineral found in the human body in the greatest quantity. Body need is increased for calcium during periods of growth and is the single most influential factor determining the efficiency of calcium absorption.
   A.   Additional factors favoring the absorption and utilization of calcium are presence of adequate vitamin D, acidity of duodenal intestinal environment, favorable intake ratio for calcium and phosphorus at 1 to 1, and presence of amino acids and lactose.
   B.   Factors which reduce absorption and utilization of calcium are the deficiency of vitamin D, excessive dietary fat intake, high phosphorus to calcium intake ratio, increased gastrointestinal motility, stress, and immobilization.
   II.   Calcium is required for normal formation and maintenance of bones and teeth, absorption of other nutrients, proper neuromuscular function, normal blood clotting, and activation of various enzymes.
   A.   Serum calcium levels are *not* regulated by calcium intake but rather by a balance of necessary hormones and vitamin D.
   B.   All disease conditions associated with a deficient calcium intake or inadequate absorption and utilization of calcium are also accompanied by a deficiency of vitamin D, inadequate absorption, utilization of phosphorus, and/or hormonal imbalances.
      1.   Rickets (develops in childhood) and osteomalacia (develops in adulthood) are diseases resulting from abnormal calcium and phosphorus absorption and metabolism due primarily to a deficiency of vitamin D.

2. Osteoporosis, a condition of reduced skeletal bone content, especially in elderly women, is a multifactorial disease related to prolonged reduced calcium intake, increased protein intake, type of hormone production, and reduced activity.

III. High protein intake, as found in the average American diet, causes increased calcium excretion and results in decreased absorption and utilization of dietary calcium and the loss of calcium from bone stores.

IV. Foods high in calcium are principally milk and milk products, dark green vegetables, and fish eaten with bones.

    A. Oxalic and phytic acid interfere with the availability of calcium from grains, legumes, and some green vegetables.

    B. Adult RDA for calcium is 800 mg/day.

V. Although the optimal *intake* ratio of calcium to phosphorus is accepted as 1 to 1, the calcium to phosphorus ratio *present in the body* is 2 to 1.

VI. Calcium and phosphorus are in a constant state of deposition into and resorption from bones.

VII. Phosphorylation (the combining of a substance with phosphorus) is a reaction necessary for energy metabolism, enzyme activation, and the absorption and transportation of various nutrients. Phosphorus-containing compounds serve as buffers which help to regulate the acid-base balance of the blood.

VIII. Absorption and utilization of phosphorus is influenced by many of the same factors affecting the absorption and utilization of calcium: presence of vitamin D, hormonal controls, oxalic and phytic acids in food, calcium:phosphorus intake ratio, and intestinal motility.

    A. Foods high in phosphorus are cheeses, meats, fish, milk, and many soda drinks.

    B. The adult RDA for phosphorus is 800 mg/day.

Questions: Calcium and Phosphorus

1. The mineral present in the largest amount in the human body is _____ .

2. The small percentage of calcium present in the body but not involved in the structure of bones and teeth is found where?

3. Pregnancy, lactation, and growth periods increase the body's need for many nutrients. The body absorbs (more/less) than the normal 30 percent of its dietary intake of calcium during these periods.

4. The small intestine provides a generally alkaline environment. However, calcium is absorbed from the small intestine even though calcium becomes insoluble in an alkaline medium. Where in the small intestine does most calcium absorption occur and why?

5. Review Table 10-1 (Mineral Composition of Some Foods) and the factors enhancing calcium absorption. Identify four factors which enhance the absorption of milk fortified with vitamin D.

6. Meats provide important sources for phosphorus. The American diet is generally high in meat content. Keeping in mind the advantage of a diet with a calcium: phosphorus ratio of 1:1, what could be the result of a diet high in meat and other sources of phosphorus in relation to calcium absorption?

7. Keeping in mind the greater solubility of calcium in an acid environment, what could one do when cooking soups or stews or roasts, which include meat bones,

to increase the availability of the calcium from the bones for human consumption?

8. Phytic and oxalic acids form insoluble calcium compounds in the intestine. These compounds are not able to be absorbed and are excreted from the body in the:
    a. urine
    b. perspiration
    c. feces

9. Bones are not static storage for calcium. There is a dynamic state of exchange between the calcium in bones and the calcium in the blood plasma.
    a. Which hormone regulates the mobilization of calcium from bones into the blood as needed?
    b. This hormone is secreted by which glands?
    c. Which hormone depresses calcium extraction from bones into blood serum?
    d. Which vitamin increases absorption of calcium from the intestine to maintain serum calcium levels?

10. Calcium is lost from bones during periods of immobilization or lengthy bedrest.
    a. True
    b. False

11. Ionized calcium stimulates the release of thromboplastin which also in the presence of calcium catalyzes the conversion of prothrombin to thrombin. Thrombin, also activated by ionized calcium, then aids in the conversion of fibrinogen to fibrin.
    a. What is fibrin?
    b. What is its function?

12. Thrombin is:
    a. a mineral.
    b. an enzyme.
    c. a blood clot.

13. What food sources for calcium can you recommend to a friend who does not like milk, has difficulty digesting milk, or is allergic to milk?

14. During the course of a day, a boy drinks two glasses of milk, eats one-half cup of ice cream in a cone, one-half cup of cottage cheese, and a slice of cheddar cheese (about 1½ oz) for a snack. What amount of calcium has he consumed in terms of glasses of milk?

15. Susan is a girl who did not have available to her as a child adequate food sources for calcium and phosphorus or exposure to sunshine for a source of vitamin D. She is very short, her legs are bowed, she has a hollow chest, and she has enlarged ankles and wrists. What deficiency disease did she apparently develop?

16. Many elderly adults have fragile bones and experience fractures of their bones which take a long time to heal. Describe what changes may have taken place in their dietary habits over a period of years.

17. Match the following symptoms to the disease listed:

    _____ 1. osteoporosis
    _____ 2. osteomalacia
    _____ 3. rickets

    a. a disease of childhood resulting in stunted growth, bowed legs, hollow chest, and enlarged wrists and ankles
    b. a softening of bones due to the reduction in the mineral content of the bone
    c. an actual diminishing of total bone amount in the skeleton

18. Although optimum absorption of calcium and phosphorus occurs when the di-

etary intake is a 1:1 proportion, the ratio of calcium to phosphorus in bones is:
a. 1:2
b. 2:1
c. 2:2

19. Since the recommended daily calcium allowance for healthy adults is 800 mg per day and it is recommended that a 1:1 proportion of calcium to phosphorus be consumed for maximum efficiency of absorption, what would you conclude the RDA for phosphorus is for healthy adults?

20. Match the following compounds and terms to the appropriate function of phosphorus:

_____ 1. process which facili-   a. phosphorylation
        tates absorption and   b. ADP-ATP
        transportation of   c. TPP
        various nutrients   d. DNA-RNA
_____ 2. is part of these essen-   e. lipoproteins
        tial body compounds
_____ 3. regulates the release of
        energy through for-
        mation of these phos-
        phorus-containing
        substances
_____ 4. is part of these com-
        pounds which facili-
        tate the transportation
        of fatty substances in
        blood

21. Refer to Table 10-1. In examining the items listed, what food categories can you identify as good dietary sources of phosphorus?

22. Phosphorus is also an important component of phosphoric acid and phosphate. These compounds aid in maintaining the acid-base balance of the body. Such compounds are termed _____ .

23. Oxalic and phytic acids render phosphorus and calcium unavailable for absorption by forming _____ .

24. Refer to the diagram showing a balance between calcium and phosphorus (Figure 11-2). Would you expect vitamin D and parathormone to influence phosphorus absorption as they do calcium absorption?

25. Whole grain cereals contain phytic acid. Whole grain cereals are also relatively high in phosphorus content. What may be the result of the interaction between the calcium, phosphorus, and phytic acid in the cereal?

26. Serum calcium levels are *not* regulated by dietary calcium intake.
a. True
b. False

Answers: Calcium and Phosphorus

1. calcium
2. in body fluids, soft tissue, and membrane structures

3. more
4. the duodenum, the first section of the small intestine after the stomach, where the digestive mass is still fairly acidic from mixing with HCl in the stomach
5. Fortified milk contains:
    a. vitamin D
    b. Ca/P ratio of approximately 1:1
    c. amino acids in its protein
    d. lactose
        all of which enhance calcium absorption.
6. The absorption of calcium is lowered due to the increased phosphorus intake.
7. You can add a little vinegar (acetic acid) to the cooking meat/broth mixture to dissolve some of the calcium from the bone. Thus, the calcium is available for consumption in the broth.
8. c
9. a. parathormone
    b. parathyroid
    c. calcitonin
    d. vitamin D
10. a
11. a. blood clot
    b. to plug the area of cell injury and prevent blood loss
12. b
13. firm cheeses, cottage cheese, yogurt, cream cheese, fish eaten with bones such as canned salmon and anchovies, broccoli, orange juice, dark green leafy vegetables which are low in oxalate such as turnip greens and kale, peanuts, some whole grains
14. 3½ to 3⅔ cups milk
15. rickets
16. The probably have reduced their calcium intake, especially through a reduction in intake of milk and dairy products, and/or experienced reduced calcium absorption and/or increased calcium excretion due to a variety of other factors including a prolonged high protein intake.
17. 1. c
    2. b
    3. a
18. b
19. 800 mg/day
20. 1. a
    2. c, d
    3. b, c (because TPP is the phosphorylated form of the vitamin thiamin necessary in energy metabolism)
    4. e
21. milk products and high protein foods (meat, fish, and eggs)
22. buffers
23. insoluble compounds
24. yes
25. They may combine to form insoluble compounds which reduce the availability of phosphorus and calcium from the grain source.
26. a

POTASSIUM

A 150 pound man contains about 120 grams of potassium of which at least 95 percent is located within body cells.[6] Dietary potassium is readily absorbed by the body. Normally, potassium excesses are efficiently excreted by the kidneys. *Aldosterone, a hormone produced by the cortex of the adrenal glands, signals the kidneys to increase potassium excretion.*

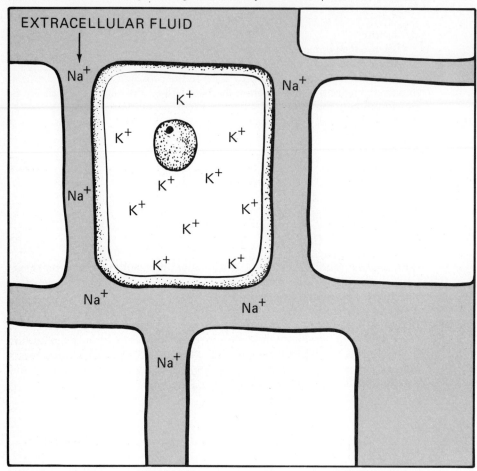

Figure 11-8. Potassium is the chief cation of the intracellular fluid. *It functions to balance the extracellular sodium to maintain normal osmotic pressures and water balance.*

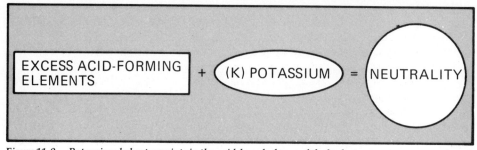

Figure 11-9. Potassium helps to maintain the acid-base balance of the body.

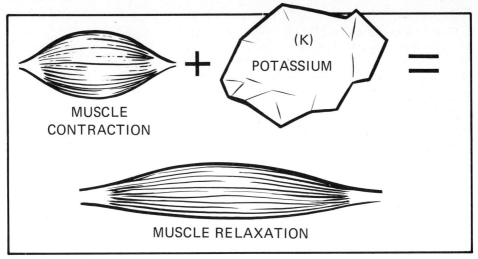

Figure 11-10.   Potassium helps to regulate muscle activity.

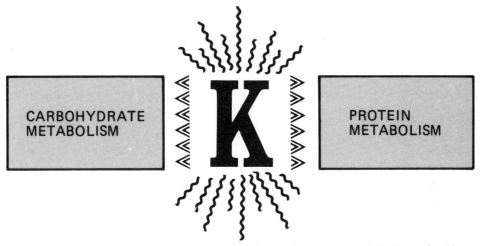

Figure 11-11.   Potassium acts as a catalyst in many biological reactions, especially those related to protein and carbohydrate.

The 1980 RDA gives a safe and adequate daily dietary intake between 1875 to 5625 mg potassium. It is also noted in the text of the RDAs that the average American diet supplies from approximately 2 to 6 g potassium daily.[7]

Hyperkalemia (elevated serum potassium). Certain conditions such as renal failure and severe dehydration can cause serum potassium to rise to toxic levels. Hyperkalemia results in a characteristic weakening of heart action which can lead to heart failure, mental confusion, poor respiration, and numbness of extremities.

Hypokalemia (low serum potassium). Hypokalemia can be the result of starvation, chronic use of diuretic drugs,[8] or a consequence of diabetic acidosis. Hypokalemia can result in overall muscular weakness, loss of appetite, nausea, vomiting, and rapid heart beat (tachycardia) leading to heart failure.

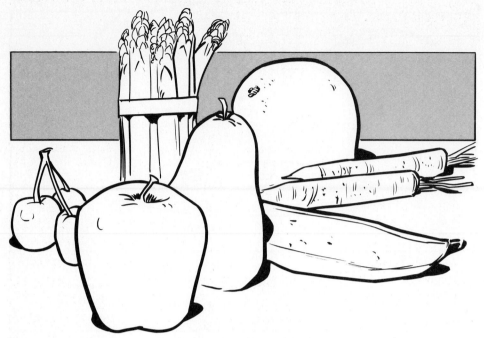

Figure 11-12.   Potassium is widely distributed in foods. In addition to meat and milk, fruits and vegetables are especially rich in this mineral.

SODIUM

A 150 pound man contains about 90 grams of sodium of which 35 to 40 percent is in the skeleton.[9] Only about ten percent of body sodium is contained within body cells. More than half of body sodium is located in extracellular[10] fluids of the body.

Sodium absorption and excretion. Sodium is the major electrolyte in the extracellular fluids, including the vascular system. The kidneys normally excrete sodium proportionately to intake and need. Some sodium is also excreted in the feces and perspiration. Large amounts of sodium can be lost in perspiration during periods of heavy energy expenditure when environmental temperatures are high. Sodium is also lost in large quantities from gastric secretions during periods of repeated vomiting. The use of diuretics can increase the loss of sodium in urine. *Aldosterone, an adrenal cortical hormone, stimulates the reabsorption of sodium by the kidneys to conserve sodium in times of increased need.*

When the serum sodium level is increased, water is retained and blood volume is increased. An increase in blood volume causes a corresponding increase in blood pressure.

Functions of sodium. Sodium functions in many ways similar to potassium. Sodium is important to the maintenance of osmotic pressures and water balance, maintenance of the acid-base balance of the body, regulation of nerve irritability and muscle contraction, and regulation of carbohydrate and amino acid absorption.

The 1980 RDAs give an estimated safe and adequate daily dietary intake range for sodium between 1100 and 3300 mg (approximately 1 to 3 grams). Since the major source of dietary sodium is common table salt, and salt is 40 percent sodium, the allowance can be interpreted as between 2.5 and 8.5 grams of salt per day. However, considerable sodium is also obtained from dairy foods, shellfish, fish, meat, poultry, eggs, and processed foods containing salt, baking powder, baking soda, and preservative additives. Some sources of drinking water are high in sodium content.

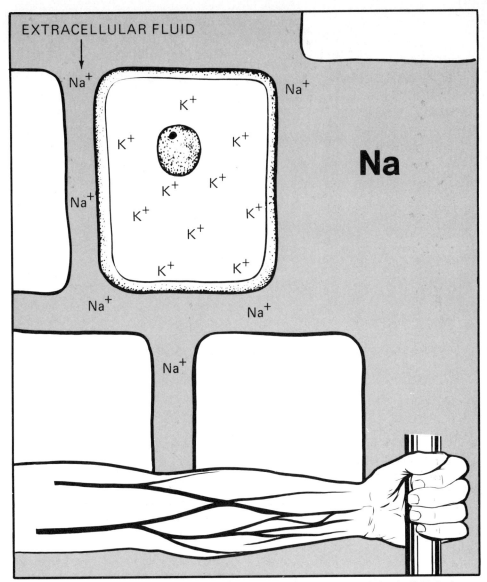

Figure 11-13. **Sodium is the major cation of the extracellular fluids.** *This includes the fluids in the vascular system as well as that surrounding the cells. The vascular system: blood vessels, veins, arteries, and capillaries.*

Deficiency due to inadequate intake is uncommon. Deficiency can be caused by unusually large losses incurred from severe vomiting episodes, very heavy perspiring, and certain disease conditions such as cystic fibrosis and Addison's disease. Deficiency symptoms include nausea, vomiting, disturbances in the acid-base balance, and diarrhea. The 1980 RDAs recommend replacement of sodium by addition of sodium chloride (table salt) to drinking water in amounts ranging between 2 to 7 grams salt per liter of extra water loss (depending on severity of the losses) when losses due to sweat are greater than three liters per day.[11]

Hypertension and sodium intake. Sodium intake has been examined in relation to the

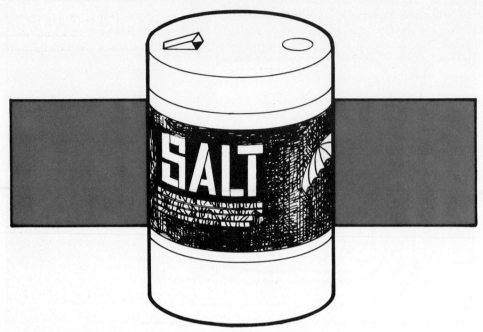

Figure 11-14.   Table salt is the major source of sodium in the American diet.

occurrence of hypertension (high blood pressure). It has been found that societies with very low sodium intakes have far less incidence of hypertension than those societies with high sodium intakes. This association has also been demonstrated in studies with rats. These associations in man have been made through epidemiological studies and are not proof of a cause and effect relationship.

Hypertension is also related to obesity, genetic predisposition, smoking, personality type, and stress. It has been found that loss of excess weight can significantly reduce hypertension without diet modifications or the use of drugs. However, some persons are less sensitive to blood pressure changes and excretion of sodium by their kidneys is inadequate to maintain normal sodium serum levels. Other persons consume such a high level of salt that they exceed their body's ability to adequately excrete excess sodium and water. Still others are more sensitive to the presence of sodium and respond with a constriction of blood vessels resulting in a higher than normal blood pressure.

For those persons who are at a greater risk of developing hypertension, especially those for whom hypertension is common among family members or who are very sensitive to the effects of sodium, a reduced sodium intake may be advisable and beneficial.[12] Often this reduction can be satisfactorily accomplished by the simple elimination of salt added to food either at the table or during preparation, and the elimination of pre-salted meats and snack foods from the diet.

CHLORINE

Chlorine is found in the body almost exclusively as the chloride anion (Cl^-) in extracellular fluid. The largest amounts of body chloride are found in gastric secretions and cerebrospinal fluid.

Chloride is readily and efficiently absorbed in the gastrointestinal tract. Body levels are chiefly controlled by the kidneys which excrete chloride excesses above body needs. As is the case with sodium, significant losses of chloride are sustained during periods of heavy perspiration, diarrhea, and vomiting.

Functions of chloride. In addition to performing significant roles in the fluid-electrolyte balance of the body and the acid-base balance of the body, chloride is the chief anion of gastric hydrochloric acid. Consequently, chloride plays an important role in the digestion and absorption of various nutrients.

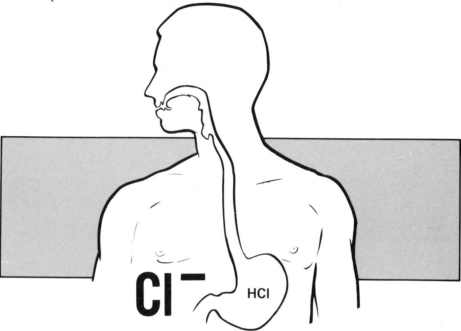

Figure 11-15. Chloride is the chief anion in extracellular fluids *and is found in large amounts in gastric secretions due to its presence in hydrochloric acid (HCl).*

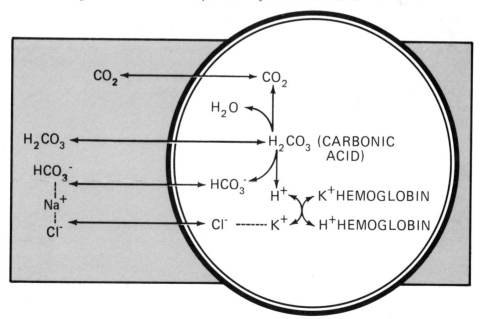

Figure 11-16. A summary of the chloride shift between red blood cells and blood plasma.

Chloride is also an important buffer necessary for the proper maintenance of blood pH (the chloride shift). When CO_2 tension in the blood increases, Cl^- goes into the red blood cell which allows more carbonic acid to be shifted out of the red blood cell to form bicarbonate ion (HCO_3^-). Bicarbonate ions can be carried as sodium bicarbonate in the plasma. When CO_2 tension decreases, Cl^- passes back into the plasma and out of the cell. Thus, the chloride shift allows for an increased carriage of CO_2 and neutralization as it forms carbonic acid until CO_2 is expelled by the lungs.[13]

Chloride is most commonly and adequately obtained from table salt (NaCl), as is sodium. Various meats, seafoods, milk, and eggs provide additional sources for chloride. The 1980 RDAs give an estimated safe and adequate daily dietary intake for chloride of between 1700 and 5100 mg. When large amounts of chloride are lost due to excessive vomiting chloride replacement is necessary to prevent disturbances in the acid-base balance of the body.

MAGNESIUM

Most of the magnesium in the human body is found in the bones and muscle tissue. The remainder is located in soft tissues, body fluids, and red blood cells. Magnesium is one of the most predominant cations of the intracellular fluids. Excesses of magnesium above body needs are normally excreted in the urine. Interestingly, the excretion of magnesium appears to be an inverse function of calcium excretion: as calcium excretion diminishes, magnesium excretion increases, and as calcium excretion increases, magnesium excretion decreases.

Functions of magnesium. Magnesium performs many varied and necessary functions. Magnesium, along with calcium, phosphorus, and vitamin D, is necessary for proper bone formation and metabolism. Magnesium is the required activator for many different enzymes. Magnesium is necessary for the metabolism of carbohydrates, fats, and proteins, and is also important for energy production as it is necessary for the formation of ATP. Magnesium ions play an interdependent role with calcium, sodium, and potassium ions in the control of nerve cell transmission and muscle contraction.

The 1980 RDAs for magnesium are 300 mg for healthy adult women and 350 mg for healthy adult men. Magnesium is a vital component of the green pigment chlorophyll in plants. Consequently, green vegetables are a good source of this mineral. Grains, soybeans, meats, milk, and poultry are additional good sources of magnesium either because of its relatively high content in those foods or because of the consumption frequency of those foods. Because magnesium can be obtained from a wide variety of food sources dietary deficiency of magnesium is rare.

SULFUR

Sulfur is present in every cell of the body. The greatest concentrations occur in the hair, skin, and nails because these tissues contain keratin, a sulfur-containing protein.

Sulfur intake and metabolism is associated with protein intake and metabolism because the amino acids methionine, cysteine, and cystine contain sulfur. Approximately one percent of dietary protein is sulfur. Most sulfur is absorbed in organic compounds, amino acids, though almost all sulfur is excreted as inorganic sulfates in the urine.

Functions of sulfur. Sulfur is an important component of sulfur-containing amino acids, and is contained in certain compounds which are important for the detoxification of toxic substances. Sulfur forms certain high energy bonds important in energy metabolism and is a constituent of some vitamins such as thiamin and biotin, and vitamin-like factors, such as lipoic acid, and the coenzyme vital to energy metabolism, coenzyme A. Sulfur is also contained in such body compounds as the hormone insulin, the pigment melanin, and

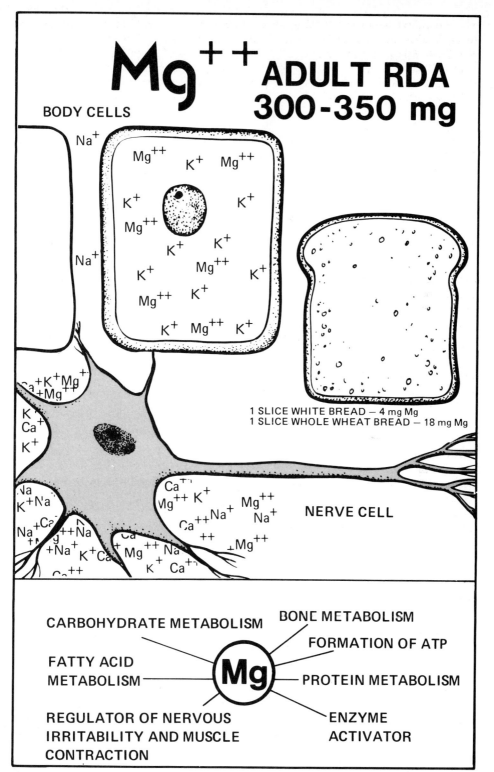

Figure 11-17.   Magnesium.

the bile acid taurocholic acid. There is no RDA for sulfur nor an estimated safe and adequate daily dietary intake range. Diets sufficient in protein are also sufficient in sulfur to meet body needs.

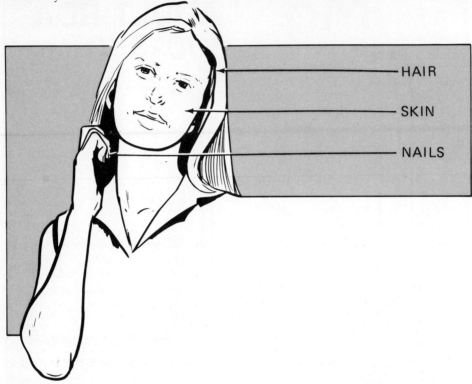

Figure 11-18.   *Highest concentrations of sulfur are found in the hair, skin, and nails due to the presence there of keratin, a sulfur-containing protein.*

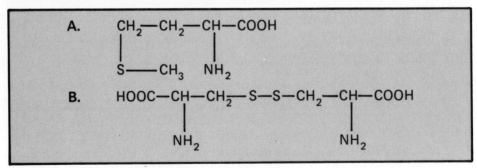

Figure 11-19.   *A. The sulfur-containing amino acid, methionine.*
B. The amino acid cystine which contains a disulfide linkage important for the maintenance of structural proteins.

Key Points: Potassium, Sodium, Chlorine, Magnesium, and Sulfur

I. Potassium is the chief cation of intracellular fluids. Potassium is readily absorbed and its excretion by the kidneys into urine is increased by the hormone aldosterone.

II. Potassium functions include the regulation of osmotic pressures and water balance, regulation of body acid-base balance, regulation of neuromuscular activity, and as a catalyst in reactions related to protein and carbohydrate metabolism.

III. A wide variety of foods contain potassium. Deficiency is more often the result of prolonged vomiting, diarrhea, use of diuretics, kidney failure, and dehydration.

IV. Most body sodium is located in extracellular fluids of the body. Sodium is conserved when needed by the action of aldosterone, a hormone, which causes the kidneys to reabsorb sodium.

V. Serum sodium draws water into the blood which causes a corresponding rise in blood pressure.

VI. Sodium functions to maintain osmotic pressures, water balance, acid-base balance, and to regulate neuromuscular activity and carbohydrate and amino acid absorption.

VII. The chief source of sodium in the American diet is table salt (NaCl) though significant amounts are supplied in dairy foods, seafood, meat, poultry, eggs, and processed foods.

VIII. A deficiency of sodium is most likely due to fluid loss in prolonged vomiting, heavy sweating, and some disease conditions.

IX. Sodium intake is associated through animal studies and epidemiological studies with the occurrence of hypertension (high blood pressure). Although low sodium diets are beneficial to persons suffering from hypertension their use is not *known* to reduce the chances of *developing* hypertension. Sodium restriction may be most beneficial in reducing the development of hypertension in persons predisposed to this condition.

X. Chlorine is found chiefly in the extracellular fluids of the body as the chloride ion (Cl^-). Excess chloride is excreted by the kidneys. Large losses of chloride occur during periods of vomiting because of the chloride contained in gastric hydrochloric acid.

XI. Chloride is important in maintaining the acid-base balance of the body, especially of blood through the chloride shift process, and for the digestion and absorption of various nutrients.

XII. Table salt, meats, seafood, milk, and eggs are sources of dietary chloride.

XIII. Magnesium is a predominant cation in intracellular fluids of the body. Excess magnesium is excreted in the urine; magnesium absorption and excretion appear to be an inverse function of calcium absorption and excretion.

XIV. Magnesium is necessary for proper bone metabolism, neuromuscular functioning, enzyme activation, carbohydrate and fatty acid metabolism, and formation of ATP.

XV. Magnesium is found in grains, meat, milk, soybeans, poultry, and green vegetables.
A. Magnesium is a component of chlorophyll, the green pigment of plants.
B. The adult RDA for magnesium is 300 mg for women and 350 mg for men.

XVI. Sulfur is contained in several amino acids. Consequently, sulfur intake and metabolism are related to protein intake and metabolism.

XVII. Sulfur is a component of many necessary body compounds such as some amino acids, some vitamins, insulin, melanin (a bile pigment), metabolic detoxification compounds, and keratin, the structural protein found in hair, skin, and nails. Sulfur forms high energy bonds in some sulfur-containing compounds.

XVIII. Diets sufficient in protein supply sufficient sulfur to the body.

Questions: Potassium, Sodium, Chlorine, Magnesium, and Sulfur

1. Potassium is the chief cation of the _____ fluid.
   a. extracellular
   b. intracellular

2. Is potassium a base-forming or acid-forming mineral? (Hint: Refer to Figure 10-10.)

3. Potassium plays a significant role in regulating the activity of muscles. Potassium exerts a _____ effect on muscles.
   a. relaxing
   b. stimulating

4. Explain why hyperkalemia could result in a weakening of heart action.

5. Potassium is required for the storage of nitrogen as muscle protein. Therefore, potassium plays a significant role in _____ .

6. Potassium is stored with glycogen which is synthesized from blood glucose. When insulin is administered to a diabetic person his blood glucose uptake by cells is increased along with an increase in his production and storage of glycogen.
   a. If a large insulin dose is rapidly given what would happen to the serum potassium level?
   b. What term is used to describe this state of serum potassium level?

7. Actually, potassium deficiency most frequently occurs as a result of large losses of body fluids. What body conditions would contribute to large losses of body fluids?
   a. diarrhea
   b. vomiting
   c. constipation

8. Refer to Table 10-1.
   a. Does potassium appear to be readily available from many different food sources?
   b. Are all food groups represented as showing potassium content?
   c. Does potassium deficiency appear to be a likely result of dietary lack?
   d. Which groups of foods are especially rich in potassium?

9. Sodium is the major cation of the _____ fluid.
   a. intracellular
   b. extracellular

10. Sodium functions with potassium to:
    a. maintain water balance and osmotic pressure
    b. maintain acid-base balance
    c. regulate protein and carbohydrate absorption

11. An increase in body sodium would tend to draw water _____ the body cells.
    a. into
    b. out of

12. Keeping in mind the influence of sodium on osmotic pressure and water balance, explain why individuals *suffering from high blood pressure* are advised to restrict their sodium intake as well as to avoid excess weight gain.

13. What are some of the risk factors associated with *development* of hypertension which are not related to diet?

14. Refer to the illustrated examples of the specific functions of minerals in general.

Sodium is particularly important in regulating cell permeability to what nutrient?
a. vitamin B_{12}
b. fatty acids
c. glucose

15. Sodium excretion is regulated by a hormone, aldosterone, secreted by the adrenal gland. This hormone influences the excretion or reabsorption of sodium by the kidney according to body need. If sodium intake has been low in conjunction with states of vomiting and diarrhea, the kidneys would increase sodium (excretion/retention) under the influence of aldosterone.

16. Chloride is the chief anion of what gastric substance?
a. KCl
b. HCl
c. NaCl

17. The main dietary source of chlorine is table salt (NaCl). Table salt in the average American diet generally provides about eight to ten times the quantity of sodium that the body needs for maintenance of sodium balance. Also, chlorine is stored in the body in the same ratio as sodium. Therefore, would you expect the intake of chloride through the use of table salt to be adequate for humans?

18. What condition would cause a loss of gastric chloride?
a. excessive urination
b. excessive perspiration
c. excessive vomiting

19. Refer to Figure 11-16. H_2CO_3 is carbonic acid. The shift of bicarbonate to the plasma and the shift of Cl^- into the RBC allows for the formation of sodium bicarbonate, a salt. The chloride anion is neutralized by the potassium cation inside the RBC. This system allows for the increased carriage of CO_2 as it effectively maintains the _____ balance in the blood.

20. In the chloride shift system, hemoglobin acts as _____ .
a. an acid
b. a base
c. a buffer

21. Magnesium is _____ .
a. an anion
b. a cation

22. Magnesium is chiefly located in the _____ fluid.
a. intracellular
b. extracellular

23. Magnesium is needed in balance with calcium, potassium, and sodium in the extracellular fluid for the normal _____ .

24. Magnesium is a catalyst in the reactions which release energy through glucose oxidation. Magnesium is also necessary for the activation of amino acids so that they can be incorporated into protein molecules. Therefore, magnesium is important to the metabolism of both _____ and _____ .

25. The greatest percentage of magnesium in the body is located in muscle tissue and with calcium and phosphorus in the _____ .

26. Magnesium is a regulator of muscle contractions. Magnesium acts as a muscle _____ . (Hint: refer to the specific functions of minerals in Chapter Ten.)
a. relaxant
b. stimulant

27. In plant life, magnesium is an essential part of the green pigment chlorophyll, which differs from the hemoglobin of blood only in that magnesium replaces iron as the mineral in its structure. Given this information, what vegetables would you expect to be a good source of magnesium?
    a. potatoes
    b. carrots
    c. dark green, leafy vegetables

28. Calcium and magnesium compete for the same carrier sites in the intestinal mucosa. In addition, reduced calcium excretion in urine is associated with increased magnesium excretion in urine. Would you expect a high calcium intake to increase or decrease the requirement for magnesium?

29. Magnesium is one mineral reduced by the processing of grains which is not restored by enrichment.
    a. True
    b. False

30. Many of the factors which inhibit calcium absorption also inhibit the absorption of magnesium. What would you expect to be the result of magnesium and phytic or oxalic acid interaction?

31. Magnesium is available from dairy products, protein sources, nuts, legumes, grains, fruits, and vegetables. Would you expect magnesium deficiency to be primarily the result of inadequate dietary intake?

32. Magnesium deficiency can occur when there is a poor food intake along with fluid loss and lowered absorption. Identify the following items which could produce a deficiency of magnesium.
    a. severe diarrhea
    b. severe vomiting
    c. excess oxalic and phytic acids
    d. a diet high in nuts, grains, and vegetables
    e. high calcium diet

33. Most of the sulfur in the body originates from the amino acids methionine, cysteine, and cystine. Amino acids are the building blocks of protein. Consequently, intake and utilization of sulfur are related to _____ .

34. Disulfide linkages are important to the maintenance of _____ .

35. The highest concentration of sulfur is found in the hair, skin, and nails. Why?

36. Some compounds containing sulfur act to render toxic substances harmless. This process is an important function of sulfur and is termed:
    a. intoxication
    b. detoxification

37. The sulfhydryl group is able to form high energy bonds and is, therefore, important in _____ metabolism.

38. Cystine is an amino acid formed by the combination of two cysteine amino acids through the formation of a _____ linkage.

39. Why do you suppose the sulfur-containing amino acid methionine is considered an essential amino acid while cysteine and cystine are not?

Answers: Potassium, Sodium, Chlorine, Magnesium, and Sulfur

1. b

2. base-forming
3. a
4. Hyperkalemia is a state of high serum potassium which would have a more powerful relaxing effect on muscular contractions and results in weakened heart actions.
5. protein metabolism
6. a.   It would rapidly decrease
   b.   hypokalemia
7. a, b (also extended use of diuretics and severe burns which increase fluid loss)
8. a.   yes
   b.   yes
   c.   no
   d.   fruits and vegetables
9. b
10. a, b
11. b
12. Because an increase in the use of table salt would increase the body intake of sodium. The increased sodium would draw water into the vascular system causing increased hypertension and added burden on the heart. Loss of excess weight can significantly reduce hypertension. Treatment of hypertension involves the control of body weight to desirable levels.
13. Genetic predisposition, smoking, personality type, and stress.
14. c
15. retention
16. b
17. yes
18. c
19. acid-base
20. c
21. b
22. a
23. transmission of nerves
24. carbohydrate; protein
25. bones
26. a
27. c
28. increase
29. a
30. Phytic and oxalic acids would form insoluble magnesium compounds reducing magnesium absorption.
31. no
32. a; b; c; e
33. protein intake and utilization
34. structural proteins
35. Sulfur is found in keratin, the protein of nails, hair, and skin
36. b
37. energy
38. disulfide
39. Methionine must be obtained from the diet because it cannot be manufactured in the body. However, the body can manufacture cysteine and cystine from methionine when adequate methionine is present.

REFERENCES

[1] Avioli LV: Major minerals. Chapter 7, A. Calcium and Phosphorus, *In* Goodhart RS and Shils ME (eds): Modern Nutrition in Health and Disease, 6th ed. Philadelphia, Lea and Febiger, 1980, pp. 299-302

[2] Linkswiler HM: Calcium. *In* Present Knowledge in Nutrition, 4th ed. New York and Washington, D.C.; The Nutrition Foundation, Inc., 1976

[3] A good review and update on osteoporosis and its treatment can be found in: Marx JL: Osteoporosis: New help for thinning bones. Science, 207, February 1980, pp. 628-630

[4] Latinen O: Osteoporosis: Nature, treatment and possible future trends. Public Health Reviews, 7, 1978, p. 177

[5] Marsh AG, Sanchez TV, Mickelsen O, Keiser J, and Mayor G: Cortical bone density of adult lacto-ovo-vegetarian and omnivorous women. Journal of the American Dietetic Association, 76, February 1980, pp. 148-151

[6] Randall HT: Water, electrolytes and acid-base balance. *In* Goodhart RS and Shils ME (eds): Modern Nutrition in Health and Disease, 6th ed. Philadelphia, Lea and Febiger, 1980, p. 363

[7] Recommended Dietary Allowances, Ninth Revised Edition. Food and Nutrition Board, National Academy of Sciences-National Research Council, Washington, D.C., 1980, p. 172

[8] **Diuretics** are drugs which cause increased excretion of urine.

[9] Randall HT: Water, electrolytes and acid-base balance. *In* Goodhart RS and Shils ME (eds): Modern Nutrition in Health and Disease, 6th ed. Philadelphia, Lea and Febiger, 1980, p. 362

[10] **Extracellular** refers to locations outside of a cell.

[11] Recommended Dietary Allowances, Ninth Revised Edition. Food and Nutrition Board, National Academy of Sciences, National Research Council, Washington, D.C., 1980, p. 170

[12] A good review of the current literature on the relationship of sodium intake and development of hypertension can be found in: Cullen RW, Paulbitski A, and Oace SM: Sodium, hypertension, and the US dietary goals. Journal of Nutrition Education, 10, April-June 1978, pp. 59-60

[13] Harper HA: Review of Physiological Chemistry, 14th ed. Los Altos, California; LANGE Medical Publications, 1973, pp. 214-215

12
THE MICROMINERALS

IRON (Fe)

Iron is a metal of remarkable biologic versatility. Iron readily accepts and gives up electrons, and is a necessary constituent of the electron transport and respiratory enzyme systems. Iron enters the body usually as ferric iron (Fe^{+++}) in food. *In the acid medium of the stomach ferric iron is reduced to ferrous iron (Fe^{++}), the form necessary for absorption.*

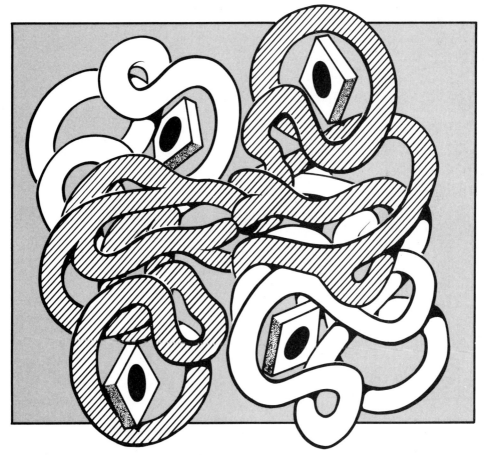

Figure 12-1. **Hemoglobin.** *A schematic representation of the hemoglobin molecule: there are two pairs of polypeptide chains each with subunits of alpha and beta chains—the alpha which is shown as lined and beta which is shown as plain—intertwine four protoporphyrin molecules, the squares, each of which holds an atom of iron, shown as a solid oval.*

Approximately three-fourths of the iron in the body is functioning iron. The remainder is storage iron which is in the form of *ferritin* or *hemosiderin*. Most of the functioning iron is contained in *hemoglobin*. Iron circulates in the plasma as *transferrin*. *Myoglobin* is an iron-protein complex in the muscle which stores some oxygen for immediate use by the cell.

Iron is complexed with a variety of protein molecules. The way it combines with each of the various proteins confers specific function to that protein. If the protein is globin, the resultant molecule is hemoglobin. Hemoglobin is the principal component of the red blood cell, and it accounts for most of the iron in the body. It also acts as a carrier of oxygen from the lungs to the tissues and indirectly aids in the return of carbon dioxide to the lungs.

Iron absorption. Soluble iron enters the cells of the duodenal mucosa. Part of the iron

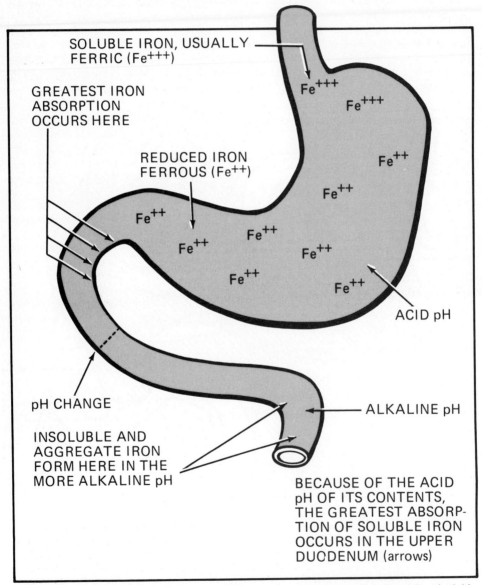

SOLUBLE IRON, USUALLY FERRIC (Fe^{+++})

GREATEST IRON ABSORPTION OCCURS HERE

REDUCED IRON FERROUS (Fe^{++})

Fe^{+++}

Fe^{+++}

Fe^{++}

Fe^{++}

Fe^{++}

Fe^{++}

Fe^{++}

Fe^{++}

Fe^{++}

Fe^{++}

ACID pH

pH CHANGE

ALKALINE pH

INSOLUBLE AND AGGREGATE IRON FORM HERE IN THE MORE ALKALINE pH

BECAUSE OF THE ACID pH OF ITS CONTENTS, THE GREATEST ABSORPTION OF SOLUBLE IRON OCCURS IN THE UPPER DUODENUM (arrows)

Figure 12-2. Iron absorption. *Because of the acid pH of its contents, the greatest absorption of soluble iron occurs in the upper duodenum.*

passes through the mucosal cells into the plasma. Any unneeded iron combines with a protein, *apoferritin*, to form *ferritin* within the mucosal cell. This excess iron remains in the mucosal cell until it is exfoliated (sloughed-off) and excreted in the feces (about every two to three days). The amount of ferritin present in the mucosal cells exerts a regulating effect on iron absorption: the greater the ferritin content, the lower the quantity of iron absorbed.

Measurements in man indicate that food iron absorption usually ranges from five to 15 percent of that available from intake. Approximately two to ten percent of the iron in vegetables can be absorbed while approximately ten to 30 percent of the iron from animal protein can be absorbed.

Generally, about ten percent of the iron in a mixed diet is absorbed. In other words, for every 10 mg of iron ingested about 1 mg is absorbed. Excretion averages about 1 mg/day. *For the healthy adult, daily iron intake needs are based upon the replacement of daily iron losses.* The 1980 RDA for iron in adult men is 10 mg and for adult women it is 18 mg. Women's needs are higher because their losses due to menstruation are greater.

Absorption of nonheme iron[1] is enhanced by the presence of ascorbic acid. In fact, the 1980 RDA for ascorbic acid for adults was raised from 45 mg to 60 mg primarily due to its enhancing effect on iron absorption. In addition to the more readily absorbed heme iron

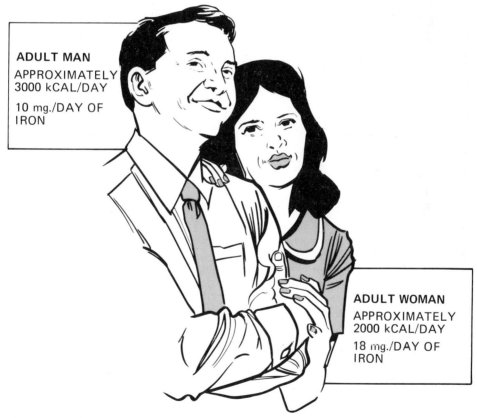

ADULT MAN
APPROXIMATELY
3000 kCAL/DAY

10 mg./DAY OF
IRON

ADULT WOMAN
APPROXIMATELY
2000 kCAL/DAY

18 mg./DAY OF
IRON

Figure 12-3.   Of all the nutrients, the iron allowance is the most difficult to meet through diet for women of childbearing age. The iron content of typical diets adequate in other respects is estimated to be 6 mg per 1000 kcal. Thus, men and boys with their higher caloric intake can easily meet their iron needs. But, girls and women with their lower caloric intake have difficulty in meeting their iron needs even with a good selection of diet. Girls and women have higher iron intake needs due to menstrual losses which total about 20 mg/month.

found in animal tissue, there appears to be a factor in meat, fish, and poultry (referred to as MFP) which enhances the absorption of nonheme iron. Consequently, when a food containing ascorbic acid or an animal tissue protein is consumed with other foods the total iron absorption is increased. The best sources of dietary iron are meats, enriched grain products, legumes, and dried fruit. Milk is a very poor source of iron.

Table 12-1.   Factors affecting iron absorption.

Factors facilitating iron absorption	Factors inhibiting iron absorption
Body need	Surgical removal of stomach tissue which decreases the production of HCl acid
Ascorbic acid	
Hydrochloric acid	Malabsorption syndromes
Calcium (removes binding agents found in the intestines which bind iron, such as phytic acid)	Diarrhea
	Severe infection
	Presence of binding agents: phosphate, phytate, oxalate
Presence of heme iron from animal protein*	Presence of dietary foods such as: egg, bran, tea*
Presence of "meat factor" in meat, fish, and poultry (MFP) which enhances the absorption of nonheme iron**	

 * Cook JD: Food iron availability. Food and Nutrition News, 49, February 1978
** Monsen ER: Simplified method for calculating available dietary iron. Food and Nutrition News, 51, March-April 1980

Iron cycle in the body. There is a constant flow of iron to the erythroid bone marrow (red-blood cell producing) where it is incorporated into hemoglobin in new red blood cells. These cells circulate for about 120 days after which they are destroyed by the reticuloendothelial cells of the liver, spleen, and bone marrow. The iron that is separated from its hemoglobin is returned to the plasma. The small amount of iron normally found in blood plasma is in transit.

Iron, therefore, circulates from the reticuloendothelial cell to the erythron (red blood cell) repeatedly, and with very little loss. Some dietary iron is needed daily to replace the small amount of iron lost in excretion. However, the overwhelming majority of body iron is constantly recycled and reused in an efficiently conservative system.[2] See Figure 12-4.

Nutritional Anemia. Nutritional anemia is a result of inadequate iron in the diet. A deficiency of iron results in a hypochromic microcytic anemia (the red cells are small in size and very pale in color). Infants, preschool children, adolescent girls, and pregnant women are particularly susceptible to this type of anemia.

Hemosiderosis. Hemosiderosis is a disorder of iron metabolism in which large deposits of iron are made in the liver. It is believed to be caused by an overload of dietary iron and can also result from hemolytic anemia.[3] The iron overload leads to iron deposition because the transferrin of the circulation becomes saturated and is unable to bind all of the iron that is absorbed. Cells in which the iron is deposited become distorted and cellular death occurs damaging the organ involved.

Table 12-2.   Iron content of selected foods.

	mg/100g/3½ oz
Almonds, dried	4.7
Apple, raw (one small)	.3
Apricots, dried	5.5
Apricots, raw (2 to 3 medium)	.5
Bananas	.7
Beans, common white cooked	2.7
Beans, lima, cooked and drained	2.5
Beef, round, broiled	3.7
Beef, hamburger, cooked	3.5
Bread, white, enriched	2.4 (0.6 mg/slice)
Bread, whole wheat	2.3 (0.5 mg/slice)
Chicken, dark meat, cooked	2.0
Cod, cooked, broiled	1.0
Cowpeas (blackeye), cooked, boiled, drained	2.1
Eggs, poached (2 medium)	2.2
Heart, calf, cooked	4.4
Liver, cooked	8.8
Milk, whole fluid	trace (0.1 mg/cup)
Oysters, canned	8.1
Peas, cooked	1.8
Pork, lean and cooked	3.5
Potato, baked in skin (one medium)	.7
Prune juice	4.1
Raisins	3.5
Soybeans, cooked and drained	2.5
Tuna, drained	1.9
Vegetables, mixed, cooked, drained	1.3
Wheat flakes, cereal	4.4 (1.3 mg/cup)

Source: Composition of Foods, Agriculture Handbook No. 8, Agricultural Research Service, U.S. Department of Agriculture, 1963

COPPER (Cu)

Though copper is present in all body cells it is concentrated in the liver, brain, heart, and kidney tissues where it is most metabolically active. Absorption of copper takes place in the intestine, especially in the duodenum. Zinc and other trace metals interfere with the absorption of copper.

Copper is sometimes referred to as the "iron twin" because it shares many functions with iron. Copper, like iron, is involved in the cytochrome oxidation system of tissue cells for energy production. Copper is essential, together with iron, to the formation of hemoglobin. Copper promotes the absorption of iron from the gastrointestinal tract and is involved in iron transport from the tissues into the plasma. In addition to its iron-related functions, copper is involved in three other major areas of metabolism: bone formation, brain tissue formation, and maintenance of myelin in the nervous system, and is an essential component of certain enzymes.

The 1980 RDAs recommend a safe and adequate daily intake range of 2 to 3 mg for copper based on copper balance studies. A wide variety of foods supply varying amounts

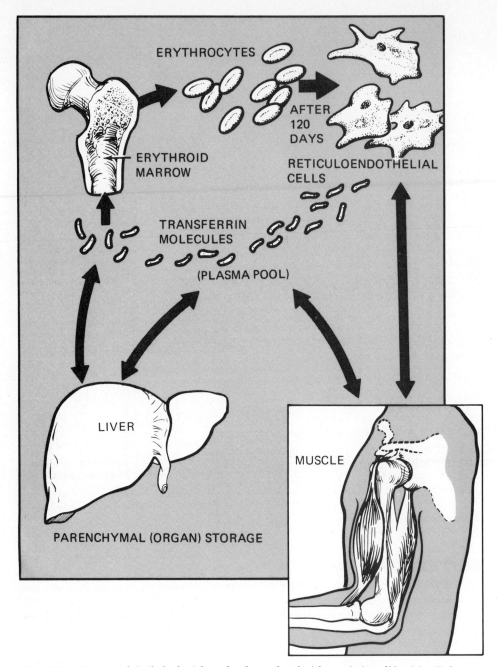

ERYTHROCYTES

AFTER
120
DAYS

ERYTHROID
MARROW

RETICULOENDOTHELIAL
CELLS

TRANSFERRIN
MOLECULES

(PLASMA POOL)

LIVER

MUSCLE

PARENCHYMAL (ORGAN) STORAGE

Figure 12-4.   Iron's cycle in the body. Adapted and reproduced with permission of Nutrition Today Magazine, 703 Giddings Ave., Annapolis, MD, 21404, © Summer 1969.

of copper. However, in order to meet the RDA for copper, diets must be consumed that contain more energy value than ordinarily consumed in the United States, as well as foods seldom selected such as organ meats and shellfish.[4] Those foods especially rich in copper are oysters, lobster, nuts, legumes, and corn oil. The potato can be a good source of copper

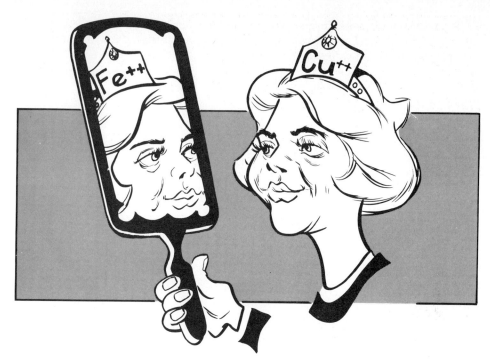

Figure 12-5.   Copper as the so-called twin of iron.

for some people because of the frequency with which it is eaten. Cow's milk is a poor source of copper but human milk contains significant amounts of copper.

    Dietary deficiency of copper sometimes occurs in association with kwashiorkor and with iron-deficiency anemia. A deficiency causes some depigmentation of hair and skin as well as textural changes to hair.[5] Copper is toxic to man when ingested in large amounts.

    Zinc/copper ratio. Zinc is antagonistic to copper and reduces copper absorption and storage in the liver. Relatively high zinc intake with resultant copper deficiency has been associated with increased serum cholesterol levels. Some epidemiological studies have produced information *suggesting* a positive correlation between the zinc-to-copper ratio in the diet and the incidence of cardiovascular disease.[6,7]

Key Points: Iron and Copper

   I. Interaction between the various microminerals substantially affects the absorption and utilization in man of an individual micromineral.

  II. An acid environment greatly enhances the absorption of iron. Thus, ascorbic acid (vitamin C) is a nutrient useful for increasing the absorption of iron from a meal of mixed foods when consumed with that meal.

 III. Daily iron intake needs for healthy adults are based upon the replacement of daily iron losses.

 IV. Heme iron obtained from animal tissue protein and an additional factor obtained from meat, fish, and poultry (MFP) increase the absorption of total iron available from a meal of mixed foods.

  V. Though nutritional anemia is a result of inadequate iron in the diet, iron deficiency is increasingly being recognized as a state of reduced or absent body iron *stores.*

 VI. Copper shares many of the same functions of iron: involvement in cellular oxidation of energy nutrients, involvement in the formation of hemoglobin necessary for proper red blood cell formation, enhancement of iron absorption, involvement in iron transport from tissues into plasma.

VII. Foods high in copper content are those infrequently selected for consumption such as organ meats, shellfish, and nuts.

VIII. Dietary deficiency of copper is often associated with kwashiorkor and iron-deficiency anemia.

IX. There may be a correlation between an increased zinc-to-copper intake ratio of a population group and the increased incidence of cardiovascular disease.

Questions: Iron and Copper

1. Iron is absorbed in its bivalent form.
   a. The term to describe this iron ion is (ferric/ferrous).
   b. The chemical symbol for this ion is (Fe^{++}/Fe^{+++}).
   c. Is this a cation or anion?

2. Most of the body iron is storage iron.
   a. True
   b. False

3. Each hemoglobin molecule carries how many atoms of iron? (Refer to Figure 12-1)

4. Most functioning iron is contained in what protein complex?
   a. hemoglobin
   b. myoglobin
   c hemosiderin

5. This protein complex in question 4 is the principal component of what type of body cell?

6. Hemoglobin aids directly in the carriage of _____ from the lungs to body tissues, and indirectly in the carriage of _____ from the tissues to the lungs.

7. The protein-iron complex which occurs in the plasma and provides for the transport of iron in the body is:
   a. hemosiderin
   b. transferrin
   c. ferritin

8. Where in the body does the greatest absorption of soluble iron occur? Why?

9. Achlorhydria is an absence of hydrochloric acid from gastric juice. Would you expect this condition to favor or inhibit iron absorption?

10. In which body state does the greatest percentage of iron absorption occur:
    a. normal
    b. iron overload
    c. iron deficiency

11. The greater the ferritin content of the mucosal cell, the (greater/lesser) the iron absorption.

12. In the normal adult not experiencing growth states, the dietary intake needs actually equal the daily _____ amounts of iron.

13. Generally, about ten percent of the iron in a mixed diet is absorbed. If a woman has an intake of 18 mg of iron in a day, what is the amount of iron she probably absorbs?

14. Which of the following enhance iron absorption:
    a. diarrhea
    b. ascorbic acid
    c. calcium
    d. hydrochloric acid
    e. severe infection
    f. iron deficiency anemia
    g. phytic and oxalic acids
    h. presence of heme iron and "meat factor"

15. Menstruation (increases/decreases) the need for iron by women.

16. Refer to Table 12-2, the iron content of selected foods.
    a. Which is the best source of iron, fresh or dried fruits?
    b. Which food listed gives the greatest amount of iron per 100 grams?
    c. Are cereals and whole wheat bread relatively good sources of iron?
    d. What might render the cereals and whole wheat breads less satisfactory as iron sources?
    e. Are legumes (beans, peas) relatively good sources of iron?
    f. Is milk a good source of iron?

17. If milk (cow and human) is a poor source of iron, and there are limited reserves of iron storage in an infant's body, what are the implications for meeting infant needs for dietary iron?

18. Joey is two years old. Joey's mother makes sure that Joey drinks eight ounces (one glass) of milk at each meal. His mother feels he must be getting very nutritious meals which should maintain his good health. However, Joey's pediatrician says he is anemic. What can you conclude about Joey's eating habits? What are some things that you can suggest to his mother to help her to get him to meet his calcium and iron needs for each day?

19. a. Hypochromic microcytic anemia results in what type of red blood cells?
    b. The size and color of these blood cells indicates (increased/decreased) hemoglobin content.
    c. This results in (increased/decreased) oxygen carrying capacity of the red blood cells.

20. Hemolytic anemia results in great destruction of the red blood cells. Refer to Figure 12-4 showing the iron cycle of the body. How could the destruction of a large number of red blood cells lead to hemosiderosis, a disorder of iron metabolism in which large deposits of iron are made in the liver?

21. In previous years cooking pots were commonly made of iron. Would you expect the use of iron cooking utensils to increase the iron content of the foods prepared in them?

22. Match the phrases on the right to the terms on the left which they best describe:
    _____ 1. apoferritin
    _____ 2. reticuloendothelial system
    _____ 3. hemoglobin
    _____ 4. myoglobin
    _____ 5. functioning iron
    _____ 6. ferrous (Fe^{++})
    _____ 7. hemosiderosis

    a. iron-protein complex in the muscle
    b. the protein in mucosal cells which complexes with excess iron from intestines
    c. excessive iron storage in liver due to iron overload or hemolytic anemia
    d. special cells of the liver, spleen, and bone marrow for dismantling old, red blood cells
    e. most of the iron in the body
    f. reduced iron in the form needed for optimum body absorption
    g. iron-containing protein of red blood cells

23. Review Table 12-2, the iron content of foods chart, and the list of food sources high in copper. Are many of the best sources of these two minerals the same?

24. In some areas the use of copper cooking utensils increases the copper intake of the population. Would you expect the use of copper pipes in water systems to provide a source of copper in the diet?

25. Fecal loss of copper and iron represents the (absorbed/unabsorbed) dietary copper and iron.

26. Copper is essential, along with iron, for the formation of hemoglobin. Therefore, copper has a role in the prevention of some types of anemia.
   a. True
   b. False

27. A dietary deficiency of copper is not likely because _____ .

28. The theory associating the zinc:copper ratio to the incidence of cardiovascular disease is based upon a:
   a. correlation of low copper levels with increased cholesterol levels.
   b. positive correlation of high zinc levels to low copper levels with the incidence of cardiovascular disease.
   c. correlation of low zinc/high copper ratio with the incidence of cardiovascular disease.

29. Copper is necessary for the proper absorption and utilization of iron as well as for reactions involving energy production.
   a. True
   b. False

30. Which of the following conditions might be related to copper deficiency:
   a. certain nervous disorders
   b. reduced eye vision
   c. fragility of bones
   d. altered senses of taste and smell
   e. altered enzyme activity in metabolism

Answers: Iron and Copper

1. a. Ferrous
   b. Fe^{++}
   c. cation
2. b
3. four
4. hemoglobin
5. red blood cell (erythron)
6. oxygen; carbon dioxide
7. b
8. in the upper duodenum because of its acid pH which favors iron absorption
9. inhibit
10. c
11. lesser
12. excretion
13. 1.8 mg
14. b, c, d, f, h
15. increases

16. a. dried
    b. liver
    c. yes
    d. the presence of binding agents such as phosphates and phytic acid as well as fiber
    e. yes
    f. no
17. Infant diets must be fortified with iron supplements about 3-4 months of age and, later, with iron-fortified cereals.
18. Milk offered to Joey at the beginning of a meal depresses his appetite so that he consumes only small amounts of solid food, which are not providing adequate amounts of iron. His mother can serve milk in solid food forms such as casseroles and puddings; serve milk as a refreshing drink and snack between meals; serve vegetables high in calcium and iron; serve dried fruits as snack foods to Joey; and serve organ meats, especially liver, to him.
19. a. red blood cells that are small in size and pale in color
    b. decreased
    c. decreased
20. Almost all the iron in the body is recycled. When the red blood cells are destroyed more quickly than new red blood cells are formed, the excess iron is stored in muscle and liver tissue.
21. yes
22. 1. b
    2. d
    3. g
    4. a
    5. e
    6. f
    7. c
23. yes
24. yes
25. unabsorbed
26. a
27. copper is present in varying amounts in a wide variety of foods.
28. a, b
29. a
30. a, c, e

IODINE (I)

Iodine is present in every living cell of the body. However, this essential trace mineral is present in the body by weight in very small amounts, approximately 25 to 50 mg. About three-fourths (75%) of the body's iodine is concentrated in the thyroid gland. Dietary iodine is absorbed into the bloodstream where about one-third of it is captured by the thyroid gland. The excess is taken up by the kidney and excreted in the urine.

The only known function of iodine is as a component of the thyroid hormones, thyroxine and triiodothyroxine. Thyroxine, with iodine as a necessary component, functions as a regulator of the growth and development of the body and its rate of metabolism. The stimulating effect of thyroxine on metabolism is appreciable. It is because thyroxine increases the rate of the body's biochemical reactions that it causes an increase in total body oxygen utilization and metabolic rate.

The adult RDA for iodine is only 150μg (micrograms). Both food and water provide iodine in the human diet. The amount of iodine in water generally parallels that of the soil of the same area from which it is obtained. Because of the presence of iodine in seawater, fish and other seafoods are good sources of iodine. Seaweed is able to concentrate iodine from seawater and provides a rich source of iodine for such countries as Japan where seaweed is a major dietary item. The iodine content of vegetables varies with the soil in which they were grown. The leaves of plants generally provide the highest iodine content. Corn is especially low in iodine content.

The use of iodized salt supplies a regular source of dietary iodine and has been responsible for significantly reducing the incidence of endemic goiter in noncoastal geographic locations. In addition, breads in which iodine-containing dough conditioners are used also contribute significant amounts of iodine to the diet.

Iodine deficiency. Iodine deficiency results in simple or endemic goiter which is characterized by an enlargement of the thyroid gland. Endemic goiter usually occurs in areas where the iodine content of the soil is so low that insufficient iodine is obtained from food and water. Sea water is rich in iodine and inland soils and water are poor in iodine content.

Cretinism. Cretinism is a condition characterized by stunted growth, dwarfism, and varying degrees of mental retardation. Cretinism frequently occurs where the soil is poor in iodine and where iodine deficiency has been prevalent for years accompanied by endemic goiter. Cretinism occurs in the infant who was deprived of iodine as a developing fetus because his or her mother was severely iodine deficient.

Goitrogens. Certain foods contain substances called goitrogens which block the absorption or utilization of iodine. Goitrogens can predispose a person who has marginal iodine intake to the iodine deficiency disease, goiter. Foods of the cabbage family, such as rutabagas, turnips, and cabbage, contain goitrogens which can be inactivated by heat during the cooking process. Refer to the section on goitrogens in Toxicants Occurring Naturally in Foods (Chapter 15) in this text for additional information about goitrogens.

Excess iodine intake. Iodine is one of the nutrients that produces similar symptoms in man if the dietary intake is deficient or excessive. Enlargement and hyperactivity of the thyroid gland occurs as a reaction to excessive intake of iodine and results in a condition termed "iodide goiter."

In the U.S. many processed foods contain additives which have iodine as a constituent. Also, dairy cattle are often fed iodine-supplemented feed or iodized salt which results in a production of milk with increased iodine content.[8] Because of the greater availability of iodine-containing foods, and the fact that iodine is readily absorbed by man, concern has arisen about possible excessive iodine intake in the U.S.

A recent Market Basket Survey conducted by the FDA found total iodine content of foods comprising a reference intake of 2800 kcal to be four times the U.S. RDA for iodine.[9] Though it considers the present level of iodine consumption in the U.S. to be safe, the Food and Nutrition Board has recommended that iodine-containing food additives be replaced where possible by iodine-free compounds as a precautionary measure against the possible excessive intake of iodine.[10]

FLUORINE (F)

Fluorine[11] is accepted as a required mineral nutrient due to its now well-established protective effect against dental caries. The effect of fluoridation of the water supply on the dental health of children in various communities has been studied. These studies showed an observed reduction of 50 to 70 percent in dental caries. The fluoride ion is incorporated into the crystalline structure of hydroxyapatite in teeth which increases the caries resistance of the teeth. Fluoroxyapatite appears to increase tooth enamel hardness and decrease enamel solubility. Fluoroxyapatite in bones also seems to reduce resorption of bone and to decrease the incidence of osteoporosis in older persons.

The homeostatic mechanism that helps to maintain blood levels of fluorine at a constant level is, in part, due to the increased excretion of fluorine with urine. In this way uptake of fluorine by the bones is retarded.

When fluorine is added to the community water supplies it is added at a rate of 1 ppm (1 part per million or 1 mg/liter). The 1980 RDA gives an estimated safe and adequate daily dietary intake range for fluorine as 1.5 to 4.0 mg for adults. This range is safely maintained when public drinking water is fluoridated to recommended amounts.[12] Notable food sources other than fluoridated water are tea and seafood. Fluorine is found in all foods though perhaps only in trace amounts.

Excess fluoride intake. Excessive fluoride intake can result in the mottled staining of the teeth evidenced by dull and unglazed areas to deep brown stains in other areas. Sometimes excessive fluoride intake can cause the development of osteosclerosis, abnormal density of the skeletal bone. Evidence of dental fluorosis (mottling) does not generally occur unless the fluorine content of water rises above 2 ppm.

SELENIUM (Se)

Selenium is part of the enzyme glutathione peroxidase which protects cells and membranes against oxidative damage. Selenium appears to work together with vitamin E in some antioxidant capacity, though this association is not yet well understood. Selenium, along with vitamin E, may also provide some protection against the toxicity of some heavy metals such as cadmium and mercury.[13]

Selenium daily intake is recommended to range between .05 to 0.2 mg for adults. Some probable toxic results from increased intakes of selenium include antagonism of sulfur metabolism, inhibition of certain enzymes, and interference with normal embryonic development. An association between increased intake of selenium and an increased incidence of dental caries has been noted.

The amount of selenium in food is a function of the amount of selenium in the soil in which it is grown. Seafoods, organ meats, meat, milk, and grains are the main sources of dietary selenium.

Children with kwashiorkor have lowered selenium levels which may indicate that selenium deficiency occurs in protein-calorie malnutrition.

MANGANESE (Mn)

Manganese has not been demonstrated as an essential nutrient in man. However, on the basis of its requirement by other mammals it is accepted as essential for man. Manganese appears to be necessary for bone growth and development, reproduction, and for the formation of mucopolysaccharides. The chief function of manganese appears to be as an enzyme activator in reactions necessary for urea formation and metabolism of protein, fat, and carbohydrate.

The recommended daily intake range for manganese is between 2.5 to 5 mg for adults. Good sources of manganese include nuts, legumes, tea, coffee, and unrefined grains. No deficiency has been demonstrated in humans.

ZINC (Zn)

Zinc functions both as a component of and an activator of enzymes necessary to many biological functions; zinc is necessary for protein synthesis; appears to be necessary to nucleic acid metabolism though its role is not well-defined; and is a component of the hormone insulin though insulin's biological activity may not depend upon zinc as a constituent.

The 1980 revised RDA now includes zinc with an adult RDA of 15 mg. The best sources of zinc are shellfish (especially oysters), dairy products, eggs, legumes, and whole grain cereals.[14] Because zinc's utilization is reduced by phytic acid and fiber, the availability of zinc is greater from animal protein. It has been suggested that the diets of poverty groups, which are low in animal products and high in cereals and other vegetable foods, may be marginal in zinc. In fact, for a vegetarian who consumes no animal derived foods, the RDA for zinc may be insufficient.[15]

Yeast fermentation during the bread-making process destroys some phytate and increases the zinc availability from whole wheat grain/bread products.[16] Indeed, zinc deficiency has been noted in countries such as Egypt and Iran where the consumption of unleavened bread is customary.[17]

The most distinct consequence of zinc deficiency is a reduction of the growth rate. Hypogeusia and hyposmia (impairment of taste and smell acuity, respectively) are in some circumstances responsive to increased zinc uptake. Some of the major features of human

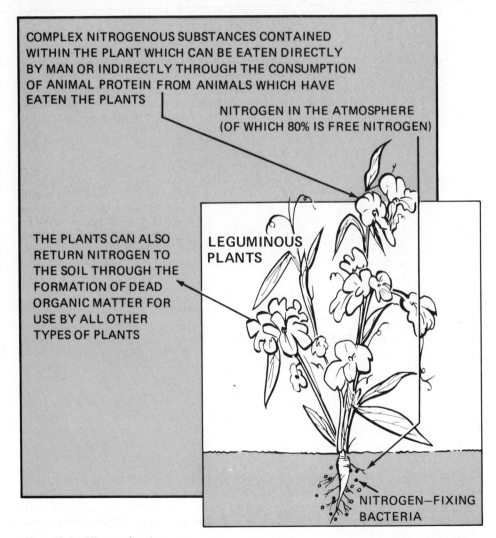

COMPLEX NITROGENOUS SUBSTANCES CONTAINED WITHIN THE PLANT WHICH CAN BE EATEN DIRECTLY BY MAN OR INDIRECTLY THROUGH THE CONSUMPTION OF ANIMAL PROTEIN FROM ANIMALS WHICH HAVE EATEN THE PLANTS

NITROGEN IN THE ATMOSPHERE (OF WHICH 80% IS FREE NITROGEN)

THE PLANTS CAN ALSO RETURN NITROGEN TO THE SOIL THROUGH THE FORMATION OF DEAD ORGANIC MATTER FOR USE BY ALL OTHER TYPES OF PLANTS

LEGUMINOUS PLANTS

NITROGEN—FIXING BACTERIA

Figure 12-6.   Nitrogen fixation.

zinc deficiency are: growth retardation and loss of appetite, delayed wound healing, hypogonadism (retardation of sexual development), flat or delayed rise in the oral glucose tolerance test, skin lesions or changes, decreased taste acuity, and response to zinc therapy and an adequate diet.

MOLYBDENUM (Mo)

Molybdenum is essential for all nitrogen-fixing bacteria. These bacteria convert atmospheric nitrogen into organic nitrogen-containing compounds which are taken up by plants, especially legumes. Nitrogen is an essential component of protein. By making nitrogen available for human consumption and utilization, molybdenum ultimately affects the synthesis of protein.

Molybdenum competes with copper for metabolic sites and even small increases in molybdenum increase loss of copper by way of urine. High sulfate intake both decreases absorption and increases the excretion of molybdenum. Molybdenum is present in body tissues in extremely low concentrations even though dietary molybdenum is readily absorbed. The enzyme xanthine oxidase and certain flavoproteins contain molybdenum. Xanthine oxidase is an enzyme that oxidizes xanthine, an intermediate product of nucleic acid metabolism, to uric acid.

Recommended daily intake ranges between 0.15 to 0.5 mg to provide adequate intake and to avoid toxicity. Legumes, whole grains, and organ meats are good sources of molybdenum.

CHROMIUM (Cr)

The total body content of chromium is small, less than 6 mg. Tissue levels are measured in parts per billion (ppb). Generally, chromium is poorly absorbed.

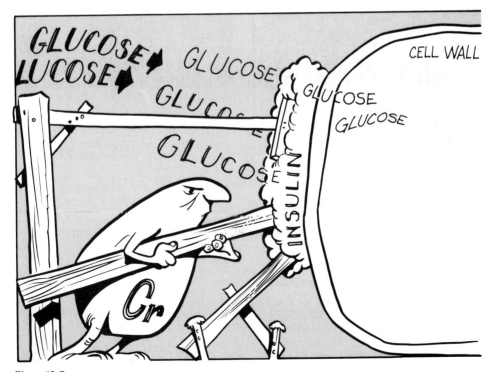

Figure 12-7.

Chromium is associated with a decrease in glucose tolerance. The usable form of chromium (Cr^{+++}) occurs in an organic complex known as the Glucose Tolerance Factor. It is thought that chromium acts to bind insulin to the receptor site on the cell wall. Insulin acts to influence the uptake of glucose by the body cell.

The amount of chromium in tissues decreases with age. This fact, along with the association of chromium deficiency with abnormal glucose tolerance tests,[18] has led some investigators to believe that chromium deficiency is related to maturity-onset diabetes. The recommended daily chromium intake ranges between 0.15 to 0.2 mg for adults. The best food sources are egg yolk, meats, brewers yeast, cheeses, beer, and whole grains.

COBALT (Co)

The only known function of cobalt in human nutrition is its necessary incorporation into vitamin B_{12}, cobalamin, which plays a vital role in red blood cell formation. A deficiency of cobalt in animal feed results in a deficient production of vitamin B_{12}. Cobalt must be obtained in the preformed vitamin B_{12} since human tissues cannot synthesize this vitamin. Vitamin B_{12} is obtained from animal food sources such as liver, muscle meat, fish, eggs, and dairy products.

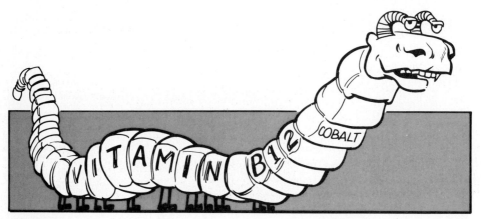

Figure 12-8.

Key Points: Iodine, Fluorine, Selenium, Manganese, Zinc, Molybdenum, Chromium, and Cobalt

I. Iodine is a necessary component of thyroxine, the hormone produced by the thyroid gland which has a stimulating effect on the body's metabolic rate.

II. Iodine content of food and water reflect the iodine content of the soils from which they are obtained; coastal soils are generally high in iodine content because of the iodine in seawater; inland soils are generally poor in iodine content.

III. The use of iodized salt supplies a regular source of iodine and is largely responsible for the decreased incidence of goiter, the iodine deficiency condition, in noncoastal areas.

IV. Iodine absorption and utilization is decreased by goitrogens found in food.

V. Increased iodine intake in the U.S. is primarily due to the increased use of iodine-containing food additives and livestock feed.

VI. Scientific tests have established the protective effect fluorine exerts against dental caries.

VII. Fluorine added to public drinking water supplies at the rate of 1 mg/liter (1 ppm) is safe for consumption, adequate to provide dental protection, and low enough to avoid the mottling of teeth.

VIII. Selenium, perhaps in association with vitamin E, protects cells and membranes of the body against oxidative damage.

IX. Animal protein foods are the best dietary sources of selenium.

X. Zinc functions both as a component and activator of various enzymes; is important for protein synthesis; and is a constituent of other body compounds including insulin.

XI. Molybdenum ultimately affects protein synthesis through its role as a required substance by nitrogen-fixing bacteria which convert atmospheric nitrogen into organic nitrogen-containing compounds.

XII. Chromium contained within an organic compound termed the Glucose Tolerance Factor enhances the action of insulin to effect the cellular uptake of glucose.

XIII. Cobalt is a vital component of vitamin B_{12}. However, vitamin B_{12} must be obtained preformed in the diet since the body cannot manufacture it.

Questions: *Iodine, Fluorine, Selenium, Manganese, Zinc, Molybdenum, Chromium, and Cobalt*

1. Where does the greatest concentration of iodine occur in the human body?

2. Which organ in the human body provides protection against the accumulation of toxic levels of iodine in tissues other than the thyroid gland?

3. The thyroid gland is normally the size of a lima bean. A disease of iodine deficiency characterized by a greatly enlarged thyroid gland weighing 1 to 1½ and more pounds is (goiter/cretinism).

4. Severe restriction of iodine intake during pregnancy and early childhood, or long-term iodine deficiency in an iodine-poor area where goiter is endemic, can produce a condition of severe mental retardation accompanied by dwarfism. This condition is (goiter/cretinism).

5. What is the most influential factor regarding the amount of iodine content in vegetables?

6. Iodine requirements are measured in:
   a. milligrams
   b. grams
   c. micrograms

7. What are some of the factors contributing to increased iodine intake in the U.S.?

8. Match the phrases on the right to the words on the left which they best describe:

   _____ 1. coastal areas
   _____ 2. table salt
   _____ 3. goitrogen
   _____ 4. thyroxine
   _____ 5. mountains and plains

   a. iodine-containing hormone of the body which speeds up the metabolic rate of the body
   b. generally having soils low in iodine content
   c. generally having soils high in iodine content
   d. food which is iodized to provide a reliable source of iodine
   e. substance interfering with iodine absorption, uptake, or utilization

9. When consumed in minute amounts this trace mineral provides protection against dental caries:
    a. iodine
    b. fluorine
    c. selenium

10. In the consideration of dental caries, this mineral consumed in minute amounts provides protection against dental caries: _____ ; and, this mineral taken in excess may predispose a person towards the development of dental caries: _____ .

11. Match the phrases on the right to the items on the left which they best describe:
    _____ 1. fluoroxyapatite   a. a mottled staining of teeth
    _____ 2. seafood and tea   b. development of abnormal density of
    _____ 3. dental fluorosis   skeletal bone
    _____ 4. osteosclerosis   c. increases tooth enamel hardness and
    _____ 5. urine   decreases enamel solubility
                                     d. substance in which excess fluorine is
                                         excreted from the body
                                     e. notable dietary sources of fluorine

12. The amount in which fluorine can be safely added to the community water supply is 1 mg/liter or:
    a. 1 ppm
    b. 2 ppm
    c. 4 ppm

13. Since the main sources for selenium are protein foods, especially those of animal origin, selenium deficiency may occur as a deficiency and complicating factor in kwashiorkor. Kwashiorkor is a deficiency disease due to _____ .

14. This mineral somehow works in conjunction with vitamin E to prevent oxidative damage to various membranes and compounds.
    a. chromium
    b. zinc
    c. selenium

15. The central role of manganese is as an enzyme activator for many reactions necessary for normal body metabolism.
    a. True
    b. False

16. Why might vegetarians who eat only plant-derived foods, and other persons whose diet chiefly consists of plant-derived foods, be at an increased risk of consuming diets marginal in zinc content or of developing zinc deficiency?

17. By forming complex nitrogenous substances within leguminous plants, how do nitrogen-fixing bacteria contribute nitrogen to the human diet?

18. a. What type of plants support growth of the nitrogen-fixing bacteria?
    b. How might you deduct that these plants contribute nitrogen necessary for all plant growth?
    c. Molybdenum, then, is a key participant in the ultimate formation of _____ .

19. Xanthines are chemical derivatives from the metabolism of nucleic acids RNA and DNA. Xanthine oxidase is an enzyme that oxidizes xanthines to uric acid which is excreted from the body in urine. Which is the mineral contained in the enzyme xanthine oxidase?

20. Match the phrases on the right to the terms on the left which they best describe:

_____ 1. zinc
_____ 2. cobalt
_____ 3. manganese
_____ 4. selenium
_____ 5. molybdenum
_____ 6. chromium

    a.   mineral that is part of the enzyme glutathione peroxidase which protects cells against oxidative damage

    b.   mineral necessary for growth, reproduction, and enzymes involved in urea formation and energy nutrient metabolism

    c.   mineral whose deficiency causes retarded growth and sexual development, delayed wound healing, and skin changes

    d.   mineral which is necessary for all nitrogen-fixing bacteria

    e.   mineral present in the Glucose Tolerance Factor whose deficiency causes an abnormal glucose tolerance test

    f.   mineral which is an integral part of vitamin B_{12}

21. Chromium somehow makes the action of insulin more effective in increasing cellular permeability to glucose.
    a. True
    b. False

22. Vitamin B_{12} is necessary to prevent:
    a. nutritional anemia
    b. sickle cell anemia
    c. pernicious anemia

23. What are the advantages of consuming cobalt in its free state?

Answers: *Iodine, Fluorine, Selenium, Manganese, Zinc, Molybdenum, Chromium, and Cobalt*

1. in the thyroid gland
2. the kidneys
3. goiter
4. cretinism
5. the level of iodine in the soil in which they were grown.
6. c
7. iodine is readily absorbed by man; increased use of livestock feed containing iodine; increased use of iodine-containing food additives
8. 1. c
   2. d
   3. e
   4. a
   5. b
9. b
10. fluorine; selenium

11. 1. c
     2. e
     3. a
     4. b
     5. d
12. a
13. protein deficiency
14. c
15. a
16. Because of the high content of phytate and fiber in plant-based diets which decrease absorption and the utilization of dietary zinc.
17. Man obtains the nitrogen directly by eating the plants or indirectly by consuming the animal protein of animals which have eaten the plants.
18. a. legumes
     b. By being returned to the soil as organic matter which is decomposed and contributes nitrogenous compounds to the soil, which can be used by all other types of plants.
     c. protein
19. molybdenum
20. 1. c
     2. f
     3. b
     4. a
     5. d
     6. e
21. a
22. c
23. None, since human tissues cannot synthesize vitamin B_{12}, the only known need for cobalt.

REFERENCES

[1] Nonheme iron is iron obtained from sources other than hemoglobin and myoglobin. Heme, however, is iron contained in hemoglobin and myoglobin and obtained in the diet from those two sources.

[2] Finch CA: Iron metabolism. Nutrition Today, 4, Summer 1969, p. 5

[3] **Hemolytic anemia** results from the excessive destruction of red blood cells.

[4] Mertz M: Mineral elements: New perspectives. Journal of the American Dietetic Association, 77, September 1980, p. 261

[5] O'Dell BL: Copper. In Present Knowledge in Nutrition, 4th ed. New York and Washington, D.C.; The Nutrition Foundation, Inc., 1976, p. 307

[6] Recommended Dietary Allowances, Ninth Revised Edition. Food and Nutrition Board, National Academy of Sciences-National Research Council, Washington, D.C., 1980, p. 151

[7] Forbush J: Copper and coronaries: The hidden risk factor. CNI Weekly Report (Consumer Nutrition Institute), 5, December 18, 1975; pp. 4-5

[8] A good review on iodine and a discussion of the merits of iodized salt can be found in: Cullen RW and Oace SM: Iodine: Current status. Journal of Nutrition Education, 8, July-September 1976, pp. 101-102

[9] Harland BF et al: Calcium, phosphorus, iron, iodine, and zinc in the total diet. Journal of the American Dietetic Association, 77 July 1980, p. 20

[10] Recommended Dietary Allowances, Ninth Revised Edition. Food and Nutrition Board, National Academy of Sciences-National Research Council, Washington, D.C., 1980, p. 150

[11] Fluorine is used to designate elemental fluorine; fluoride designates the fluoride ion. Both terms are used interchangeably.

[12] Refer to the section in this text on dental health in Chapter Three, Carbohydrates, for references to interesting articles which address the fluoridation of public water controversy.

[13] Suitor CW and Hunter MF: Nutrition: Principles and Application in Health Promotion. Philadelphia, J. B. Lippincott Company, 1980, pp. 169-170

[14] Willis BW and Mangubat AP: Zinc in foods. Family Economics Review, Spring 1975, pp. 16-17

[15] Mertz W: Mineral elements: New perspectives. Journal of the American Dietetic Association, 77, September 1980, p. 259

[16] Position Paper on the Vegetarian Approach to Eating. Journal of the American Dietetic Association, 77, July 1980, p. 65

[17] Sanstead HH et al: Current concepts on trace minerals: Clinical considerations. Medical Clinics of North America, 54, November 1970, pp. 1514-1520

[18] Refer to the section on Blood Glucose Levels in Chapter Three, Carbohydrates, for information on the glucose tolerance test.

13
WATER AND ELECTROLYTES

The storage capacity for the different nutrients varies. Carbohydrate (glycogen) can be stored to a limited capacity in the human body. When its stores are depleted, both fats and proteins can fulfill the important energy production function of carbohydrates. Fat can be stored in adipose tissue in unlimited amounts providing a long term concentrated source of energy for the body. Though the supply of amino acids available from the metabolic pool is limited, lean body tissue can be broken down to provide required amino acids for essential body functions during periods of restricted protein intake. Many vitamins and minerals can be stored in appreciable amounts in the body; it may take from days to years for deficiency symptoms from a lack of these nutrients to appear.

However, the body can only survive for a few days in the absence of water intake. Water provides the environment necessary for each living cell to carry out its essential functions. Water is also a participant in some of the chemical reactions necessary to the life of each cell. We frequently take water for granted until we are faced with the need to obtain uncontaminated water during unexpected periods of short supply.

Body water distribution. Water is divided into two general body locations: inside the body cells *(intracellular fluid—*ICF), and outside the body cells *(extracellular fluid—*ECF). Intracellular fluid (ICF) accounts for the largest percentage of body water volume. All cells contain water: those of hard tissues such as bones and teeth as well as those of soft tissue such as muscle. However, the amount of water in various cells differs.

Extracellular fluid (ECF) encompasses fluid in several different locations:

1. Plasma is the fluid within the heart and blood vessels.[1] Though more apparent than other body water, plasma fluid provides only a small percentage of body water volume.

2. Interstitial fluid is the fluid which surrounds the outside of the cells. It provides the medium for transfer of substances into and out of cells. Interstitial fluid is in a state of constant exchange with the vascular fluid of the blood and lymph systems, and it is held in balance with vascular fluid by numerous interacting factors.

3. Extracellular fluid is also found in secretions of the various glands, gastrointestinal tract, and mucous membranes as well as in the cerebral spinal fluid and eye space fluid.

Muscle tissue is relatively high in water content while adipose (fat) tissue is relatively low in water content. Approximately 65 percent of the weight of an adult man is due to water. The percentage of water in an adult woman is less because of the normal increase in fat to muscle ratio in women compared to men. Due to the difference in water content of muscle and adipose tissues, the normal percentage of body water varies within men and women according to the amount of body fat they have. Obesity results in a lowered percentage of total body weight provided by body water. Older persons normally experience a decrease

251

in total body water content. On the other hand, an infant has a high percentage of total body weight contributed by body water.

Water regulation. Daily water intake and water excretion are regulated to maintain a close balance. There are often slight imbalances which occur. However, these imbalances are generally corrected within a few days. Under normal circumstances about 2½ liters of water are taken in and excreted daily by the body.

WATER BALANCE

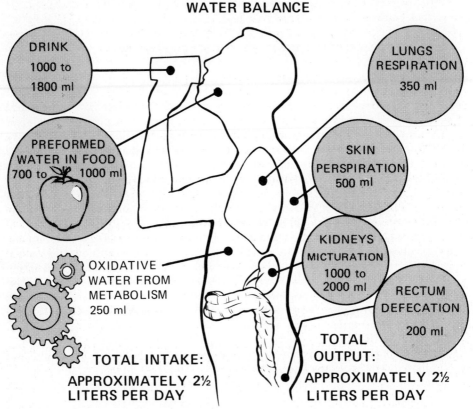

DRINK
1000 to
1800 ml

LUNGS
RESPIRATION
350 ml

PREFORMED
WATER IN FOOD
700 to   1000 ml

SKIN
PERSPIRATION
500 ml

OXIDATIVE
WATER FROM
METABOLISM
250 ml

KIDNEYS
MICTURATION
1000 to
2000 ml

RECTUM
DEFECATION
200 ml

TOTAL INTAKE:
APPROXIMATELY 2½
LITERS PER DAY

TOTAL
OUTPUT:
APPROXIMATELY 2½
LITERS PER DAY

Figure 13-1.   Daily water balance according to water intake and excretion showing sources, location, and approximate amounts.

There are times when conditions such as heavy perspiring and compensatory intake will increase normal total excretion/intake amounts. There are also times of decreased excretion and intake which lower normal total excretion/intake amounts. The minimum urine volume necessary to excrete body waste products varies according to different expert nutrition sources. However, a minimum urine excretion between 600 to 900 mL (approximately ¾ to 1 liter) seems necessary. Consumption of extra water helps to flush out waste products contained in urine with greater ease and provides for greater dilution of toxic products. Water drawn into feces also helps to facilitate elimination.

Functions of body water. Water is necessary for the processes of body metabolism. *By providing the medium into which participants of the various chemical reactions of metabolism are dissolved, water enables the chemical reactions to take place. Water is also a participant in the chemical reactions involving energy production and synthesis of carbohydrates, lipids, and protein.* (Refer to the condensation reactions involving these nutrients in Chapters Three, Four, and Five.)

Water is also necessary for the digestion of food. Mechanically, water is necessary for saliva production, for the mixing of intestinal contents, for the passage of intestinal contents, and the flow of digestive juices. Chemically, water participates in the breaking down of carbohydrates, fats, and protein during digestion. (Refer to the hydrolysis reactions described in Chapters Three, Four, and Five involving carbohydrates, fats, and proteins.) The total amount of gastrointestinal fluid involved in digestion and absorption is variously estimated between 7,500 to 10,000 mL daily.[2] As you can deduce by examining the amount of water excreted in feces in Figure 13-1 most of this gastrointestinal fluid is reabsorbed.

One of the most obvious functions of body water is the transportation it provides for all the various body nutrients and metabolic products within the blood system, the lymph system, and the interstitial fluid. Transportation of waste products out of the body is also accomplished by body water in urine and feces as well as by water in the mucous membranes of the gastrointestinal tract.

Water in the mucous secretions throughout the body, in tears, in saliva, and water surrounding body joints all perform an important lubrication function. Water is very important in the regulation of body temperature. Cooling is accomplished by the evaporation of water from the lungs and skin.[3] Warming is accomplished, in part, by body water absorbing the heat released from energy production reactions within the cells and carrying this heat throughout the body, just as the heated water in an ordinary household radiator circulates warmth to the different rooms of a home.

Electrolytes. An electrolyte is any substance that dissociates into its component ions when dissolved in water. Ions are charged particles. Cations are ions with a positive charge; anions are ions with a negative charge. The different electrolytes vary widely in their percentage of dissociation. Strong electrolytes are those which have a high percentage of dissociation.

An atom is the smallest particle of an element which retains the characteristics of that element. Atoms have a nucleus consisting of protons which are positively charged particles, and neutrons which are neutral particles. Electrons which are negatively charged particles circulate around the nucleus. The number of electrons in an atom equals the number of protons in the nucleus. Their respective negative and positive charges are equal. However, an electron (or electrons) can be separated from an atom leaving the atom with a total +1 charge (or more if more electrons are involved). *Each electron* which joins another

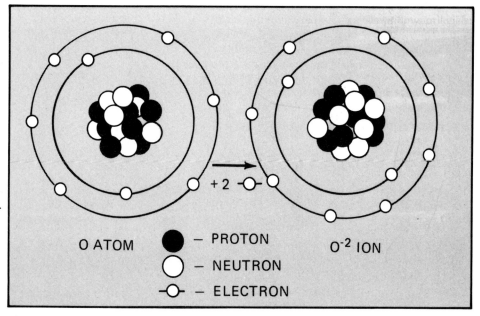

O ATOM   ● — PROTON   O⁻² ION
           ○ — NEUTRON
          –○– — ELECTRON

Figure 13-2.   Formation of the negatively charged oxygen ion.

atom causes that atom to take on a -1 charge. These are the charged atoms referred to as ions. An ion can also be composed of several atoms in an associated group which collectively have a net charge such as the hydroxide ion (OH^-).

Electrolytes are so named because when they dissociate into ions in solution the solution is capable of conducting an electric current. *An important concept to remember is that electrolytic solutions are always balanced in their total number of positive and negative charges.* In other words, the solutions are balanced according to the chemical combining abilities of their solute particles.

Electrolytes are extremely important to the regulation of water balance between the intracellular and extracellular fluids. Electrolytes are solutes in these two fluids and help to control water balance between them through their influence on osmotic action (see below for an explanation of osmosis). The electrolytes of the extracellular and intracellular fluids are divided as follows:

Extracellular fluid:
Cations:
    Sodium ion (Na^+)} largest amount

    Potassium (K^+)
    Calcium (Ca^{++}) } collectively, a small amount
    Magnesium (Mg^{++})
Anions:
    Chloride (Cl^-)} largest amount

    Bicarbonate ions (HCO_3^-)
    Phosphate ions ($HPO_4^=$)
    Sulfate ions ($SO_4^=$) } collectively, variable small amounts
    Organic acids
    Protein
Intracellular fluid:

Cations:
    Potassium (K^+)} largest amount

    Magnesium (Mg^{++})
    Sodium (Na^+) } collectively, a small amount
    Calcium (Ca^{++})
Anions:
    Phosphate (HPO_4^-)} largest amount

    Bicarbonate ions (HCO_3^-)
    Chloride (Cl^-) } collectively, small variable amounts
    Sulfate ions ($SO_4^=$)
    Proteins

Mechanism for control of water balance between cellular membranes. A dissolved substance spreads from an area of high concentration to that of lesser concentration leading to its uniform distribution throughout a solution. This can even occur between fluids separated by membranes such as cellular membranes. This solute movement is called *diffusion.* See Figure 13-4.

The cell membrane is a semi-permeable membrane which means it does not allow the free transport of all substances through it. Thus, the cell membrane is selectively perme-

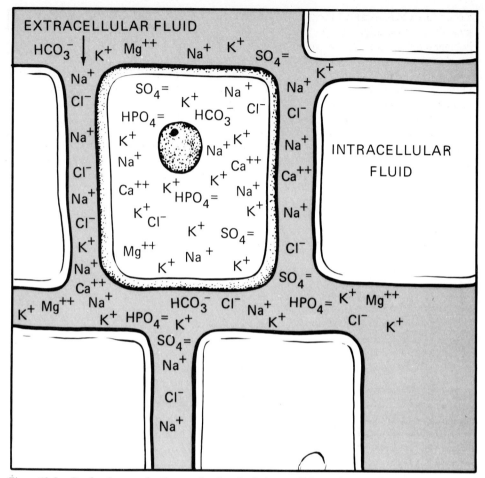

Figure 13-3.   Predominance of cations and anions in the intracellular and extracellular fluids.

able. Water can freely cross through the cell membrane. Potassium and sodium do not pass across the cell membrane by diffusion alone but seem to require a pump system.[4] The pump consists of proteins capable of selectively transporting potassium and sodium across the cellular membrane. Such a pump system is termed *active transport*.

The concentration of solutes on opposite sides of the semi-permeable cellular membrane exert respective pressures. The difference between the pressures created is called the *osmotic pressure*. The more concentrated solution exerts a greater pulling force on the water on the other side of the cell membrane. Consequently, water flows across the membrane until the concentration of solutes on either side of the membrane equalizes. This flow of water through a semi-permeable membrane is termed *osmosis*. Therefore, it is the regulation of electrolyte concentration, intracellularly and extracellularly, which largely determines water flow into or out of cells. See Figure 13-5.

Hormonal influence on water and electrolyte balance. There are two major hormonal systems which operate to regulate body water. Though they both accomplish water control they differ in their means.

1.   The antidiuretic hormone (ADH) secreted by the posterior lobe of the pituitary gland signals the distal collecting tubules of the kidneys to increase water reab-

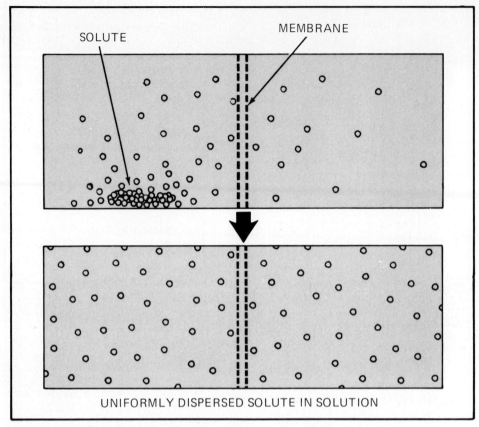

Figure 13-4.   Uniform distribution of a solute within a solution and even across a membrane after the passage of sufficient time by diffusion.

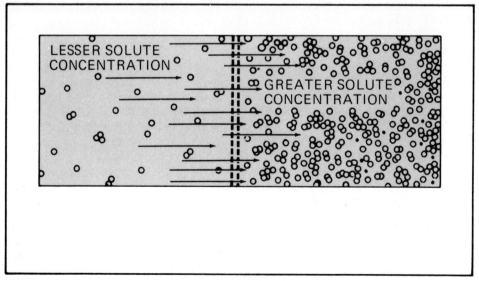

*Figure 13-5.   **Osmosis** is the movement of water across a semipermeable membrane from an area of lesser solute concentration to an area of greater solute concentration.*

sorption during periods of perceived diminished blood volume.[5]

2. Aldosterone secreted by the adrenal cortex stimulates the reabsorption of sodium in the distal tubules of the nephrons. The hormone aldosterone is produced as a result of a complicated series of reactions. Refer to Figure 13-6.

Fluid and electrolyte imbalance. Imbalances can occur for a variety of reasons. Increased water and electrolyte losses occur from prolonged vomiting, diarrhea, fever of extended duration, burns, and excessive perspiration. Hemorrhage decreases total blood volume and, therefore, body water. Intake of water to replace these losses needs to be accompanied by electrolyte replacement as well.

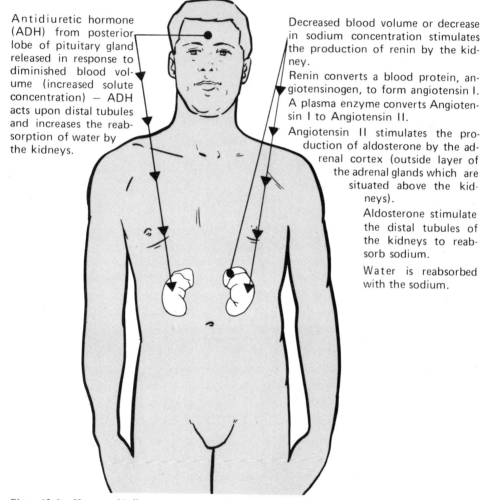

Antidiuretic hormone (ADH) from posterior lobe of pituitary gland released in response to diminished blood volume (increased solute concentration) — ADH acts upon distal tubules and increases the reabsorption of water by the kidneys.

Decreased blood volume or decrease in sodium concentration stimulates the production of renin by the kidney.

Renin converts a blood protein, angiotensinogen, to form angiotensin I. A plasma enzyme converts Angiotensin I to Angiotensin II.

Angiotensin II stimulates the production of aldosterone by the adrenal cortex (outside layer of the adrenal glands which are situated above the kidneys).

Aldosterone stimulate the distal tubules of the kidneys to reabsorb sodium.

Water is reabsorbed with the sodium.

Figure 13-6.   Hormonal influence on water and the electrolyte balance.

Temporary retention of body water is no cause for alarm. The body usually corrects these excesses within a few days. When retention of extra water within extracellular and intracellular fluid spaces occurs suddenly, or for a lengthy period of time, edema results. *Edema produces tissue swelling and can tax the effort of the heart in pumping the fluid of the circulatory system.*

Dehydration results in an imbalance involving too great a water loss. Infants are susceptible to dehydration because of their greater percentage of body water as compared to an adult. Fluid replacement is a more immediate need than food intake during periods of infantile diarrhea, vomiting, and fever. Because elderly persons have decreased body water content they, too, are especially vulnerable to the negative effects of dehydration.

Water intake regulation. Body excretions such as saliva contain water. Water travels from areas of lesser solute concentration to areas of greater solute concentration due to osmotic action. Therefore, it is reasonable to conclude that salivary gland secretion is reduced when:

1. The body is dehydrated
2. The blood plasma volume is diminished or its solute concentration is high causing water to be drawn into the circulatory system from other body areas.

These situations do indeed reduce salivary gland secretions which, in turn, produce the feeling of a dry mouth or thirst. This is the body's way of signaling the need for increased water intake.

Also, there are special receptors located in the hypothalamus of the brain which perceive an increase in the concentration of solutes in the blood and initiate a desire to drink.[6] In at least these two ways the body regulates water intake to meet its individual and changing body water needs.

Key Points: Water and Electrolytes

I. The human body can only survive for a few days in the absence of water intake.

II. Body water is contained in two general locations: intracellular fluid (ICF) and extracellular fluid (ECF).

III. All cells contain water: muscle tissue is relatively high in water content; adipose tissue is relatively low in water content.

IV. Total body water is in excess of half of total body weight.

V. Daily water intake and water excretion are closely balanced: approximately 2.5 liters daily.

VI. Body water functions include:
A. Providing the medium in which body chemical reactions take place.
B. Participating in certain body chemical reactions.
C. Enabling the digestion of food.
D. Transporting body nutrients and waste products.
E. Lubricating body tissues and joints.
F. Regulating body temperature.

VII. Electrolytes are substances which dissociate into their component ions when dissolved in water.
A. Ions are charged particles.
B. Cations have a positive charge and anions have a negative charge.
1. Major extracellular cation: Na^+
2. Major intracellular cation: K^+
3. Major extracellular anion: Cl^-
4. Major intracellular anion: $HPO_4^=$
C. Electrolytic solutions are always balanced in their total number of positive and negative charges.

VIII. Control of water balance between cellular membranes is obtained by the following mechanisms through their effects on solute and water flow.
A. Diffusion: solute spreads from an area of high concentration to an area of lesser concentration until uniformity is reached.

B.   Active transport: an energy-requiring pump system for various solutes.

C.   Osmosis: water flow from an area of lesser solute concentration to an area of greater solute concentration.

D.   Hormonal controls
1.   Antidiuretic hormone (ADH): increases water resorption by the kidneys.
2.   Aldosterone: increases resorption of sodium by the kidneys which produces a secondary effect of increasing water retention.

IX.   Loss of large amounts of body water requires replacement of water and electrolytes.

X.   Edema is excessive tissue swelling from water retention.

XI.   Sensation of thirst increases during periods of dehydration due to decreased saliva production and stimulation of the hypothalamus when blood solute concentration increases, blood volume decreases, or extracellular osmotic pressure increases.

Questions: Water and Electrolytes

1.   The nutrient for which we have the most frequent and constant intake need in order to sustain life is _____ .

2.   Most body water is contained within _____ fluid.
a.   intracellular
b.   extracellular

3.   All body cells contain water including those of bones and teeth.
a.   True
b.   False

4.   List the following individuals in declining order according to their body water percentage (that is, from most to least).
a.   an obese middle-age woman
b.   a healthy adult male of "ideal" body weight
c.   a one-month old infant
d.   a healthy adult woman of "ideal" body weight

5.   Extracellular fluid includes: 1. _____ 2. _____
3.   _____.

6.   The more concentrated the urine the greater the work load of the kidneys, and the greater the exposure of the kidneys to toxic substances.
a.   True
b.   False

7.   Water is necessary for the intake, digestion, absorption, and metabolism of food because:
a.   water provides the medium in which the chemicals involved are dissolved and react.
b.   water is a necessary participant in many chemical reactions of digestion, energy production, and synthesis.
c.   water in saliva and gastrointestinal tract secretions facilitate mechanical movement of food from the mouth through the remainder of the gastrointestinal tract, as well as the mechanical breakdown of food and the mixing of gastrointestinal contents.
d.   all of the above.

8.   Most of the gastrointestinal secretions are lost from the body in the elimination of feces.
a.   True
b.   False

9. Identify the following according to whether they contain intracellular (ICF) or extracellular (ECF) fluid.
   a. _____
   b. _____
   c. _____
   d. _____

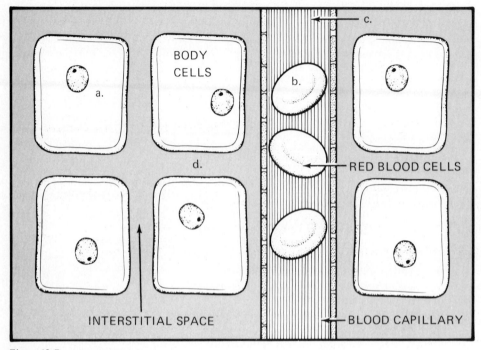

Figure 13-7.

10. Match the items on the right to the terms or symbols on the left which they best describe:

    _____ 1. a proton   a. has a −1 electrical charge
    _____ 2. Na^+ b. an electrolyte
    _____ 3. a neutron   c. an anion
    _____ 4. an electron   d. has no charge
    _____ 5. NaCl   e. balanced in the positive and negative
    _____ 6. OH^- charges of its solute particles
    _____ 7. electrolyte solutions   f. has a +1 electrical charge
           g. a cation

11. Fill in the name of the ion which each phrase best describes:
    a. principle cation of ECF: _____
    b. principle cation of ICF: _____
    c. principle anion of ECF: _____
    d. principle anion of ICF: _____

12. A solute in solution slowly spreads from an area of high concentration to an area of lesser concentration until the solute is uniformly spread throughout the solution. This solute movement is termed _____ .

13. A pump system requiring energy which is necessary for the carriage of a certain

substance   through   a   cellular   membrane   performs   the   function   of
_____ .

14. The cell membrane is:
    a. slightly permeable to all substances.
    b. a semi-permeable membrane.
    c. only permeable by the action of active transport systems.

15. Potassium ions must be pumped continually into the cells and sodium ions
     pumped continually out of the cells by active transport systems in order to main-
     tain proper ICF and ECF cation concentration balance.
    a. True
    b. False

16. The flow of water through a semi-permeable membrane in order to equalize the
     concentration of solutes on both sides of the membrane is termed
     _____ .

17. Would you expect that a person suffering severe hemorrhage would experience
     ADH secretion? Why?

18. Aldosterone primarily causes the reabsorption of sodium in the distal tubules of
     the nephrons. What is the secondary influence of this action?

19. The temporary weight gain experienced by a young woman at the beginning of
     her menstruation periods is generally serious in nature.
    a. True
    b. False

20. Excessive perspiration necessitates the increased consumption of
    a. electrolytes
    b. water
    c. water and electrolytes

21. Edema is tissue swelling due to the excess accumulation of tissue water and can
     be a serious condition requiring medical attention.
    a. True
    b. False

22. Dehydration is especially dangerous for persons with a high percentage of body
     weight due to body water such as _____ , and persons with a low
     percentage of body weight due to water such as _____ .

23. What are two methods the body uses to regulate water intake?

Answers: Water and Electrolytes

1. water
2. a
3. a
4. 1. c   greatest percentage of body water
    2. b
    3. d
    4. a   lowest percentage of body water
5. 1. plasma
    2. interstitial fluid
    3. secretions of glands, gastrointestinal tract and cerebral spinal fluid and eye
        space fluids
6. a
7. d
8. b

9. a. ICF
    b. ICF
    c. ECF
    d. ECF
10. 1. f
    2. g
    3. d
    4. a
    5. b
    6. c
    7. e
11. a. sodium (Na^+)
    b. potassium (K^+)
    c. chloride (Cl^-)
    d. phosphate ($HPO_4^=$)
12. diffusion
13. active transport
14. b
15. a
16. osmosis
17. Yes; because the posterior lobe of the pituitary gland secretes ADH during periods of *perceived* decreased blood volume and hemorrhage decreases total blood volume.
18. reabsorption of water which follows the reabsorption of sodium
19. b
20. c
21. a
22. infants; the elderly
23. Reduction of salivary secretion which produces a dry mouth and a desire to drink; high solute concentration detected by special receptors in the hypothalamus which stimulates thirst so water intake will be increased and blood solute concentration will be diluted.

ACID-BASE BALANCE

Acids are substances which donate protons. Protons are designated by the hydrogen ion (H^+). Hydrochloric acid (HC1) is a strong acid because it almost completely dissociates into H^+ and Cl^- in solution. *Bases are substances which combine with or accept protons.* Examples of substances which readily accept protons and are, therefore, bases include chloride, Cl^- ($Cl^- + H^+ \rightarrow HC1$); hydroxide, OH^- ($OH^- + H^+ \rightarrow H_2O$); ammonia, NH_3 ($NH_3 + H^+ \rightarrow NH_4^+$).

The charged ions in body fluids participate in the regulation of pH (acidity) of the fluids.[7] Blood pH is and must be maintained at a relatively constant narrow range for the proper functioning of the body. Blood is normally slightly alkaline at approximately pH 7.4. An increase above pH 7.45 results in alkalosis and a decrease below pH 7.35 results in acidosis.

Acidosis and alkalosis cause malfunctions in body metabolism. If you refer back to the denaturation of proteins you will realize that acidosis and alkalosis greatly affect the proper functioning of enzymes (catalytic proteins). When enzymes do not function properly the whole series of chemical reactions involved in body metabolism is impaired. Energy production is slowed and the undesirable intermediaries of metabolic reactions are inefficiently cleared. *Many of the end products of body metabolism are acidic in nature:* carbonic acid, lactic acid, pyruvic acid, keto acids, amino acids, uric acid, sulfuric acid, and phosphoric acid. Neutralizing mechanisms for these products are necessary in order for the body to maintain a constant blood pH.

Normally, there are several forces operating to control blood pH. The kidneys are able to respond to blood filtrate pH and can selectively excrete ions according to body pH regulation needs at any given time. Refer to Appendix C: The Kidneys. The kidneys generally conserve bicarbonate (HCO_3^-) and excrete hydrogen ions (H^+). The kidneys also generate ammonia (NH_3) from certain amino acids. Ammonia can be combined with hydrogen ions (H^+) to form the ammonium ion (NH_4^+). The ammonium ion then combines with certain salts such as NaCl and displaces the basic ion (Na^+) to form an ammonium salt (NH_4Cl) which is excreted. The basic ion (Na^+) is diffused back into the blood supply. In these two ways the kidneys tend to conserve basic electrolytes and excrete acidic electrolytes (H^+). Consequently, the kidneys are able to increase blood pH effectively.

Another means by which the body controls pH is through the action of the lungs. Carbon dioxide is a potential acid because it forms carbonic acid when it is dissolved in water:

$$CO_2 + H_2O \rightleftharpoons H_2CO_3 \text{ (carbonic acid)}$$

Carbonic acid is a weak acid since it dissociates in solution slightly. When carbon dioxide is held in the body, as when you hold your breath or decrease your normal rate of breathing (hypoventilate), more carbonic acid is formed in the blood causing the blood to become more acidic:

$$CO_2 + H_2O \rightleftharpoons H_2CO_3$$

When carbon dioxide is greatly released, such as when you breathe rapidly (hyperventilate), the carbonic acid concentration in the blood is decreased which reduces blood acidity:

$$H_2CO_3 \rightleftharpoons CO_2 + H_2O$$

The body automatically sets the pace for breathing rate according to blood pH. For example, during heavy exercise excess CO_2 is produced which increases carbonic acid in the blood and, consequently, lowers blood pH. But both heavy exercise and lowered blood pH (acidosis) produce rapid breathing (hyperventilation) which helps to quickly excrete the additional CO_2. A build-up of blood bases (alkalosis) produces a depression in breathing rate (hypoventilation) which helps to increase the blood pH by holding in more CO_2. Therefore, the direction of the chemical reactions of carbonic acid toward uptake and excretion or release of hydrogen ions into the blood is directly related to the action and efficiency of the lungs.

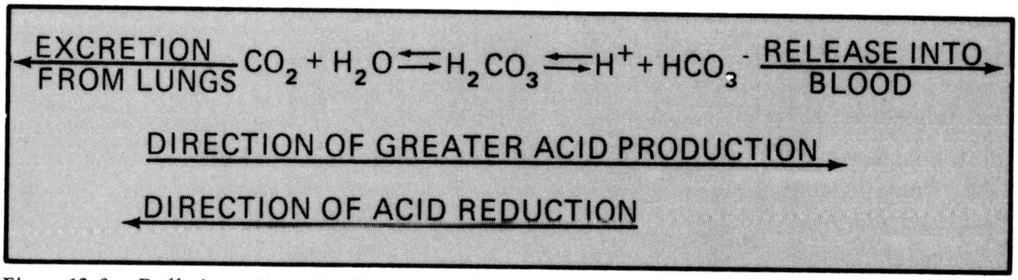

Figure 13-8.   *Buffering action of carbonic acid.*

Buffers also participate in the regulation of acid-base balance. Buffers are substances which act to alter hydrogen ion concentration in solution. They can both accept or release hydrogen ions (H^+). Consequently, they effect the maintenance of a relatively constant pH despite the addition of significant quantities of acid or base. Buffer systems are generally composed of a weak acid and its salt.[8] Physiologically, carbonic acid and its sodium salt, sodium bicarbonate, perform very important buffering functions:

H_2CO_3 (carbonic acid; weakly dissociates)
$NaHCO_3$ (sodium bicarbonate; strongly dissociates)

If a strong acid (remember, strong acids are those with a high degree of dissociation in solution) is added to a solution of sodium bicarbonate and carbonic acid the following reaction partially occurs.

$$(Na^+ + HCO_3^-) \quad + \quad (H^+ + Cl^-) \rightarrow (Na^+ + Cl^-) \quad + \quad H_2CO_3$$

sodium   strong acid   neutral salt   weak acid
  bicarbonate

A neutral salt is formed along with a weak acid (remember, a weak acid is only slightly dissociated) and only a slight change in blood pH occurs.

If a strong base is added, the following reaction partially occurs.

$$H_2CO_3 \quad + \quad NaOH \quad \rightarrow \quad NaHCO_3 \quad + \quad H_2O$$

carbonic   strong   salt   water
acid   base

The products of this reaction are essentially neutral and blood pH is only slightly altered.

Proteins are also buffers. The elements within the various side chains of the bonded amino acids have different abilities to either pick up or release hydrogen ions. Plasma proteins are important acid-base buffers for the regulation of blood pH. Hemoglobin, an important protein in red blood cells, is not only important for its ability to bind and transport carbon dioxide, but also for its buffering ability which aids in the maintenance of proper blood pH.

Respiratory acidosis or respiratory alkalosis results from a reduced or excessive carbon dioxide output by the lungs, respectively. Metabolic acidosis results from an excess or organic acids produced from various metabolic processes (an increase in total hydrogen ion concentration). Metabolic alkalosis results from a loss of hydrogen ions, excessive bicarbonate intake, or abnormal electrolyte shifts between intracellular and extracellular fluids.

Various foods contain elements which produce predominately acid or alkaline metabolic end-products. Although the healthy person seldom needs to worry about his or her food source intake as it relates to acid-base balance, there are some health conditions which do necessitate dietary modifications. Figure 13-9 illustrates the acid-base properties of various foodstuffs. The very fact that certain foods do have an effect on the production of acid or base compounds should be recognized as another valid reason to consume a mixed diet without the excessive intake of any one nutrient or food.

Key Points: Acid-Base Balance

I.   Acids are substances which donate protons (hydrogen ions): H^+Cl^-

II. Bases are substances which combine with or accept protons: Cl^-, OH^-, NH_3

III Blood acidity level must be closely maintained at approximately pH 7.4 (slightly alkaline).

IV. Conditions of body acidosis and alkalosis alter normal body functioning, that is, enzymes and hormones malfunction.

    A. Most metabolic body reactions produce acidic end-products.

    B. The body has several neutralizing mechanisms:

        1. The kidneys tend to excrete H^+ ions and retain Na^+ and HCO_3^- which raises blood pH. A malfunction in normal kidney action leads to metabolic alkalosis or acidosis.

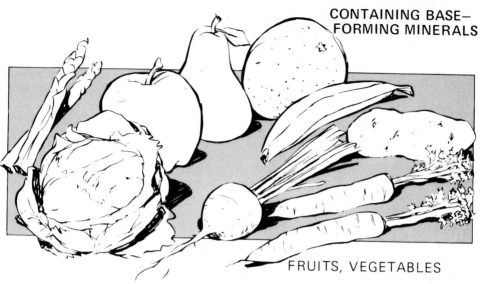

CONTAINING BASE—
FORMING MINERALS

FRUITS, VEGETABLES

Certain fruits which contain
acids that cannot be metabolized
are: Plums
        Cranberries
        Prunes

The base—forming elements
Sodium (Na)   Magnesium (Mg)
Potassium (K) Iron (Fe)
Calcium (Ca)

Fats, sugars and starches
do not form either predominantly
acid or base metabolic
end products

CONTAINING ACID—
FORMING MINERALS

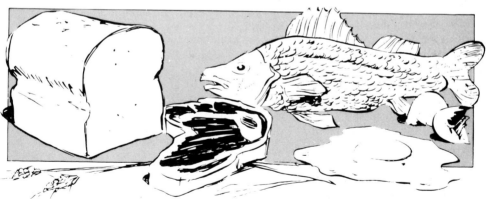

CEREAL PRODUCTS, PROTEIN FOODS

The acid—forming elements
Sulfur (S)
Phosphorus (P)
Chlorine (Cl)

Figure 13-9.   Base- and acid-forming foods.

2. The lungs excrete CO_2 which reduces the formation of H_2CO_3 (carbonic
    acid) in the blood. A malfunction in normal lung action leads to respiratory
    acidosis or alkalosis.

3. Buffer compounds which chemically neutralize strong acids and bases: a weak acid plus its salt and various proteins.

Questions: Acid-Base Balance

1. On the pH scale, which direction indicates
   a. acidity?
   b. alkalinity?
   c. neutrality?

2. Identify the items on the left as acid or base.
   _____ 1. proton acceptors   a.   acid
   _____ 2. proton donors   b.   base
   _____ 3. H^+
   _____ 4. OH^-
   _____ 5. NH_3
   _____ 6. HC1

3. The hydrogen ion (H^+) is a:
   a. neutron
   b. proton
   c. electron

4. Normal pH of blood is _____ .

5. The body may function properly within a wide range of blood pH values.
   a. True
   b. False

6. The largest percentage of metabolic intermediary and end-products are
   _____ .
   a. acidic
   b. basic
   c. neutral

7. Enzymes are especially sensitive to the pH of body fluids, and the various enzymes require the maintenance of a restricted pH range for their individual proper functioning.
   a. True
   b. False

8. A high base to acid proportion results in _____ .
   a. alkalosis
   b. acidosis

9. A high acid to base proportion results in _____ .
   a. alkalosis
   b. acidosis

10. Identify the three general devices which the body uses to control body pH.

11. The net effect of the kidney's conservation of bicarbonate (HCO_3^-) and excretion of hydrogen ion (H^+) is:
    a. reduction in blood pH (more acid)
    b. reduction in urine pH (more acid); rise in blood pH (more alkaline)
    c. rise in urine pH (more alkaline)

12. Excretion of ammonium salts such as NH_4Cl results in a net effect of:
    a. conservation of basic electrolytes; excretion of acidic electrolytes.
    b. conservation of acidic electrolytes for reabsorption into blood.
    c. reduction of blood pH.

13. Carbonic acid (H_2CO_3) is a _____ acid.
     a. weak
     b. strong

14. *Hypo*ventilation results in _____ blood pH.
     a. lowered (more acidic)
     b. raised (more alkaline)

15. *Hyper*ventilation results in _____ blood pH.
     a. lowered (more acid)
     b. raised (more alkaline)

16. Buffers can:
     a. only accept protons (H^+)
     b. only release protons (H^+)
     c. accept or release protons (H^+)

17. Buffer systems are generally composed of _____ .

18. Buffers allow only a slight variation in pH value to occur.
     a. True
     b. False

19. Proteins are _____ buffers.
     a. good
     b. poor

20. During periods of increased body exercise blood pH would _____ if the lungs did not increase the rate of breathing.
     a. increase (become alkaline)
     b. decrease (become acid)

21. Which condition would you expect to naturally occur in *response* to a body state of acidosis resulting from heavy excercise? Why?
     a. hyperventilation
     b. hypoventilation

22. A man fell from a ladder while house painting and suffered a severe head injury resulting in a depressed rate of breathing. What body state do you expect to result from his condition?
     a. acidosis
     b. alkalosis
         What two other devices may he have working to maintain his acid-base balance? (Hint: Refer back to question 10.)

23. What classes of foods generally produce metabolic end-products which are:
     a. acidic
     b. basic

24. Under normal body conditions which foods generally do not form acid or base metabolic end-products?

25. Why are some fruits like plums, cranberries, and prunes acid end-product formers?

26. You would expect any disease which interferes with the normal functioning of the lungs to produce conditions of:
     a. metabolic acidosis/alkalosis.
     b. respiratory acidosis/alkalosis

27. You would expect a person with uncontrolled diabetes to be in a state of metabolic _____ . (Hint: Refer back to the section on Some Malfunctions Involving Lipid Metabolism in Chapter Four, Lipids.)

28. Emphysema and pneumonia produce conditions of reduced lung surface area available for gas exchange (CO_2 and O_2). Which body condition would you expect might occur as a result of these diseases:
    a. respiratory acidosis
    b. respiratory alkalosis
    c. metabolic acidosis

29. Periods of severe vomiting cause a large loss of gastric acid, HCl. Which body condition would you expect to result from excessive vomiting?
    a. respiratory acidosis
    b. metabolic acidosis
    c. metabolic alkalosis

Answers: Acid-Base Balance

1. a. pH less than 7
   b. pH greater than 7
   c. pH 7
2. 1. b
   2. a
   3. a
   4. b
   5. b
   6. a
3. b
4. pH 7.4
5. b
6. a
7. a
8. a
9. b
10. the kidneys; the lungs; buffer compounds
11. b
12. a
13. a
14. a
15. b
16. c
17. a weak acid and its salt
18. a
19. a
20. b
21. a. hyperventilation; the lungs increase the rate of breathing in order to excrete excess CO_2 so it will not be retained in blood with the resultant increased formation of H_2CO_3 (carbonic aicd).
22. a; kidneys, buffers
23. a. proteins (meat, cheese, eggs, grains)
    b. fruits; vegetables; milk
24. fats, sugars, starches
25. Because they contain organic acids which are not metabolized by the body; therefore, these acids pass through the body unchanged and do acidify body fluids.
26. b
27. acidosis

28. a, due to the large amount of carbonic acid produced
29. c, increased loss of HCl (acid) would decrease total body acid and increase total body bases.

REFERENCES

[1] **Plasma fluid** is the liquid portion of whole blood exclusive of the red and white blood cells. It is a yellowish, viscous fluid containing numerous compounds including the circulating proteins.

[2] Williams SR: Nutrition and Diet Therapy, 3rd ed. St. Louis, The C. V. Mosby Company, 1977, p. 180.

[3] Water which evaporates immediately from the skin and is not noticeable is termed *insensible* perspiration versus the water of heavier, obvious perspiration.

[4] McNeely GR and Battarbee HD: Sodium and potassium. *In* Present Knowledge in Nutrition, 4th ed. New York and Washington, D.C.; The Nutrition Foundation, 1976, p. 261

[5] Refer to Appendix C, The Kidneys, for more detailed information on the anatomy and physiology of a working kidney.

[6] Robinson JR: Water the indispensable nutrient. Nutrition Today, 5, Spring 1970, pp. 17 and 23

[7] pH represents the percentage of hydrogen ions in a solution. The means for determining this concentration is not necessary here. What is important to understand is the relative acidity represented by the various pH values. This can be illustrated by the following scale:

0 ⎯⎯⎯⎯⎯⎯⎯⎯⎯⎯⎯⎯⎯⎯ 7 ⎯⎯⎯⎯⎯⎯⎯⎯⎯⎯⎯⎯ 14

most acid   neutral   most alkaline (base)

direction of increased   direction of increased

acidity (H^+)   alkalinity (OH^-)

[8] Anthony CP and Kolthoff NJ: Textbook of Anatomy and Physiology, 9th ed. St. Louis, The C. V. Mosby Company, 1975, pp. 523-524.

14

ENERGY BALANCE AND THE CONTROL OF BODY WEIGHT

ENERGY BALANCE AND MEASUREMENT

Energy balance is achieved when the total caloric expenditure for various body activities equals the total caloric intake. Each of us has some control over both our expenditure and intake of calories though there are some factors influencing energy balance over which we have little or no control.

Energy Measurement. Energy is measured in units called calories. A calorie (spelled with a small c) is the amount of heat required to raise 1 gram of water 1°C. However, in terms of measuring the heat energy of food or the expenditure of energy by the body, this calorie is too small to use conveniently. Therefore, when referring to calories in food or equivalents of energy expenditure of the body the large kilocalorie is used. *A kilocalorie (kcal or Calorie with a capital C) is the amount of heat energy necessary to raise 1 kilogram of water 1°C.* In the metric system the joule and kilojoule are used to express heat energy. Refer to Appendix A, The Metric System, for information about converting calories to joules.

Determination of the energy value of food. A direct method of determining the energy or caloric value of food is found by burning a food sample in the presence of oxygen, but in a closed container immersed in a liter of water. The whole apparatus is surrounded by an insulated cover to prevent heat escape. All the heat produced by the burning of the food sample is used to heat the liter of water. Each degree of heat measured on the Centigrade scale thus produced represents one kilocalorie (Calorie) or 1,000 calories.[1] An indirect method for determining the caloric value of food involves computations utilizing the measurement of the amount of oxygen consumed when the food is burned.

Obviously, a great deal of technical work goes into developing the tables of caloric values of food which most of us have used from time to time. Even the calories given for various foods in these tables represent averages rather than exact values since food naturally contains variations in its composition depending on such factors as the season of growth or production, species or variety, and changes in environmental conditions surrounding growth or production. For example, the water content of different potatoes may vary which causes a difference in the caloric values between potatoes even of the same size and variety. These values, however, are sufficiently accurate for use in estimating the energy value of various foods, diet, and intake.

Determination of energy expenditure by the body. The methods used to determine the energy expenditure of the body are similar to those used to determine the energy value of food. A direct method involves placing a person in a chamber similar in action to a bomb calorimeter, where released body heat is captured by a water-containing apparatus, and the change in degrees is measured. When the measurement is taken for a one-hour period that value can be multiplied by 24 to obtain the measured energy expenditure for one day.[2]

An indirect method for determining body caloric expenditure involves the determination of heat production according to the amount of oxygen consumed. Special portable devices which measure oxygen intake and carbon dioxide output can be worn while individuals perform various activities. These devices enable estimates of the caloric value of various types of body work to be made.

Basal Metabolism. Basal metabolism is the energy expenditure by the body at rest and in a fasting state when nutrients are being metabolized but not digested or absorbed. The basal metabolic rate, therefore, is the amount of energy required to carry on the involuntary maintenance work of the body.

Factors affecting the basal metabolic rate (BMR). Body composition and surface (skin) area have a significant effect on BMR. *The greater the proportion of muscle to fat tissue the higher the BMR.* Muscle tissue is a metabolically more active tissue than adipose (fat) tissue.[3] Since heat is lost from the body by radiation, the greater the skin area the greater the heat loss and the higher the BMR. *A tall, thin person (the ectomorph) has proportionally greater skin area and a higher BMR than the person of shorter, rounded stature (the endomorph).*

Sex has another significant affect on BMR. Women have a lower BMR than men due in part to a different body composition (women have a higher proportion of fat to muscle than men) and activity of the sex hormones.

Age causes a variation in BMR. Basal metabolic rate is highest during infancy. After a decline during childhood, and a slight increase during adolescence, the BMR begins a lifelong decline at a rate of about two percent for each decade after the age of twenty.

Body temperature also affects BMR. Maintenance of a constant body temperature when the external temperature is low (cold) requires an increase in BMR. This increase helps to keep the body warm. *A significant increase in BMR occurs with each degree of increased internal temperature (fever).*

Body state can cause variations in BMR. An increased production of certain hormones such as thyroxine from the thyroid gland increases BMR. An undernourished individual may have a decreased BMR (this is thought to be an energy conservation method of the body when energy supplies are low). Pregnancy increases the BMR because of the growth activity of building new tissues and the increased metabolic rate of the growing fetus.

Voluntary Energy Expenditure. The greater the muscular exercise the greater the caloric expenditure. The word muscular is the key to understanding how your work and recreational activities increase your caloric requirement. Doing busy mental work or paperwork such as that done sitting at a desk may be mentally fatiguing, but it is not costly in terms of caloric requirement. Refer to Table 14-1 to compare the approximate caloric values for various activities. As you can see, it is the physically strenuous activities which require the highest amount of energy. Unfortunately, most of us engage in activities requiring only very light to light energy output. Strenuous activity is generally confined only to short periods of energy surges.

Obviously, the voluntary energy expenditure of each individual will vary from day to day. Even the way in which each individual utilizes energy sources fluctuates periodically because of the internal and external influences previously discussed, such as climatic conditions, aging, and hormonal controls. A grouping of energy-requiring activities by similar energy costs as presented in Table 14-1 can be made for practical, general, rule-of-thumb reference.

Specific Dynamic Action of Food (SDA). The digestion, absorption, and metabolism of food is an energy-requiring process. (Remember the enzyme production, peristalsis activity, pumps for absorption and anabolic and catabolic processes which required sources of energy?) Protein seems to require more energy to be digested, absorbed, and metabolized than fats or carbohydrates. Why there is a difference in SDA between macronutrients is unknown. Some researchers feel that the increase in metabolic rate caused by digestion and absorption of the various macronutrients (SDA) more correctly reflects loss of heat energy incurred during the processes which convert the potential energy in food into high energy bonds within compounds, which are ultimately broken down and the captured energy released to accomplish the work of the body. Digestion and absorption may further decrease the efficiency of this energy transformation process and may be reflected as increased heat loss, that is, the specific dynamic action of food. However, most scientists agree that the overall energy cost for the digestion, absorption, transportation, and metabolism of combined nutrients due to whatever reason is ten percent of the total energy needed for basal metabolism and voluntary activities.[4]

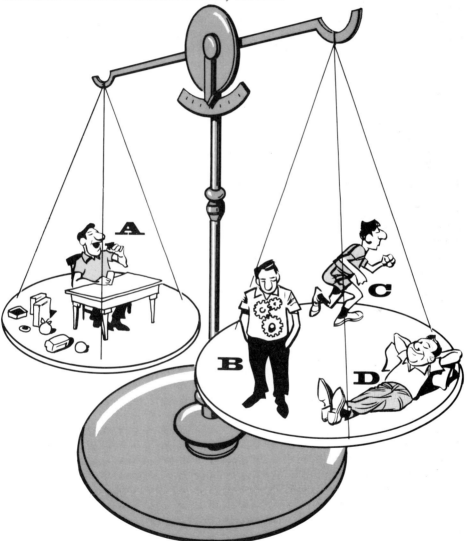

Figure 14-1.   Energy balance is achieved when food intake (A) equals basal metabolism (D), plus the SDA (specific dynamic action of food—B), plus voluntary energy activity expenditure (C). Body weight maintenance at ideal weight is achieved when the caloric balance is kept at a level appropriate for one's age, height, sex, and body frame.

Calorie need. In order to maintain a balance in body weight, the total calories expended for basal metabolism, voluntary activities, and specific dynamic action of food (SDA) must be compensated for by an equivalent caloric intake of food. Foods supply the following calories according to nutrient composition:

carbohydrates—4 kcal per gram
protein   —4 kcal per gram
fat   —9 kcal per gram
alcohol   —7 kcal per gram

Information contained in the food exchange system found in Chapter Two reveals the energy values assigned to the various exchange groups (these are rounded off average values):

Exchange group	Energy (kcal) value
Skim milk (1 cup)	80
Vegetables (½ cup cooked)	25
Fruit (generally 1 small)	40
Bread (1 slice bread or ½ cup cooked pasta)	70
Lean meat (1 oz or 1 egg)	55
Fat (1 tsp oil or solid fat)	45

Familiarization with the foods and portions contained in the above exchange groups simplifies the determination of caloric intake and diet planning. Each exchange always supplies the same *approximate* amount of calories as shown.

Table 14-1.   Approximate estimates of energy values for various types of activities.

Very light, less than 100 kcal/hour:
    Seated and standing activities such as painting, automobile driving, typing and writing, sewing, ironing, playing musical instruments
Light, between 100-200 kcal/hour:
    Walking at a normal rate on a level surface, moderate carpentry work, golfing, bicycling, light housework, volleyball
Moderate, between 200-350 kcal/hour:
    Walking briskly, swimming and skating moderately, walking upstairs, playing tennis, dancing, riding horseback at a trot.
Heavy, above 350 kcal/hour:
    Running, bicycle racing, vigorous swimming and dancing, playing basketball and football, heavy carpentry, work with a pick and shovel.

Some sources for individuals to use in determining the caloric value of foods consumed include reference tables for individual foods and nutrition labeling information. Nutrition labeling information supplies, in particular, the energy values (kcal) for processed foods which may not be listed in food composition tables such as a specific type of new breakfast pastry.

It takes 3,500 kcal to form one pound of body fat. Conversely, it takes a reduction of 3,500 kcal to lose one pound of body fat. This is a hard and fast rule in human nutrition. Therefore, in order to gain one pound of body fat you need to consume 500 extra kcal each day for a week (7 days x 500 kcal=3,500 kcal). In order to lose one pound of body fat you need have a daily deficit of 500 kcal for a week.

Quick weight loss is usually reflective of water or lean tissue (water and protein) loss rather than loss of body fat. Because body fat is less dense than water or protein, one pound of body fat is greater in volume than one pound of water or protein. Consequently, the loss of actual body fat is cosmetically more desirable as well as nutritionally more desirable than the loss of body water or protein. Loss of body fat results in a greater decrease in body size than a comparable loss of body water or protein.

Key Points: Energy Balance and Measurement

I. Energy balance is achieved when total caloric expenditure for various body activities equals total caloric intake:
    Basal metabolic rate+Specific dynamic action of food+Voluntary energy expenditure=Caloric intake

II. Energy is measured in units called calories.
    A. A calorie=the heat required to raise 1 gram of water 1°C
    B. A kcal=1000 calories=Calorie=the heat required to raise 1 kilogram of water 1°C
    C. Energy measurement in the metric system is in terms of joules: 1 kcal=4.2 kJ
    D. Energy value of food is determined using a device termed a bomb calorimeter. An indirect measure can be calculated from the amount of oxygen consumed when the food is burned.
    E. Energy expenditure by the body can be determined by a device termed a respiration calorimeter. Indirect measurement of energy expenditure can be determined by measuring the amount of oxygen consumed. The amount of oxygen consumed is directly proportional to the amount of heat liberated during a particular activity.

III. Basal metabolic rate (BMR) is the energy the body expends while at rest and in a fasting state when nutrients are being metabolized but not digested or absorbed. BMR is affected by the ratio of muscle to fat tissue, total skin area, sex, age, body temperature, and body state including hormone production, nutritional status, pregnancy, and growth.

IV. Specific dynamic action of food (SDA) is the amount of energy required for absorption and metabolism of food.

V. Caloric value of energy foods are:

    carbohydrates and protein: 4 kcal/gram
    fat: 9 kcal/gram
    alcohol: 7 kcal/gram

    The food exchange system enables the grouping of foods in portions according to similar kcal values.

VI. It takes 3,500 kcal to form one pound of body fat; it takes a deficit of 3,500 kcal to lose one pound of body fat.

Questions: Energy Balance and Measurement

1. Energy balance is achieved when:
    a. caloric intake equals the caloric expenditure for the metabolism of food (SDA) and basal metabolism.
    b. caloric intake equals the caloric expenditure for the metabolism of food (SDA) and voluntary activities.
    c. caloric intake equals caloric expenditure for the metabolism of food (SDA), basal metabolism, and voluntary activities.

2. A Calorie is equal to:
   a. a kcal
   b. a joule
   c. 1000 calories

3. A Calorie is the amount of heat energy necessary to raise _____ of water _____ .

4. Identify the following situations as normally ones of increased or decreased basal metabolic rate:

   _____ 1. a highly developed   a. increased
            muscular body of an   b. decreased
            athlete
   _____ 2. an obese individual
   _____ 3. a healthy, pregnant
            woman
   _____ 4. a starving adult man
   _____ 5. a tall, thin man
   _____ 6. a four month-old in-
            fant boy
   _____ 7. a person with an over-
            active thyroid gland

5. Women usually have higher basal metabolic rates than men.
   a. True
   b. False

6. Match the phrases on the right to the items on the left which they best describe:

   _____ 1. endomorph   a. basal metabolic rate
   _____ 2. fever   b. 4.2 kilojoules (KJ)
   _____ 3. kilocalorie (kcal) c. amount of heat energy needed to raise
   _____ 4. calorie   1 gram of water 1°C
   _____ 5. BMR   d. an apparatus used to determine the
   _____ 6. bomb calorimeter   caloric value of a food sample
   _____ 7. mesomorph   e. an insulated chamber specially con-
   _____ 8. respiration chamber   structed to determine the amount of
   _____ 9. ectomorph   heat released by the body at rest (BMR)
                               f. a large, heavy-boned, muscular-type
                                  person
                               g. a tall, thin-type body build
                               h. a short, round, stocky-type body build
                               i. causes a significant increase in BMR

7. Business and mental work which create fatigue do not appreciably increase caloric expenditure for voluntary activity.
   a. True
   b. False

8. Food composition tables give _____ figures for the energy values of various foods.
   a. exact
   b. average

9. The (muscle/fat) tissue is metabolically more active than (muscle/fat) tissue.

10. The energy expenditure by the body at rest in a post absorptive state where only involuntary maintenance work of the body is being performed is descriptive of:
    a. large voluntary muscle movement
    b. basal metabolic rate (BMR)
    c. specific dynamic action of food (SDA)

11. The calorie cost for digesting, absorbing, and metabolizing food is termed:
    a. BMR (body weight in kg X 24 hours)
    b. SDA [10 percent (BMR + voluntary activity)]
    c. voluntary activity (kcal value for the type of activity x length of time that activity performed)

12. a. Protein and carbohydrate provide _____ kcal per gram.
    b. Fat provides _____ kcal per gram.
    c. Alcohol provides _____ kcal per gram.

13. How many kcal must be consumed in, or deleted from a diet, to either gain or lose one pound of body fat, respectively?

14. Weight gain leading to overweight and/or obesity need not be the result of gluttonous behavior and, indeed, most often seems not to be. Consider the following problems where voluntary activity stays the same:
    a. How many days does it take to gain three pounds by eating just one extra three oz serving of marbled sirloin tip roast daily (140 kcal)?
    b. How much weight would be gained in six months? One year?
    c. How much weight would be gained in four weeks of just eating one extra piece of pie (350 kcal) and one 8 oz glass of whole milk (160 kcal) daily?
    d. How much weight would be gained in one year from just eating two extra cream-filled cookies (100 kcal) daily?

15. John has decided to embark upon a reducing diet and wants to combine a 700 kcal a day caloric reduction along with an hour of active tennis playing (see Table 14-1 and use tennis at approximately 300 kcal per hour).
    a. How many pounds a week will John lose if he continues with his diet and exercise program?
    b. How many weeks will it take for John to lose 20 pounds?
    c. How many pounds a week would John lose if he only increased his exercise by playing tennis one hour per day?
    d. How long will it take John to lose 20 pounds by his exercise program alone?

16. Identify the energy values (kcal) for the food categories of the exchange groups:
    a. Skim milk (1 cup) _____
    b. Vegetables (½ cup cooked) _____
    c. Fruit (generally 1 fresh, small whole) _____
    d. Bread (1 slice bread or ½ cup cooked pasta) _____
    e. Lean meat (1 oz or 1 egg) _____
    f. Fat (1 tsp. oil or solid fat) _____

17. Weight loss greater than three pounds per week generally reflects the loss of what substances?
    a. water
    b. water, lean tissue + some fat
    c. fat

18. Why is the loss of body fat cosmetically more desirable than loss of body water and/or body protein?

19. Compute the following:
    a. A loss of three pounds per week would require a daily deficit of how many kcal?
    b. A 25-year-old woman 5 feet 2 inches tall weighing 125 pounds consumes 1,800 kcal a day. In order to lose three pounds of body fat per week how many kcal would she be able to consume daily?
    c. Is a weekly loss of three pounds of body fat per week a realistic goal for this young woman?

Answers: Energy Balance and Measurement

1. c
2. a and c
3. 1 kilogram; 1°C
4. 1. a
   2. b
   3. a
   4. b
   5. a
   6. a
   7. a
5. b
6. 1. h
   2. i
   3. b
   4. c
   5. a
   6. d
   7. f
   8. e
   9. g
7. a
8. b
9. muscle; fat (adipose)
10. b
11. b
12. a. 4
    b. 9
    c. 7
13. 3500 kcal
14. a. 3500 kcal ÷ 140 kcal = 25 days to gain one pound. Therefore, 25 x 3 pounds = 75 days or a little more than two months.
    b. 6 months = 180 days, so 180 days ÷ 25 days for one pound = 7.2 pounds; one year would be 7.2 x 2 = 14.4 pounds.
    c. 350 kcal + 160 kcal = 510 kcal daily, 510 kcal x 28 days (7 days x 4 weeks) = 14,280 extra kcal ÷ 3500 kcal (to equal one pound) = 4.08 pounds.
    d. 365 days a year x 100 kcal = 36,500 kcal, 36,500 kcal ÷ 3500 kcal/lb = 10.4 lbs.
15. a. 700 + 300 = 1000 kcal deficit per day = 7000 kcal per week ÷ 3500 kcal per pound = two pounds per week
    b. 20 ÷ 2 = 10 weeks
    c. 300 kcal x 7 days = 2100 kcal per week, 2100 ÷ 3500 = .6 pounds per week
    d. 3500 kcal x 20 pounds = 70,000 total kcal to lose; 300 kcal burned per day x 7 = 2100 kcal burned per week, 70,000 ÷ 2100 = 33.3 weeks to lose 20 pounds (or 20 pounds ÷ .6 pounds per week = 33.3 weeks)
16. a. skim milk = 80 kcal
    b. vegetables = 25 kcal
    c. fruit = 40 kcal
    d. bread = 70 kcal
    e. lean meat = 55 kcal
    f. fat = 45 kcal
17. b

18.   Loss of body fat results in a greater decrease in body size which is the true goal of the individual.
19.   a.   3 x 3500 = 10,500 kcal per week; 10,500 ÷ 7 = 1500 kcal per day.
       b.   1800-1500 = 300 kcal
       c.   no

CONTROL OF BODY WEIGHT

Ideal Weight. Ideal weight is suggested by average height and weight charts with reference to body frame size and age. These charts are frequently developed by life insurance companies, and reflect weights within height and body frame references maintained throughout adult life which are related to longest life expectancy. However, average does not necessarily mean ideal for you. Also, we all have a tendency to be subjective in our determination of our frame size. We tend to overestimate frame size which makes weight ranges respective for our height and age more liberal than accurate. Body composition is more important in determination of fatness or leanness.

Some measurements which more accurately determine amounts of fat or lean body tissue are:

1.   Skin-fold thicknesses measured by calipers at specific body sites.
2.   Anthropometric measurements including body contour and skeletal measurements such as chest, thighs, and ankles.
3.   Water displacement and determination of the specific gravity of the body.
4.   Radioactive potassium count to determine lean body mass.
5.   X-ray measurement of body fat.[5,6]

A rule-of-thumb method for determining ideal weight is the following:

Women: 100 pounds per five feet of height and add five pounds for every inch over five feet.
Men: 110 pounds per five feet of height and add five pounds for every inch over five feet.

This gives an approximate ideal weight most applicable to the person of *medium* frame.

Underweight. Underweight is *generally* accepted as being below ten percent of ideal (average) weight. But, again, body composition is the best indicator. A person who appears underweight by this standard may actually have a body fat to lean tissue ratio appropriate for his or her body size and build. A person who is habitually underweight because of more limited kcal intake must choose foods high in nutrient density in order to consume nutrient amounts that approximate his or her need.

Anorexia nervosa is an example of a pathological condition involving severe weight loss due in large part to psychological problems. Anorexia nervosa is manifested as a self-starvation condition. Though anorexia nervosa is a physiological disorder, this severely underweight condition cannot be successfully corrected without psychiatric treatment.[7]

Overweight. Overweight is defined as weight 10 to 20 percent in excess of ideal (average) weight. Again, however, it is more accurate to determine body composition and judge overweight on too high a proportion of fat to lean body tissue. Overweight is probably more of a cosmetic problem than a medical problem.[8] An overweight condition elicits feelings of embarrassment due to the social stigma associated with overweight.

How do you determine if your overweight condition, as reflected by statistics on a reliable height-weight-age chart, is due to fat or muscle tissue? Are you in good physical condition? Have you been in training to play a sport or compete in a sporting event? Are you a sedentary individual with poor muscle tone? If, when you observe yourself from front, rear, and side views in a full-length mirror while undressed you appear fat, then you probably are fat.[9]

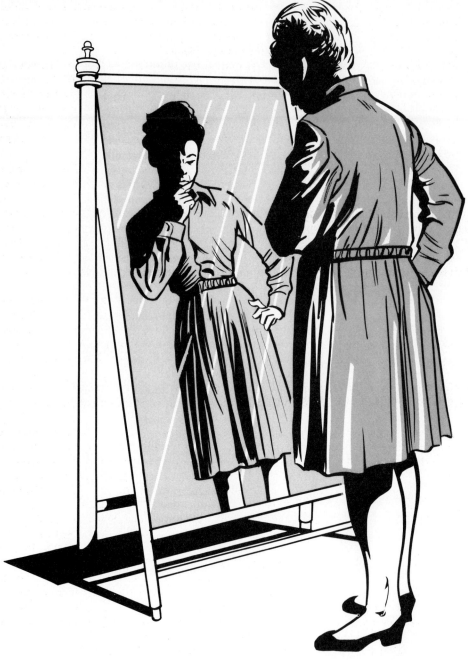

Figure 14-2.   Judging overweight and the need to reduce body weight requires being honest with one's self as to one's appearance and the setting of realistic weight achievement goals.

Obesity. Obesity is *generally* accepted as weight in excess of 20 percent of the ideal (average) weight. Again, a more accurate determination of obesity can be made from the more specific measurements of the ratio of fat to lean body tissue. The obese individual has fat much in excess of that necessary for optimal body function.[10] Obesity is more than a social embarrassment for the obese individual. Obesity has been shown to be associated with an increased propensity for development of kidney disease, heart and circulatory diseases, diabetes, liver and gallbladder disease, and, for females, complications during pregnancy and childbirth among other health problems.

The Public Health Service has stated that obesity is one of the most prevalent health problems in the U.S. today with 40 to 80 million obese individuals in the U.S.[11] Attempts to identify personality traits in the obese have failed to pinpoint a personality pattern characteristic of obesity.[12] Some investigators feel that many obese individuals eat as a means to "mother" or soothe themselves during times of stress. Also, some investigators believe that some obese individuals are unable to discriminate between a need for social company and the need for eating.[13]

For many persons obesity is a life-long condition beginning in childhood. Obesity before and during pregnancy has a significant positive association with increased fatness in newborn babies.[14] Though there are no established genetic relationships for obesity, most investigators feel that genetics do play some role in the development of obesity.[15] It was once felt that simple over-indulgence in food consumption was the single most important factor contributing to the development of obesity. *It is more accepted now by most researchers that obesity is the result of several factors of which increased caloric intake is one.* Other factors seem to be reduced activity and altered metabolism with contributing underlying social and psychological forces.[16]

Some investigators have proposed the hypercellular or hyperplastic (excess fat cells) and hypertrophic (enlarged fat cells) concepts of fatness. That is, fatness is derived from an excessive number of fat cells formed during infancy as a fat baby which remain constant throughout life, and which the body tends to try to keep filled (with fat). Or, fatness is derived from a normal number of fat cells which simply greatly enlarge or "over-fill" with fat deposits; or, a combination of an excess number of fat cells with some fat cells which tend to overfill. It has also been postulated that some obese individuals have a malfunctioning response center in the brain which fails to signal appropriately the feeling of satiety when blood glucose is high.

Unfortunately, there is a low incidence of weight loss *with* the resulting maintenance of normal weight by obese persons. Treatment with appetite-depressing drugs has not been shown to achieve long-term weight loss with the maintenance of weight reduction.[17] Diuretics, drugs that cause increased water excretion, have limited value for weight control as they stimulate weight loss principally by water rather than by fat loss. The use of diuretics by some individuals may be hazardous to their health.

Fad Diets. A great obstacle to the efficient management of overweight and obesity is the dependence upon reducing diets based upon faulty reasoning and just plain wishful thinking.[18] The reason there are so many of these diets (such as "Eat-All-You-Want", "Calories Don't Count", "Quick-Weight-Loss-Diet") is that they continue to fail. There is no quick, easy, and safe way to lose weight. It took weeks, days, and sometimes years to put on weight and it takes time to take if off.[19] If there were quick and easy methods to lose weight, success would be easily achieved and there would be no need for the limitless "overnight" weight-loss methods or guides printed by the popular press. Many of these diets are not only unsuccessful when followed but dangerous to use.[20]

A weight reducing diet severely restricted in calories tends to cause the body to break down body protein (lean tissue) as well as some body fat. Following the resumption of normal eating habits, the body tends to replace the lean tissue which it has broken down.

For every pound of protein regained three pounds of water are necessarily retained. This, in part, explains the ease in regaining weight which has been too quickly lost. *A weight loss of one to two pounds weekly usually indicates loss of body fat.*

Reducing diets based upon food guides used for normal meal planning are a successful means for losing weight and maintaining weight loss. Use of these food guides encourages the development of good food habits based on sound principles of nutrition. Many overweight and obese individuals find greater success in losing weight when behavior modification techniques are also learned and used. Increasing exercise also contributes to increased body energy expenditure (that is, the burning of more calories) and the overall feeling of well-being. Exercise alone, however, is seldom effective in promoting weight loss. A quick review of Table 14-1 discloses moderate exercise activities which must be maintained for an hour to use approximately 300 kcal, the number of kcal in three ounces of well-marbled sirloin steak. However, *increasing exercise while reducing caloric intake is an effective means for creating a significant total daily calorie deficit.*

Only the reduction of caloric intake below caloric (energy) expenditure will result in loss of body fat. Development of food habits which provide for the intake of nutrients essential to good health and energy to meet, but not exceed, body energy needs can safely and effectively maintain body fat weight loss. Employing the use of diet "tips" to help reduce caloric intake is helpful to some persons. But there is no magical, mystical way to lose weight (body fat) other than reducing calorie consumption below calorie expenditure. *In order to maintain weight loss, the loss needs to occur gradually and previous poor food habits need to be abandoned for food habits based upon the proven principles of good nutrition.*

Table 14-2.   Some behavior modification techniques and "tips" to achieve weight control.

---

1. Bring eating to a conscious level. Do not eat while participating in other activities such as watching television, reading, talking on the telephone, playing cards.

2. Restrict food to the kitchen and eating to a designated place such as the breakfast room or dining room.

3. Serve food pre-portioned in small helpings on the plate and do not take second helpings. Do not place service plates with food on the table.

4. Eat slowly and chew food thoroughly. Give your brain time to sense the fullness of your stomach. Eating a large amount of food quickly does not allow time for feelings of satiety to be recognized before over-consumption has occurred.

5. Try starting meals with salads, carrot and celery sticks, or broth. These foods help to create a feeling of fullness with the consumption of few calories.

6. Save an item from your last meal or choose a very low calorie food to munch on between meals if you must snack. Snacking, however, is not a desirable food habit as it tends to hinder efforts toward weight loss and maintenance of weight loss.

7. Learn to identify and avoid foods with a high calorie concentration: candies, desserts, butter, margarine, gravies, cream sauces, nuts, syrups, jellies, honey, well-marbled meat, cream, high-fat cheeses, bacon, processed luncheon meats.

8. Learn to identify and avoid food preparation methods which increase the caloric value of food: frying, breading, sautéing, pastry wrapping.

Table 14-3.   Some cooking tips for preparing lower calorie foods.

1. Substitute low-fat plain yogurt or buttermilk made from skim milk in recipes calling for sour cream.
2. Substitute soy flour for up to one-third of the wheat flour called for in a recipe. It is higher in protein and somewhat lower in calories than wheat flour.
3. Substitute evaporated *skim* milk for the heavy cream in a recipe.
4. Use chocolate extract as a flavoring agent instead of either cocoa or unsweetened baking chocolate.
5. Use cornstarch as a thickening agent instead of flour because less cornstarch is needed to thicken a food product.
6. Use lemon juice, extracts, spices, and herbs as flavoring agents instead of butter, margarine, or oil.
7. Use low-calorie salad dressings as marinades for meats and fish.
8. Remove skin from poultry and excess fat from other meats before cooking and/or serving.
9. Use skim milk in cooked and baked foods.
10. Use small amounts of tomato juice, lemon juice, or vinegar on tossed salads instead of regular salad dressings.
11. Use canned fruits packed in water or juice instead of heavy syrup.
12. Broil or roast meats using an elevated metal rack to allow fat to escape rather than to fry or sauté.
13. Use low-calorie vegetable spray on sauce pans, fry pans, and casserole dishes to eliminate the use of fat to prevent sticking of foods.

Table 14-4.   Comparison of various amounts of food in 100 kcal portions.

Cookies
  chocolate chip—2 small
  doughnut (raised yeast)—½
  oatmeal—1½ (3″ diameter)
  sugar wafers—2
  thin butter—2
  macaroon—1

Candy
  milk chocolate kisses—4
  Almond Joy (1¾ oz)—½
  gum sticks—(10)
  life savers—10
  marshmallows—4
  milk chocolate bars—⅓ small size
  vanilla fudge (20 pcs per lb)—1

Vegetables
  avocado—⅕-¼
  beans (green)—2½ cups
  beets (sliced)—1½ cups
  lettuce, iceberg—2 lbs
  peas—1 cup
  potatoes—1 medium
  tomatoes—3 average

Miscellaneous
  baked beans—⅓ cup
  bread—1½ slices
  cheddar cheese—1 oz
  crackers-Saltines—8
  egg, boiled—1½ small
  jelly—2 tbsp
  ice cream—⅓ cup

Table 14-4.   Comparison of various amounts of food in 100 kcal portions (continued).

Miscellaneous (continued).

Drinks

   coke—8 oz
   whole milk—5 oz
   orange drink—8 oz
   scotch—(1½ oz + water)
   beer—8 oz

Fruits

   apricots (dried)—7
   apple (medium-large fresh)—1
   banana—1 small
   orange—1 large
   prunes, dried—4 large
   strawberries, raw and stems
     removed—2 cups

ice milk—½ cup
mayonnaise—1 tbsp
mushrooms, raw—15 large
noodles cooked—½ cup
peanut butter—1 tbsp
popcorn, plain popped—2 cups
potato chips—9 chips
rice—½ cup
sugar—2 tbsp
syrup—2 tbsp

Table 14-5.   Some low calorie snacks.*

Black Coffee
Broth, clear
Carrot Sticks
Celery Stalks
Cucumber
Diet Drinks
Diet Jello
Dill Pickles
Green Pepper Strips
Ice Tea
Mushrooms
Popcorn (without margarine or butter added)
Radishes
Tomato Juice
V-8 Juice

---

*Some of the foods listed are relatively high in sodium content.

Table 14-6.   How to *estimate* total daily energy (caloric) needs for an adult to attain and maintain ideal weight.

1. Basal calories: (1 kcal/hour/kg body weight)
    Desirable body weight in kg x 24 =   _____

2. Add voluntary activity calories (use one category):
    a.   Sedentary—most Americans are sedentary. For
          adults over age 76 use 20% basal calories to determine
          voluntary activity calories.
          30% basal calories (.30 x #1)   _____
    b.   Moderate:
          40% basal calories (.40 x #1)   _____
    c.   Strenuous:
          50% basal calories (.50 x #1)   _____

3. Add 10 percent of basal calories plus voluntary activity calories
    to cover the caloric value of the specific dynamic action of
    foods (calorie cost for the metabolism of foods):
    .10(#1 + #2) =   _____

4. Total kcal allowance
    (Check: Does kcal allowance fall within kcal range given in
    mean Heights and Weights Table of RDAs?)   _____

5. Add calories for conditions of growth:
    a.   Pregnancy: Add 300 kcal   _____
    b.   Lactation: Add 500 kcal   _____
    c.   Desirable weight gain: For each gain of one pound
          per week add 500 kcal (that is, for a gain of two
          pounds per week add 1000 kcal).   _____

6. Computation of calories for desirable weight loss:
    a.   Calculate basal calories to maintain *present* weight:
          Present weight in kg x 24 =   _____
    b.   Add voluntary calories calculated as in #2 above (.3 x
          basal kcal for sedentary; .4 x basal kcal for moderate;
          .5 x basal kcal for strenuous) =   _____
    c.   Add 10 percent of basal calories plus voluntary
          calories to cover the value of the specific dynamic
          action of foods: .10 (#a + #b) =   _____
    d.   Total kcal allowance required to maintain *present*
          weight: _____
    e.   Subtract calories for desirable weight loss: For each
          one pound per week weight loss subtract 500 kcal per
          day (suggested limit of loss for women = 1-2 pounds
          per week; for men = 2-3 pounds per week)   _____

                                                      Total   _____

Adapted from: A Guide for Professionals: The Effective Application of 'Exchange Lists for Meal Planning.' Prepared by committees of The American Diabetes Association, Inc. and The American Dietetic Association, 1977, pp. 17-18.

Recent Advances in Therapeutic Diets, 3rd ed. Staff, Dietary Department, University of Iowa Hospitals and Clinics, Iowa City (Ames, Iowa; Iowa State University Press), 1979, p. 87.

Table 14-7.   Desirable weights per height and body frame.

Weight in Pounds According to Frame (In Indoor Clothing)

	HEIGHT (with shoes on) 1-inch heels Feet Inches		SMALL FRAME	MEDIUM FRAME	LARGE FRAME
	5	2	112-120	118-129	126-141
	5	3	115-123	121-133	129-144
	5	4	118-126	124-136	132-148
	5	5	121-129	127-139	135-152
	5	6	124-133	130-143	138-156
Men	5	7	128-137	134-147	142-161
of Ages 25	5	8	132-141	138-152	147-166
and over	5	9	136-145	142-156	151-170
	5	10	140-150	146-160	155-174
	5	11	144-154	150-165	159-179
	6	0	148-158	154-170	164-184
	6	1	152-162	158-175	168-189
	6	2	156-167	162-180	173-194
	6	3	160-171	167-185	178-199
	6	4	164-175	172-190	182-204

	HEIGHT (with shoes on) 2-inch heels Feet Inches		SMALL FRAME	MEDIUM FRAME	LARGE FRAME
	4	10	92- 98	96-107	104-119
	4	11	94-101	98-110	106-122
	5	0	96-104	101-113	109-125
	5	1	99-107	104-116	112-128
	5	2	102-110	107-119	115-131
Women	5	3	105-113	110-122	118-134
of Ages 25	5	4	108-116	113-126	121-138
and Over	5	5	111-119	116-130	125-142
	5	6	114-123	120-135	129-146
	5	7	118-127	124-139	133-150
	5	8	122-131	128-143	137-154
	5	9	126-135	132-147	141-158
	5	10	130-140	136-151	145-163
	5	11	134-144	140-155	149-168
	6	0	138-148	144-159	153-173

For girls between 18 and 25, subtract 1 pound for each year under 25.

Source: Metropolitan Life Insurance Company, New York.

Table 14-8   Some suggested food exchange choices for daily caloric patterns.

Exchanges	1,000 Calories	1,200 Calories	1,500 Calories	1,800 Calories	2,000 Calories	2,200 Calories	2,500 Calories
Milk, skim	2	2	3	3	3	3	3
Vegetable	2	2	3	3	3	3	3
Fruit	3	3	4	5	6	7	8
Bread	3	5	6	8	9	11	12
Fat	2	2	4	5	5	6	7
Meat	5	6	6	7	8	8	10
Total calories	995	1,204	1,510	1,804	1,985	2,206	2,505

Key Points: Control of Body Weight

I. Ideal weight is suggested by average height/weight charts with reference to body frame and size and is related to longevity.
   A. Body fat to lean tissue measurements are more accurate in determining "fatness" or "leanness."
   B. Some measurements for determining body composition are
      1. Skin-fold thickness measurement by calipers.
      2. Anthropometric measurements.
      3. Water displacement and determination of specific gravity of the body.
   C. Rule-of-thumb measurement for persons of medium frame for determining ideal weight:
      women: 100 lbs per five feet height + five lbs for every inch over five feet
      men: 110 lbs per five feet height + five lbs for every inch over five feet

II. Underweight is generally accepted as 10 percent below ideal (average) weight though the determination should consider individual body composition and appearance.

III. Overweight is generally accepted as 10 to 20 percent in excess of ideal (average) weight though the determination should consider individual body composition and appearance. Overweight is usually a social embarrassment for an individual.

IV. Obesity is generally accepted as body weight in excess of 20 percent of the ideal (average) weight. Obesity is more than a social embarrassment, it is a health problem.
   A. Obesity is a result of social, psychological, and physiological forces as well as excess nutrient intake above total body caloric expenditure.
   B. Obese persons may have an altered metabolic process.
   C. Weight loss and maintenance of weight loss is seldom achieved on a permanent basis.

V. So-called fad diets are not successful in promoting safe loss of body fat.
   A. A severe restriction of caloric intake promotes loss of body lean tissue and water.
   B. A weight loss of about two pounds per week generally reflects a loss of body fat.

VI. Weight loss is most satisfactorily achieved when diets are planned around nutritionally sound food guides, behavior modification techniques are used, and physical exercise is increased. Total caloric intake must be less than total caloric expenditure.

Questions: Control of Body Weight

1. Identify the following methods for determining proportion and amounts of fat and lean tissue.
   a. use of calipers to determine amounts of fat tissue
   b. comparisons of body contour and skeletal measurements to standards
   c. determination of specific gravity of the body

2. Identify the probable conditions of the following persons:
   _____ 1. John is 5 ft. 9 in. tall, of medium frame, and weighs 275 pounds.
   _____ 2. Mary is 5 ft. 5 in. tall, of medium frame, and weighs 150 pounds.
   _____ 3. Joan is 5 ft. 5 in. tall, of medium frame, and weighs 105 pounds.
   _____ 4. Jennifer is 5 ft. 5 in. tall, of medium frame, weighs 87 pounds, is a teenager, and stubbornly refuses to eat due to a deep-seated, probably unreasonable, fear of gaining weight and appearing fat.

    a. underweight
    b. overweight
    c. anorexia nervosa
    d. obese

3. Why does a person who is underweight and consuming calories on the low side of average need to choose foods of high nutrient density?

4. A healthy, muscular football player is 5 ft. 11 in. tall and weighs 230 pounds. Is this man overweight?

5. The Public Health Service has stated what condition related to eating habits to be one of the most prevalent health problems in the U.S. today?

6. Most obesity is probably the result of:
    a. gross over-eating
    b. glandular disorders
    c. a combination of genetic, physiological, social, and psychological factors

7. By rule-of-thumb calculation, what is the ideal weight of a woman of medium frame who is 5 ft. 3 in. tall?
    a. 120 pounds
    b. 115 pounds
    c. 110 pounds

8. By rule-of-thumb calculation, what is the ideal weight of a man of medium frame who is 5 ft. 7 in. tall?
    a. 145 pounds
    b. 155 pounds
    c. 165 pounds

9. Kevin is a man of medium frame who is 5 ft. 7 in. tall. He only weighs 126 pounds. Is he underweight?

10. What is one personal method of determining whether you in particular are overweight due to body fat?

11. There is an increased occurrence of some disease conditions such as gallbladder disease, diabetes, and heart and circulatory disease among obese individuals.
    a. True
    b. False

12. Being overweight during infancy and childhood often extends to being overweight in adulthood. Research has indicated that most overweight and obese children are less active than children of average weight, and they grow up to be less active adults than adults of average weight. Consequently, overweight and obesity are now recognized as being due in part to a level of _____ .

13. Some overweight individuals seem to utilize food differently than persons of average weight. It can be said, then, that overweight may be due in part to an _____ reflective of an abnormal utilization of food.

14. The fat cell theory of obesity involves basically two types of fat cell conditions: one, there is an excessive number of fat cells which continually try to "fill-up" with fat; and two, there are a normal number of fat cells which continually try to remain filled or "over-filled."
    a. What is the term (s) which describes an excess number of fat cells?
    b. What is the term which describes fat cells that tend to "over-fill?"

15. What is the crux of the theory involving blood glucose level and satiety?

16. Treatment success for weight loss involving the use of appetite depressant drugs is high.
    a. True
    b. False

17. Diuretics increase the loss of body _____ .
    a. fat
    b protein (lean tissue)
    c. water

18. An overweight individual has been successful in losing weight (body fat) and is presently at his or her ideal weight. Identify the following principles applicable to this person:
    a. This person should not consider himself or herself as cured of overweight problems, but rather as having the conditions causing overweight under control.
    b. This person can relax now and freely choose favorite foods for mealtime and snacks.
    c. This person must identify the caloric level at which present weight can be maintained; then choose foods and a food plan using a nutritionally sound food guide which will allow appetizing and nutritious meals to be planned and eaten within the limitations of his or her calorie level.

19. Eating a varied diet from the different groups of food helps to avoid overconsumption of foods which are high in caloric (energy) value and low in nutrient value.
    a. True
    b. False

20. Mary prides herself on her cooking ability. However, she is worried about the tendency of all her immediate family members to be overweight. Tom, her husband, is obese and his doctor has advised him many times to lose weight. Mary thought about this while she fixed cream gravy to accompany her traditional Sunday fried chicken and mashed potatoes dinner.

    Janie, Mary's 12 year-old daughter, stopped her sewing project and helped to set the table. She put food on the serving platters and carried them to the table. She helped herself to a piece of sweet chocolate in the refrigerator while she took out the beverages and sour cream/roquefort dressing to put on the salad. She eyed the lemon meringue pie on the kitchen counter which was to be for dessert. Mark, Janie's little brother, came into the kitchen and threw away the empty cookie bag he had been eating from his desk in his room while he did his homework.

    Everyone was very hungry and eagerly sat down to dinner at 6 p.m. Though they loved their meal they all hurried to get done in time for Dad to watch his favorite Sunday evening television show at 6:30 p.m. By 6:30 p.m. all the dishes were cleared from the table and dish washing started. Everyone elected to eat their pie later while watching television.

    Refer to Tables 14-2 and 14-3.
    a. What are some food preparation methods that would lower the caloric value of this meal?
    b. What improvements in snacking patterns could be made to help Janie and Mark avoid consumption of high-calorie snacks?
    c. Describe the apparent activity level of this family.
    d. Does this family seem to allow sufficient time for meals?

21.   Study the list of foods in 100 kcal portions in Table 14-4.
a.   Choose three foods seemingly high in caloric value because of the small quantity allowed.
b.   Choose three foods seemingly low in caloric value because of the large quantity allowed.
c.   How would you classify the high calorie foods? Low calorie foods?

22.   Complete the following activities:
a.   Pick out your desirable weight from the height/weight/age chart (Table 14-7) and compute your kcal allowance (use Table 14-6).
b.   Most Americans are of what activity level (see Table 14-6)?
c.   A 5 ft. 5 in. woman 22 years-old weighs 143 pounds (65 kg) and is a sedentary individual. She has maintained this weight for two years. What is her present caloric requirement? How many calories a day must she delete to lose two pounds per week? What will her reducing diet calorie level be?

23.   Compose a day's meals (breakfast, lunch, and dinner) in food exchanges within a 1200 kcal meal plan.

Answers: Control of Body Weight

1.   a.   skin-fold thickness measurements
b.   anthropometric measurements
c.   water displacement measurement methods
2.   1.   d
2.   b
3.   a
4.   c
3.   Because his (or her) total daily calorie intake is limited and he (or she) cannot afford to use part of that calorie allotment on foods of high energy, low nutrient value. Also, high calorie foods tend to be high in carbohydrate or fat which tend to further depress the appetite.
4.   Probably overweight by statistical standards but not "over-fat"
5.   obesity
6.   c
7.   b
8.   a
9.   By statistical calculation Kevin is underweight (weight below 10 percent of ideal weight). However, we are not given further details of his body build, eating patterns, or condition of health. It is possible that Kevin is in good health, eats food that meets his nutritional needs, and appears visually to have weight appropriate for his body size.
10.   Observe yourself in a mirror while undressed. If from the rear, side, and front views you appear fat, then you probably are overweight due to body fat.
11.   a
12.   reduced activity
13.   altered metabolism
14   a.   hypercellular or hyperplastic
b.   hypertrophic
15.   A center in the brain senses blood glucose level. High blood glucose levels tend to decrease appetite and increase the feeling of satiety. Low blood glucose levels tend to increase appetite and diminish feelings of satiety. Obese persons may have a malfunction in this brain center.

16. b
17. c
18. a, c
19. a
20. a. Broil or bake the chicken; make gravy with skim milk or omit gravy; use lemon juice and crushed herbs for a salad dressing; serve chicken skinless; use fresh fruit or canned fruit packed in water or juice for dessert instead of pie.
    b. Limit snacks to kitchen area; limit snacks to times when other activities are not being performed such as homework or television watching; keep low calorie snacks in the refrigerator ready to eat (see Table 14-5 for suggestions) and keep high calorie snacks out of sight or easy reach (if present at all).
    c. Activities such as cooking, sewing, homework, and television watching indicate a sedentary activity level.
    d. Meal times appear hurried and eating is probably excessive in a short time span so feelings of satiety are not reached while family members are still at the table.
21. a. Examples: candies; dried prunes; cheese; sugar; syrups; peanut butter; ice cream
    b. Examples: fresh, unsweetened strawberries; green beans; lettuce; tomatoes; beets; plain, popped popcorn; raw mushrooms.
    c. High calorie foods seem to be concentrated sweet and fat foods; low calorie foods seem to be most fresh fruits and vegetables.
22. a. Did you check the calorie level with the RDA table for appropriate energy values?
    b. sedentary
    c. 65 kg x 24 = 1560 basal kcal plus 468 (1560 x .3) kcal = 2028 kcal, plus 10 percent of 2028 for 203 kcal SDA of food = 2231 kcal; 1000 kcal; 2231 − 1000 = 1231 kcal (or 1200 kcal diet plan)
23. Breakfast: Lunch:
    1 fruit   1 milk
    2 bread   1 fruit
    1 fat   2 bread
    1 meat   2 meat
    Dinner:
    1 milk
    1 fruit
    2 vegetables
    1 bread
    1 fat
    3 meat

REFERENCES

[1] This apparatus used for the determination of the caloric value of a food sample is called a *bomb calorimeter*.
[2] This apparatus used for determining caloric expenditure by the body is called a *respiration calorimeter*.
[3] The *mesomorph* is representative of the person with a large heavy-boned, muscular body type.
[4] Guthrie HA: Introductory Nutrition, 4th ed. St. Louis, The C. V. Mosby Company, 1979, p. 115

[5] Williams SR: Nutrition and Diet Therapy, 3rd ed. St. Louis, The C. V. Mosby Company, 1977, p. 503

[6] Guthrie HA: Introductory Nutrition, 4th ed. St. Louis, The C. V. Mosby Company, 1979, p. 507-509

[7] Mitchell HS et al: Nutrition in Health and Disease, 16th ed. Philadelphia, J. B. Lippincott Company, 1976, pp. 392-393. An interesting study of anorexia nervosa and related emotional/psychological conditions can be found in: Bruch H: Anorexia nervosa. Nutrition Today, 13, September-October 1978, pp. 14-18.

[8] Deutsch RM: Realities of Nutrition. Palo Alto, California, Bull Publishing Company, 1976, p. 75

[9] Mayer J: Obesity. *In* Goodhart RS and Shils ME (eds): Modern Nutrition in Health and Disease. Philadelphia, Lea and Febiger, 1980, p. 721

[10] Ibid

[11] Abramson EE: A review of behavioral approaches to weight control. Behaviour and Research Therapy, 11, November 1973, 547-556

[12] Johnson SF et al: Personality characteristics in obesity: Relation of MMPI profile and age of onset of obesity to success in weight reduction. The American Journal of Clinical Nutrition, 29, June 1976, 626-632

[13] Kruskemper G: Maternal food intake and weight of grown-up offspring. The New England Journal of Medicine, 295, November 4, 1976, p. 1084

[14] Udall JN et al: Interaction of maternal and neonatal obesity. Pediatrics, 62, July 1978, pp. 17-21

[15] Weil WB: Current controversies in childhood obesity. The Journal of Pediatrics, 91, August 1977, p. 180

[16] Ibid

[17] Experts weigh reducing potions. FDA Consumer, 13, October 1979, p. 11

[18] Fineberg SK: The realities of obesity and fad diets. Nutrition Today, 8, July-August 1972, pp. 23-26

[19] A dozen diets for better or worse. California Dietetic Association, Los Angeles District, November 1973

[20] A critique of low-carbohydrate ketogenic weight reduction regimens—a review of Dr. Atkins' diet revolution. Journal of the American Medical Association, 224, June 4, 1973, pp. 1415-1419

15
PROTECTION AND SAFETY OF THE FOOD SUPPLY

FOODBORNE ILLNESSES

Certain organisms can be transmitted to man through food that can cause illness and even death. Modern food technology and knowledge of sanitation and safe food-handling practices have greatly reduced the threat to health from commercial food contamination. However, the personal use of many unsafe food-handling practices persists. The following is a review of some pathogenic organisms which can contaminate food and some safe food-handling procedures recommended for use at home.

PARASITES

Round worms (nematodes). An example of a round worm which is disease-producing in man is the Trichina worm *(Trichinella spiralis).* Hogs which eat uncooked, unsanitary feed (such as garbage) transmit the tiny trichina worm to humans. The worms ingested with the contaminated feed produce larvae which invade the pork muscle. If this pork meat is not cooked thoroughly and is consumed by a human the larvae survive and grow within that human's body. The mature females deposit new larvae which travel by way of the circulatory and lymph systems to muscle tissue which they again invade. Trichinosis causes muscular pain, chills, fever, and even death. Prevention can be accomplished by:

1. Cooking hog feed.
2. Cooking pork meat to at least 170°F.
3. Freezing pork meat for three or more days at temperatures of 0°F (− 18°C) or below.

Tapeworms (cestodes). Infestation of tapeworms occurs by a cyclic fecal-oral route. Mature worms (that are segmented) and eggs are eaten by livestock along with feed from sewage-polluted areas. These larvae also survive in the animal's intestine where they grow; some migrate to other organs and muscle tissue where they form cysts. When this animal flesh is eaten raw or only partially cooked, the larvae survive and grow in the human intestines. Because they use up nutrients consumed by the human which they inhabit they cause weight loss, anemia, and nutrient deficiencies. Strict sanitation regulations for disposal of human feces (sewage) is necessary to control infestation by such tapeworms. Fish tapeworms can infest the human body when fish is eaten raw or undercooked. Prevention can be accomplished by:

1. Separating sewage areas from livestock feed areas.
2. Practicing good personal hygiene principles such as washing hands following defecation or handling of soil.

3.   Consuming well-cooked meats.

4.   Freezing meats for three or more days at temperatures of 0°F (−18°C) or below.

Amebae (parasitic protozoa). Amebic dysentery is caused by pathogenic protozoa of the species *Entamoeba histolytica.* They are transmitted to humans by way of infected food and water using a cyclic fecal-oral route. Once in the human intestine they burrow into the intestinal lining which then becomes eroded and ulcerated. They may also travel by way of the blood and lymph to other tissues such as the liver, lungs, and brain which they subsequently invade. Medical treatment is essential to avoid serious threat to health or possibly death. Prevention can be accomplished by:

1.   Separating human fecal sewage from food and water sources.

2.   Following good principles of personal hygiene.

3.   Preventing human carriers from handling food.

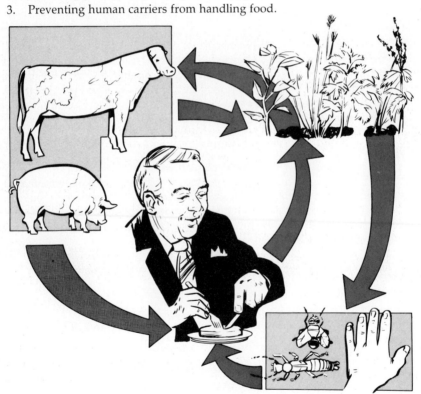

Figure 15-1.   The oral-fecal route. The route is cyclic and results from human consumption of infected meat which is poorly cooked; deposition of contaminated feces in livestock feeding areas; consumption of infectious organisms by livestock; and contamination of livestock muscle tissue by infectious organisms. The cycle is also continued with contact of food by hands, insects, or flies which carry infectious organisms from contaminated feces to food to mouth.

BACTERIAL INFECTIONS

Salmonellosis. This infection is caused by numerous species of the Salmonella bacilli. These bacteria are capable of surviving cold and relatively long periods of time in water, soil, and various foodstuffs. However, the bacilli are easily destroyed by heat. Salmonella are most commonly found in raw meats, poultry, eggs, milk, fish, and products made from them. Other sources can be pets such as dogs, cats, birds, and fish. Typhoid fever is caused by a species of Salmonella.

Symptoms of Salmonella infection are fever, headache, diarrhea, abdominal discomfort, and occasionally vomiting. These symptoms generally appear about 24 hours after eating contaminated food. Most people recover in two to four days. Infants, small children, elderly persons, and people already weakened by disease are more seriously affected by Salmonella infection. Observe the following precautions in order to avoid Salmonella infection:

1.   Cook foods thoroughly.
2.   Reheat leftovers thoroughly. Bring broths and gravies to a rolling boil for several minutes. Serve food promptly following heating.
3.   Follow good principles of personal hygiene and food-handling procedures.
4.   Store foods below 40°F or cook and hold above 140°F.

Clostridium perfringens. These bacteria are widely distributed in nature. They can be found naturally in the soil, dust, on food, and in the intestinal tracts of man and other warmblooded animals. They are one of the most widespread, disease causing micro-organisms. These bacteria are destroyed by heat but their spores are heat resistant. Favorable conditions can allow the spores to grow producing large numbers of bacteria.

Disease outbreaks frequently occur when foods are held in large quantities at improper temperatures for extended periods of time. Perfringens outbreaks are closely associated with restaurants or other large feeding establishments where foods are held for long periods of time on steam tables or other warming devices. Symptoms include diarrhea and abdominal pain.

Some effective controls which prevent the growth of *Clostridium perfringens* include:

1.   Thoroughly cooking food and then holding (if necessary) above 140°F.
2.   Storing leftovers in small containers at temperatures below 40°F in order to effect a rapid cooling period.
3.   Reheating foods to temperatures well above 140°F.
4.   Avoid holding foods at room temperature. Refrigerate leftovers immediately following a meal.

BACTERIAL TOXINS

Staphylococci food poisoning. This foodborne disease is quite common in the United States. Staphylococci bacteria are normally present in the respiratory passages and on the skin of humans. Contamination of food frequently occurs from a minor skin infection on the hand of a food service worker.

Symptoms of staphylococci intoxification ensue rapidly following ingestion of the tox in produced by the bacteria: severe cramping, vomiting, diarrhea, headache, and fever. Symptoms usually subside within a day or two from their first appearance.

Staphylococci grow in a wide variety of foods: all meat, poultry, eggs and egg products, tuna, chicken, potato and macaroni salads, cream filled pastries, and sandwich fillings. If staphylococci bacteria multiply to high levels they form significant amounts of toxin which cannot be destroyed by heat. Prevention of poisoning by staphylococci bacterial toxin can be attained by:

1.   Observing good principles of personal hygiene.
2.   Immediately refrigerating prepared foods until ready to be served at temperatures below 40°F.

3. Thoroughly cooking foods and holding when necessary at temperatures above 140°F.

4. Refraining from tasting possibly contaminated food even though it does not appear to have spoiled.

Botulism. Clostridium botulinum bacteria produce a highly toxic poison which is usually fatal to humans. *Clostridium botulinum* is a spore-forming bacillus which grows in the absence of oxygen. Botulinum spores are found throughout the environment and are harmless. However, in the proper environment the spores divide and produce poisonous toxins. The toxins of *C. botulinum* are heat sensitive and are readily destroyed by normal cooking temperatures. Boiling for 10 to 15 minutes safely inactivates all types of these toxins. *Never taste a sample of food suspected of contamination by Clostridium botulinum before adequate heating of the food product.* In order to avoid illness it is best to discard a suspect food.

Most outbreaks of botulism have been traced to home canned vegetables, fruits, fish, and meat products. Modern commercial food preservation and canning methods have greatly decreased botulism outbreaks from commercially prepared foods. Botulism is usually associated with low-acid foods that have been given a preservation treatment, stored for some time, and consumed without appropriate heating. Open-kettle and water-bath methods of home canning are not adequate enough to prevent the growth of *C. botulinum* spores in low-acid foods. Canning needs to be accomplished by appropriate steam pressure methods.

Botulinum toxin causes paralysis starting in the face and progressing downward. When the diaphragm and chest muscles become fully involved respiration is no longer possible and death from asphyxia results. Other early signs of botulism are weakness, dizziness, double-vision, and difficulty in speaking and swallowing.[1]

BRUCELLOSIS (Undulant Fever)

This disease is caused by Brucella bacteria and is transmitted by unpasteurized milk and contact with infected animals such as cows and goats. It results in a recurrent fever that can last for only a few days to years with accompanying aching joints, general discomfort, and profuse sweating. It is a tedious and debilitating disease which creates depression, loss of ambition and general fatigue.

Pasteurization of milk is accomplished by the heating of milk to temperatures lethal to most bacteria either at a relatively low degree for a lengthy time, or at a relatively high degree for a short time. Pasteurized milk is equal to raw milk in nutritive value except for slight losses of thiamin and ascorbic acid (vitamins B_1 and C respectively).[2]

SAFE FOOD HANDLING METHODS

Even though most of us know the best ways of handling food for safe consumption, we frequently overlook them in favor of shortcuts in food preparation.[3] However, great nutrient losses occur as a result of food spoilage. These nutrients are not available to the people who need them. Disease and illness caused by food contamination add to human misery and should be avoided whenever possible. The following are some safe and simple food-handling practices which help prevent foodborne illness[4]:

1. Clean and wash hands, cutting surfaces, and cutting knives after each use. Avoid cross-contamination of meats and vegetables by washing hands, knives, and cutting boards between cutting operations. Preferably, use different cutting boards for meats and fruits/vegetables.

2. Refrigerate perishables immediately following your return home from shopping.

3. Refrigerate foods between preparation and cooking times if being held to cook later.

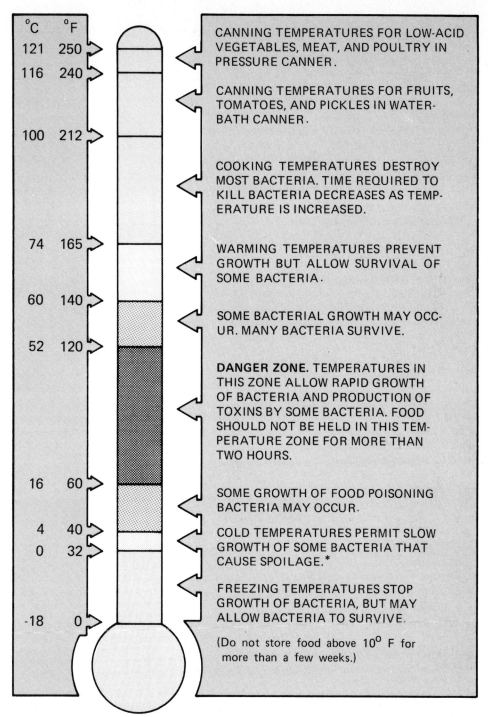

Figure 15-2. Temperature of food for control of bacteria. Adapted from: Keeping Food Safe to Eat. Home and Garden Bulletin, No. 162, U.S. Department of Agriculture, revised 1978.

4. Store leftovers promptly following meal service.

5. Keep refrigerator at 40°F or below. Use a refrigerator thermometer. Check refrigerator gaskets for adequately tight seals. If you can easily pull a dollar bill out from between the gaskets of the door and the refrigerator door frame when the refrigerator door is shut there is probably air leakage.

6. Defrost frozen foods in the refrigerator (not at room temperatures).

7. Refrigerate foods promptly in small, shallow containers in order to reduce food temperatures quickly.

8. Use meat thermometers to cook meat to appropriate, safe *internal* temperatures (about 180°F for poultry and 170°F for pork).

9. Do not taste possibly contaminated food; throw it out.

10. Clean the tops of cans before opening to prevent dust and dirt from entering contents during the opening process.

11. Wrap fresh meat loosely for refrigeration.

12. Cover leftovers tightly for refrigeration.

13. Place foods in the refrigerator in such a way as to allow for proper air circulation.

14. Do not leave perishable foods unrefrigerated for long periods of time during food preparation processes.

15. Store foods away from areas containing water pipes, heating pipes, household chemicals, and cleaning compounds.

16. Throw out, without tasting, the contents of any leaking, bulging cans of food. Report their occurrence to the market from which you purchased them.

17. When packing carry lunches or other meals use vacuum thermoses to keep liquids cold or hot as necessary, and use sandwich fillings which are less likely to become contaminated with bacteria during the period of nonrefrigeration: peanut butter, sliced cheese, canned meat and poultry products, fully cooked bologna and frankfurters.[5]

18. Wash fruits and vegetables before eating or cooking.

19. Do not stuff a turkey hours ahead of cooking. It is best to cook turkey and stuffing separately.

20. Boil leftover gravy and broths for several minutes and serve promptly.

21. Boil all home-canned, low-acid foods at least ten minutes before eating.

22. Do not eat foods with mold on it (except, of course, for the safe, intentionally mold-streaked cheeses such as Roquefort and Blue). Do not cut obvious mold off and eat the remainder of a food as unseen mold roots may go deep into the contaminated food source. Some molds themselves are toxic to humans while others produce highly potent toxins.

23. *Keep cold foods cold, below 40°F (4°C), and hot foods hot, above 140°F (60°C).*

Key Points: Foodborne Illness

I. Control of foodborne illness depends upon adherence to principles of good sanitation: proper sewage disposal, practice of good personal hygiene, especially by food handlers; cooking of foods to properly elevated temperatures; proper storage of foods.

II. Cold foods must be kept cold, below 40°F (4°C); hot foods must be kept hot, above 140°F (60°C).

III. Safe food handling practices in the home include: washing hands, food preparation utensils, and cutting surfaces; refrigerating foods as soon after purchase as possible; defrosting of frozen foods in the refrigerator; cleaning tops of canned goods before opening; refraining from tasting suspect foods and properly disposing of them; storing of food in clean, dry areas; thorough washing and cleaning of fresh fruits and vegetables.

Questions: Foodborne Illness

1. Match the phrases on the right to the items on the left which they best describe:

    _____ 1. amebae
    _____ 2. salmonella
    _____ 3. *Staphylococci*
    _____ 4. *trichinella spiralis*
    _____ 5. undulant fever
    _____ 6. tapeworm
    _____ 7. *Clostridium botulinum*
    _____ 8. *Clostridium perfringens*

    a. a roundworm capable of invading the human body tissues
    b. a segmented worm which can survive in the human intestines causing weight loss, anemia, and nutrient deficiencies
    c. a parasitic protozoa which causes erosion and ulceration of the human intestines and severe diarrhea
    d. bacteria which are frequently found in protein foods but which are easily destroyed by the thorough heating of food
    e. bacteria whose heat resistant spores easily grow in improperly heated foods such as those held in the steam tables of restaurants
    f. bacteria which produce a toxin which cannot be destroyed by heat
    g. bacteria which produce a deadly toxin that can be destroyed by proper heating
    h. disease caused by *Brucella* bacteria passed to humans through unpasteurized milk

2. What arguments could you present in favor of the consumption of pasteurized milk in a discussion with a friend who believes raw milk should be consumed because it is more nutritious and natural than pasteurized milk?

3. Describe the fecal-oral route.

4. The eating of raw garbage by hogs is favorable to infection of hog muscle by Trichinella worms.
    a. True
    b. False

5. Freezing pork or beef meat for three or more days at temperatures of 0°F (-18°C) or below is sufficient to kill larvae of Trichinella and tapeworms.
    a. True
    b. False

6. It is a good idea to sniff and taste foods that appear to be contaminated to check for spoilage.
    a. True
    b. False

7. Review the symptoms for foodborne bacterial infections. Why might accurate identification of these diseases be overlooked frequently?

8. Why is it a poor food-handling practice to mix a meat loaf with uncovered hands when a cut or sore is on your hand?
   a. It is an unappealing practice.
   b. It can cause you irritation at the site of the sore.
   c. Staphylococci bacteria could be transmitted to the meat loaf from the cut or sore where they are concentrated, then multiply and produce harmful toxin in the prepared meat loaf which is not destroyed by cooking the meat loaf.

9. *Clostridium botulinum* bacteria which produce a deadly toxin are most often associated with:
   a. canned citrus fruit juices.
   b. home-canned, low-acid foods such as corn, green beans, fish and meat.
   c. frozen meats.

10. Identify the poor food-handling practices illustrated in the following sketch:

    Mrs. Walker bought a lot of groceries Saturday afternoon for a family reunion dinner to be held on Sunday, the Fourth of July. The phone rang just as she walked through the door with the first of her ten bags of groceries. She was glad it was the bag with her frozen foods of fruit juice, ice cream, popsicles, and crushed ice because she could put them in the freezer compartment of her refrigerator while she chatted on the phone for an hour with her sister, who was going to help her cook the food for the dinner. After she hung up the telephone she unloaded and stored the remaining groceries.

    Mrs. Walker and her sister spent Saturday evening cooking for the big meal. They prepared and stuffed a turkey for cooking the next day. They were very efficient workers. They took out all the ingredients they would need and left them on the counter where they could find them easily. Mrs. Walker's sister prepared all the desserts including pumpkin custard pie. Mrs. Walker used the cutting board and sink area so she could make all the foods requiring washing, peeling, or chopping. She chopped all her ingredients for the ham salad and pineapple/carrot/apple salad before mixing either so she could wash her cutting board and put it away for the evening.

    When she put the cutting board away underneath the sink she found the canned pineapple juice she was going to use for the punch. She quickly opened them with a punch-type opener and mixed the punch.

    When all the food was prepared and the clean-up was completed, Mrs. Walker and her sister stored the foods in the refrigerator. They laughed and joked that there was so much food not even a pin could fit into the refrigerator now. The pies had to be left on the counter covered with foil wrap for the night.

    The next day they had a wonderful time with all their close family members. Mrs. Walker's great aunt brought her home-canned succotash (corn and lima beans). Her aunt still did all her canning the laborious, old-fashioned way and did not use a pressure cooker for canning. Mrs. Walker and her sister tasted the succotash even before it was heated to see if it still tasted as good as they remembered as children.

    The dinner was delicious and the cold pineapple punch tasted good on this hot July day. There were so many family tales to exchange that they all relaxed and chatted after dinner. No one wanted to miss the fun and put the food away just yet. When they did store the food Mrs. Walker used some deep, wide dishes that made the job of fitting the many leftovers into the refrigerator easier.

11. Why might the purchase of a dozen inexpensively priced cracked eggs not be a real "bargain?"

12. A rule-of-thumb to remember in order to control bacterial growth in food: keep

cold foods cold, below _____ , and hot foods hot, above _____ . (Hint: See Figure 15-2.)

Answers: Foodborne Illnesses

1. 1. c
   2. d
   3. f
   4. a
   5. h
   6. b
   7. g
   8. e
2. a. Pasteurization is only the heating of milk to temperatures lethal to most infectious bacteria.
   b. Pasteurization of milk prevents one common means of transmitting undulant fever (a debilitating disease) to man.
   c. Pasteurized milk is equal to the nutritive value of raw milk except for slight losses of two vitamins, thiamin and ascorbic acid.
3. The passage of infectious organisms from animal to man by consuming contaminated meat which is inadequately cooked; loss of eggs, organisms or larvae of infectious organisms in human and animal feces which pollute livestock feeding areas; consumption by livestock of infectious organisms in feed; contamination of livestock muscle tissue by infectious organisms.

   Also, by contact of food by hands, insects, and flies which carry infectious organisms from contaminated feces to food to the mouth.
4. a
5. a
6. b
7. Symptoms are very similar to "flu" symptoms and are frequently dismissed as such obscuring proper identification of the disease source.
8. c
9. b
10. a. perishables other than frozen goods left in the car on a warm day for more than an hour;
    b. prepared and stuffed turkey a day before cooking (bacteria could easily grow deep in the poultry cavity with warm stuffing present which would not cool for several hours);
    c. all ingredients taken out of the cupboards and refrigerator for dishes to prepare would mean even perishables would be unrefrigerated for a long period of time;
    d. cutting board not washed between the chopping of different foodstuffs—possible cross-contamination could occur;
    e. cans of pineapple juice stored under the sink near water pipes and cleaners—an unclean area where insects or rodents are likely to be found;
    f. pineapple can top not wiped before opening;
    g. some prepared foods left unrefrigerated for a long time before storage for the night in the refrigerator;
    h. custard (milk- and egg-containing) pies left unrefrigerated for the night;
    i. refrigerator so full that air circulation is likely to be inadequate;

      j.   inadequately prepared home-canned, low-acid foods tasted before boiling for ten minutes;
      k. following the meal, the food was left unrefrigerated for an extended time;
      l.   large dishes were used which would not allow for rapid cooling of leftovers.
11. Egg protein is an excellent medium in which many bacteria may grow. Bacteria could gain entrance through cracked egg shells and contaminate the egg inside.
12. 40°F (4°C) cold; 140°F (60°C) hot

TOXICANTS OCCURRING NATURALLY IN FOODS

Food contains thousands of chemical compounds of which only a relative few are nutritionally significant: fats, proteins, carbohydrates, vitamins, and minerals as well as water. Unfortunately, some of these chemical compounds which are normal constituents of both plant and animal foodstuffs are toxic to humans. These toxic agents occur naturally in varying concentrations in plant and animal foods and differ both in severity and types of effects. Even a relatively simple food such as the potato contains several hundred different compounds some of which are known to be toxic to humans.[6]

Toxicity is the capacity of a single chemical substance to harm living organisms while hazard specifies the condition of use under which a chemical can produce injury. All ingested substances are potentially toxic but vary individually in amounts required to become hazardous to health.[7] Ingestion of very small quantities of a toxic substance over a long period of time may not be hazardous (that is, be harmless) while ingestion of the same amount of the toxic substance in a single dose could prove hazardous to one's health (cause injury or death). The harmlessness of chemical substances in foods cannot be established just because they have been consumed in the human diet with no apparent ill effects for hundreds of years.

Some of the ways in which chemical substances exert a toxic effect are through their actions as:

1. Inhibitors of enzyme activity
2. Antagonists to the assimilation of vitamins
3. Hallucinogens
4. Stimulants
5. Depressants
6. Carcinogens (causing cancer)
7. Poisons
8. Producers of degenerative diseases.

It is necessary to note, however, that the action of naturally occurring toxicants in foods is minimized through various body mechanisms. Toxicity is enhanced and hazard produced when there is an imbalance of diet that results in the increased consumption of foods containing toxic substances. Such an imbalance usually occurs during such stressful periods as war and famine when alternative foods to the normal diet are consumed in relatively large amounts.

Certain body mechanisms can degrade, detoxify, and eliminate the toxic substances normally contained in a varied diet (remember the detoxification function of the liver). Modern food processing methods of heating, refrigeration, and canning help to reduce or even in some cases eliminate the effect of some toxins. Some toxins negate the toxic effect of other toxins consumed within the same meal. We generally are able to choose foods from a large selection in the marketplace which have been produced in many different areas of the world. This imported variety reduces the chance of consuming toxic substances contained in foods of a localized geographical area. Also, modern breeding programs have experienced success in reducing some toxic components of foods.[8]

A brief summary of some toxicants in foods is given in order to provide familiarity with the occurrence of such toxicants and their food sources.[9] The positive emphasis remains, however, on the ability of the body to successfully deal with such toxicants rather than on the negative effects of the toxicants themselves.

TOXINS FROM PLANT FOOD SOURCES

Protease (protein enzyme) inhibitors. These substances interfere with the activity of enzymes to break down proteins. The proteins are rendered in part or wholly unusable for body needs. These toxins are especially found in legumes.

An example:

Trypsin (a protein-digesting enzyme)—an inhibitor in raw soybeans, lima beans, and mung beans. This inhibitor can be inactivated by sufficient heating.

Hemagglutinins. These substances in plants can cause the clumping of red blood cells. Hemagglutinins are greatly destroyed or neutralized by body mechanisms and substances in the digestive tract. It appears that only a small amount of hemagglutinins are absorbed.

An example:

Hemagglutinins found in legumes such as soybeans, kidney beans, black beans, and castor beans.

Poisoning. Some plants contain substances which are poisonous to humans.

Legume examples:

1. Lathyrism is a condition of weakness and paralysis, especially of the legs, with an accompanying loss of the sensations of heat and pain. Lathyrism is caused by toxic substances in certain vetches (sweet peas) which are eaten by human populations, such as those of India and Africa, during periods of famine when other food supplies are not available.
2. Favism is a sensitivity to fava beans by certain individuals which causes hemolytic anemia (breakdown of blood components).

Mushroom examples:

Certain species of mushrooms, especially of the genus *Amanita,* produce poisons which are fatal when ingested by humans. *It is highly recommended that mushrooms be purchased from commercial sources that handle the harmless, domestically cultivated varieties.*

Herbal examples:

Hemlock, foxglove, and nightshade are a few herbs containing poisonous alkaloids.[10]

Potato example:

The green part of sprouting potatoes contains solanine, a poisonous alkaloid.[10] This greening can also occur in potatoes exposed to strong lights like those found in many supermarkets. The solanine is found in and just under the skin of the potato and is generally removed with the peeling of the potato. Solanine causes gastroenteritis, jaundice, and weakness.

Hepatotoxins. These substances are especially toxic to the liver.
Examples are:

1. *Senecio* (a genus of plants) which contain alkaloids[10] in their seeds that are potent liver toxins causing cirrhosis and cancer. These seeds are sometimes inadvertently harvested with food grains because they grow wild in the same grain fields.
2. Mycotoxins (fungal toxins) such as aflatoxins which are associated with the formation of liver cancer. These toxins are produced by molds such as those that grow on peanuts and grains which are not sufficiently dried.

Goitrogens. These substances cause hypothyroidism (decreased production of the thyroid gland) and enlargement of the thyroid gland. Although the primary cause of goiter is a deficiency of iodine, goitrogens are responsible for a significant amount of goiter incidence worldwide. The effect of goitrogens may result from various types of action: interference with the availability of dietary iodine; increased thyroid gland function in an abnormal manner; and obstruction of thyroid gland utilization of iodine.

Plants of the *Brassica* genus contain naturally occurring goitrogens: cabbage, turnips, rutabagas, mustard greens, and radishes. Cattle consuming goitrogen-containing plants may transmit goitrogens through their milk to humans. The action of goitrogens is inhibited by cooking goitrogen-containing foods. However, some bacteria often found in human intestines have been noted to activate even goitrogens subjected to heat before consumption.

Allergens. These are substances in food which cause allergic reactions when consumed by sensitive persons. The reactions are spontaneous and peculiar to sensitive individuals. Reactions often involve the skin (hives), respiratory tract (wheezing, excessive mucus production), and sometimes the central nervous system (migraine headaches).

Examples of foods often found to cause allergic reactions are:

1. Wheat, rye, oats, barley
2. Legumes
3. Strawberries, bananas, pineapple

Binders. These are substances which interfere with the absorption of certain nutrients. An example:

Oxalic acid (found in rhubarb and spinach) forms insoluble salts with calcium and iron rendering these minerals unabsorbable from the intestines.

Vitamin destroyers. These are substances which in some way destroy the activity of a vitamin.
An example:

Thiaminase is an enzyme which destroys thiamin (a B vitamin). This enzyme is contained in several vegetables and fruits, as well as bracken fern (sometimes consumed as a delicacy) and certain fish. Thiamin deficiency could result from an unusually large consumption of thiaminase-containing foods: spinach, cabbage, and blackberries.

Hallucinogens. These substances are responsible for producing distorted sensory impressions.
Examples are:

1. Some herbs used in herbal teas (jimson weed)
2. Some mushrooms
3. Some spices (nutmeg, mace)

Hypertensives. These substances can cause a rise in blood pressure (hypertension). Examples:

1.   Amines in bananas, plantains, tomatoes, avocados, and pineapples
2.   Active substance in natural licorice

Cyanogens. These substances block the utilization of oxygen by various body cells. They cause general tissue starvation for oxygen (cyanide poisoning). Some types of blindness and neurological diseases may be caused by chronic cyanide poisoning in tropical areas where the cassava is consumed as a staple food.

Examples of foods containing cyanogens are:

1.   Maize (type of corn), sorghum millet, lima beans, kidney beans, and cassava
2.   Pits and seeds of apples, apricots,[11] cherries, pears, plums, and prunes

TOXINS FROM MARINE FOOD SOURCES

Paralytic shellfish poisoning (PSP). This poisoning is caused by the eating of shellfish from waters containing dinoflagellates (microscopic organisms) which produce a poison retained by the shellfish (which are subsequently eaten by humans). Excessive amounts of dinoflagellates in marine waters cause a "red tide" condition. Symptoms of PSP are numbness and paralysis which can lead to eventual death.

Allergic reactions. These reactions seem to be caused by specific fish in sensitive individuals. The reactions can be in the forms of hives, edema, gastrointestinal disturbances, migraine, and asthma.

Mercury in fish. Mercury toxicity results in damage to brain cells, bone marrow, lymph nodes, nerve fibers, the liver, and kidneys. Shellfish and finfish seem to be able to concentrate mercury in their tissues. However, high levels of mercury in fish most often result from contamination of water by mercury pollutants rather than from naturally occurring mercury in the waters. Some experts feel that the danger of mercury in tuna (larger, older fish who have a greater exposure to mercury in waters) has been overestimated due to various factors.

TOXIC METALS

Some metals produce toxic effects on the human body even when in low concentration: mercury, selenium, arsenic, lead, and cadmium. These metals produce toxicity by several means:

1.   Inhibition of enzyme activity
2.   Precipitation of essential body metabolites (intermediaries in the chemical processes of the body)
3.   Alteration of cell permeability
4.   Rupture of body cells.

TOXINS FROM ANIMAL FOOD SOURCES

Cheese and chianti wine. The substance tyramine, contained in cheddar cheese and chianti wine, is a potent vasopressor (constrictor of circulatory vessels) normally metabolized with no ill-effects through the action of monoamine oxidases. Certain drugs such as monoamine oxidase inhibitor (MAOI), used to treat depression, reduce the metabolic breakdown of tyramine. This causes increased amounts of tyramine to remain in the body which in turn causes hypertension and headache.

Eggs. Several toxic reactions are produced by eggs:

1.   Allergic reactions in some people (hives and asthma)
2.   Trypsin inhibitor in egg white
3.   Binding of biotin (a B complex vitamin) by aviden, a basic protein (this action is potent only in raw egg whites).

NITROSAMINES

These are potent carcinogens occurring in both animal and plant foods. They are also produced within the human body. Nitrosamines are formed from nitrates and nitrites found in many foods some of which are smoked meats and fish, spinach, lettuce, celery, scotch, and beer. Nitrates and nitrites are also used as food preservatives in meats, cheeses, and poultry to deter spoilage and botulism.

Some authorities feel more nitrosamines are formed within the body than would be consumed in food. However, the USDA (United States Department of Agriculture) is currently reassessing amounts of nitrates and nitrites allowable for processing of certain foods such as smoked meats and bacon. Refer to footnotes 5 and 25 in this chapter for additional information on nitrates and nitrites.

CAFFEINE

More than 34 million pounds of caffeine were consumed in the U.S. in 1972.[12] This caffeine, along with the chemically closely related compounds theophylline and theobromine, was consumed in coffee, tea, cocoa, cola beverages, and over-the-counter drugs. Caffeine is an alkaloid.[10]

The caffeine content of natural sources fluctuates with plant variety, geographic location, climate, and cultural practices such as fermentation. The caffeine content of brewed beverages such as coffee and tea also varies with the brewing strength. The caffeine content of a cup of coffee may vary from 60 to 150 mg; caffeine in a cup of tea from 10 to 50 mg; and caffeine in carbonated soft drinks from 40 to 65 mg.[13]

Ingested caffeine is rapidly absorbed, metabolized, and excreted in urine. Little caffeine is excreted unchanged since almost all ingested caffeine is metabolized. Caffeine is a stimulant which increases alertness and physical activity. Caffeine causes constriction of cerebral blood vessels, increased urination, and prolonged stimulation of gastric secretion.

Because it is readily excreted, body concentrations of caffeine remain low. However, caffeine can cross the placenta barrier from a pregnant woman to her developing fetus. Both the pregnant woman and the fetus have slower rates of caffeine metabolism and excretion.[14]

Excessive intake of caffeine is associated with tremors, headache, arrhythmias of the heart, diarrhea, and difficulty in falling and remaining asleep. A severe headache may result when a high intake of caffeine is suddenly discontinued. A lethal dose of caffeine for man is generally estimated to be about 10 grams.

Caffeine has been implicated in the development of benign breast lumps in susceptible women. The lumps are associated with an increased risk of breast cancer.[15] Caffeine consumption from coffee has been implicated with problem pregnancies in at least one study.[16] These pregnancies had a high incidence of spontaneous abortions, stillbirths, and premature births.

The Food and Drug Administration recently conducted a review of additives placed on the GRAS list (generally recognized as safe) at the time of adoption of the Food Additive Amendment, 1958. The review was conducted by the Federation of American Societies for Experimental Biology (FASEB). In a report released in late 1980, FASEB gave caffeine, as an additive, a class 3 status: while caffeine could remain in use for a restricted period of time, additional studies testing safety of use needed to be conducted because of currently unresolved questions in research data.

Key Points: Toxicants Occurring Naturally in Foods

I. Food contains thousands of chemical compounds, some of which are nutrients and some that are toxicants to the human body.

II. Toxicity is the capacity of a single chemical substance to harm living organisms.

III. Hazard specifies the condition of use under which a chemical can cause injury.

IV. Some mechanisms by which chemical substances exert a toxic effect are as: enzyme inhibitors, vitamin antagonists, hallucinogens, stimulants, depressants, carcinogens, poisons, and producers of degenerative diseases.

V. There are body mechanisms which are generally able to degrade, detoxify, and eliminate toxic substances normally contained in a varied diet.

Questions: Toxicants Occurring Naturally in Foods

1. The capacity of a chemical substance to harm living organisms is known as
_____ .

2. When a toxic substance is used or consumed under conditions which can produce injury the substance becomes a _____ to health.

3. What conditions often produce periods of increased consumption of foods containing toxic substances?

4. Identify at least three factors which operate to reduce the harmful effects of ingested toxic substances.

5. Soybeans are a vegetable source of high protein value. However, significant protein is not available from soybeans when eaten raw because soybeans contain:
   a. a vitamin destroyer
   b. a goitrogen
   c. a trypsin (protease) inhibitor

6. Match the phrases on the right to the items on the left which they best describe:

_____ 1.	Senecio	a. substances that cause clumping of red blood cells and are found in some legumes
_____ 2.	goitrogens	
_____ 3.	hypertensives	
_____ 4.	hemlock, foxglove, nightshade	b. weakness or paralysis caused by toxic substances in vetches (sweet peas)
_____ 5.	thiaminase	c. sensitivity to fava beans causing hemolytic anemia
_____ 6.	hemagglutinins	
_____ 7.	aflatoxins	d. some herbs that contain poisonous alkaloids
_____ 8.	lathyrism	
_____ 9.	favism	e. a poisonous alkaloid found in the green portion of sprouting potatoes
_____ 10.	solanine	
_____ 11.	hallucinogens	f. poisonous plants whose seeds are sometimes harvested with food grains
		g. toxins from molds which are known to cause liver cancer
		h. substances that interfere with thyroid gland function
		i. a vitamin destroyer in spinach, cabbage, and blackberries
		j. some herbs, mushrooms, and spices which produce distorted sensory impressions
		k. foods containing substances which can cause a rise in blood pressure

7. Mushrooms are most safely purchased from a domestic, commercial grower.
    a. True
    b. False
8. Substances which interfere with absorption of certain nutrients are called
    _____ .
9. An acid in rhubarb and spinach which binds calcium and iron is
    _____ .
10. Foods which produce reactions of hives, wheezing, excessive mucus production, and migraine headaches in sensitive persons are:
    a. binders
    b. allergens
    c. hallucinogens
11. Substances which block the utilization of oxygen by body cells producing general tissue starvation for oxygen are _____ .
12. What is the actual source of paralytic shellfish poisoning (PSP)?
13. Shellfish and finfish seem to be capable of concentrating what toxic metal?
14. Mr. Jones gets a migraine headache whenever he eats oysters. Mr. Jones is most probably _____ to oysters.
15. Mercury, selenium, arsenic, lead, and cadmium are metals which are toxic to humans even in relatively small ingested amounts.
    a. True
    b. False
16. Some toxic metals exert their effects by:
    a. altering cell permeability and rupturing some body cells
    b. precipitating essential body metabolites
    c. acting as hallucinogens
    d. inhibiting enzyme activity
17. Persons taking monoamine oxidase inhibitor (MAOI) drugs should avoid what foods?
18. Why do you suppose egg yolk is introduced to an infant as a new solid food before egg whites (which are not given until late in the first year of infancy)?
19. Nitrosamines are:
    a. potent carcinogens found naturally occurring in plant and animal foods
    b. produced in the human body from nitrates and nitrites
    c. trypsin inhibitors
20. Identify which of the following statements are true:
    a. Caffeine content of a cup of coffee is variable.
    b. Ingested caffeine produces no ill-effects.
    c. Caffeine can cross the placenta barrier to the developing fetus.
    d. A lethal dose of caffeine is approximately ten grams.

Answers: Toxicants Occurring Naturally in Foods

1. toxicity
2. hazard
3. Stressful times such as war and famine, or when the normal food source is destroyed by natural disaster such as fire or flood.
4. 1. body detoxification mechanisms
    2. improved food processing methods of heating, refrigeration, and canning

3. a mixed and varied diet
4. modern breeding programs which have resulted in reduced toxic substances in some foods
5. interaction between toxic substances consumed

5. c
6. 1. f
    2. h
    3. k
    4. d
    5. i
    6. a
    7. g
    8. b
    9. c
    10. e
    11. j
7. a
8. binders
9. oxalic acid
10. b
11. cyanogens
12. dinoflagellates (microscopic organisms) which produce a poison retained by the shellfish. These organisms cause the marine condition of "red tide."
13. mercury
14. allergic
15. a
16. a, b, d
17. cheddar cheese and chianti wine (generally, aged and fermented foods)
18. because of the multiple and frequent cause of allergic reactions by egg whites
19. a, b
20. a, c, d

FOOD ADDITIVES

A discussion of food additives generally provokes an emotional response from each partici-pant. Whether the response is favorable or unfavorable depends greatly upon the level of nutrition knowledge and the political/professional perspective of the individual. A con-sumer with a limited knowledge of chemical terminology has a legitimate reason to ques-tion the reason for and safety of additives he or she identifies from the list of ingredients on a food label. Many of these additives have names that sound complex and formidable. A food technologist, on the other hand, might recognize these same additives as welcome chemicals which have enabled us to have one of the most abundant, diversified, and safest food supplies in the world.

Scare tactics sometimes employed by certain consumer advocate activists are as unfair to the consumer as the statements stubbornly repeated by some persons associated with chemical production and food processing, which imply that all food additives are safe under all conditions of present use for all persons.

The safety of any food, with or without chemical additives, is a relative concept.[17] Even certain foods which are normally well tolerated by most persons may contain particular naturally occurring constituents which are toxic to certain individuals. Foods contain hun-dreds of different inherent chemicals, many of which are known to be toxic to humans.

However, low levels of consumption, detoxification mechanisms of the body, interaction between the chemicals consumed, and the variety of foods in our diets all help to keep toxic substances in food from becoming hazardous to our health.[18]

The deliberate addition of chemicals to food deservedly warrants public concern and strict legislative controls to ensure the protection of public health.[19] In addition, there needs to be complete, unbiased, correct information reported through all the various media to educate the consumer, and to keep the consumer informed of current data obtained from scientific investigations regarding food additives.

The Food Additive Amendment of 1958 to the Food, Drug, and Cosmetic Act established that any chemical additive petitioned to be used in food processing must be pre-tested to show the safety of its use *before* it can be used and marketed in food products. These tests include the feeding of large doses of the additive over an extended period of time to at least two kinds of animals, usually rodents and dogs. These feeding studies are designed to determine whether the substance causes cancer, birth defects, or other injury to the animals. In addition, this amendment contains the Delaney Clause which forbids the use of *any* food additive in *any* amount if it is found to induce cancer when ingested by experimental animals or humans.[20]

If a chemical is not shown to cause cancer but does produce other negative effects, then the Food and Drug Administration (FDA) sets tolerance levels at which that chemical can be added based upon well-documented scientific tests. These levels are generally about one-hundredth of the amount which produce any physiological change in laboratory animals. The FDA can regulate additives only on the basis of safety. The Agency has no power to limit the number of additives approved or to judge whether a particular food color, thickener, or sweetener is really needed.[21]

Consumers can play a significant role in helping to shape FDA regulations, policies, and programs. Proposed regulations or changes in regulations are published in the Federal Register with a deadline for public comment on the specific matter. All opinions are welcomed and considered in the process of preparing a final regulation.[22] In addition, any member of the public can petition the FDA to issue or change a regulation.

Because the public does have a voice in decision-making regarding FDA regulations including regulations involving food additives, concerned individuals have a responsibility to become knowledgeable about the many aspects of chemical additives used in foods. Benefits of general use versus risks to some consumers have to be rationally weighed and responsibly reviewed in order to make a decision for use or disuse to the greatest advantage of the general public. It is an undisputed fact that food additives have increased the total food supply through increased production (use of pesticides), improved preservation (that is, shelf-life) of many foods as well as increased nutrient content of food through enrichment, restoration, and fortification with vitamins and minerals.

Certain chemicals which had been used for a long time without apparent ill-effect before 1958 were placed on a "generally recognized as safe (GRAS)" list. The substances placed on the GRAS list were reviewed by scientists qualified through training and experience to evaluate food safety. In recognition of improved testing methods and equipment, and the accumulation of more recent and in some cases conflicting scientific data regarding safety of use for some of the chemicals on the GRAS list, all GRAS substances are being systematically retested and reviewed for safety. (For more details on this review refer to the section in this book on Food Labeling Laws and Regulations, Chapter Sixteen.)

Cyclamate, a non-nutritive sweetener, is an example of a chemical substance orginally placed on the GRAS list but later removed and banned from use when certain experimental tests demonstrated its questionable safety as a food additive.[23] Saccharin is another non-nutritive sweetener currently being re-evaluated in terms of safety for human consumption in light of newer data obtained from more recent scientific experiments.

What are additives? A food additive is any substance that becomes part of a food product when added either directly or indirectly. *An intentional food additive is intended to impart a particular characteristic to a food or to facilitate food production or processing.* For example, some food additives are preservatives while some are nutrients, coloring agents, or flavoring agents which enhance the food product. *An incidental food additive is one present in a food product, usually in a trace quantity, as a consequence of some phase of production, processing, storage, or packaging.* For example, an incidental (unintentional) food additive would be a chemical substance present in food because of its migration from the packaging material or processing equipment used.

Why use additives? An additive is intentionally used for the following purposes:[24]

1. *To maintain or improve nutritional value.* This includes the addition of vitamins for enrichment, restoration, or fortification.
2. *To maintain freshness.* This includes preservatives, anti-oxidants, and natural color and flavor protectors.[25]
3. *To help in processing or preparation.* This includes thickeners, texturizers, emulsifiers, pH controllers, humectants, and leavening agents (necessary to make baked goods rise).
4. *To make food more appealing.* This includes coloring agents, natural and synthetic flavors, and flavor enhancers. These are the food additives which are the most controversial. Their use is based on subjective preference rather than necessity.

Key Points: Food Additives

I. The Food Additive Amendment of 1958 to the Federal Food, Drug, and Cosmetic Act requires the safety of food additives to be established by testing according to set standards *before* they are used and marketed in food products.
   A. This amendment also contains the Delaney Clause which states that a food additive cannot be used in *any* amount if it causes cancer when ingested by experimental animals or humans.
   B. Tolerance levels are set for additives which produce negative effects other than cancer; these levels are generally 1/100 of the minimum amount needed to produce the physiological change.
   C. Chemicals which had been seemingly safely used for a long time prior to enactment of the Food Additive Amendment were placed on a "generally recognized as safe" (GRAS) list. They are presently being re-evaluated for safety of use.
II. Intentional food additives are used to impart a special characteristic to a food or to facilitate food production or processing.
III. Incidental food additives are present in a food product in generally trace amounts and are inadvertently added to food during some phase of food production, processing, storage, or packaging.
VI. Food additives are generally used in a food product to maintain or improve nutritional value, to maintain freshness, to help in processing or preparation, and to make food more appealing.

Table 15-1. Food Additives: Why they are used, where they are used, and in what foods they are added.

Some Reasons for Using Additives	Some Additives Used	Some Foods in Which Such Additives Are Used
To impart and maintain desired consistency. Emulsifiers distribute tiny particles of one liquid in another to improve texture homogeneity, and quality, for example, oil and water mixtures. Stabilizers and thickeners give smooth uniform texture, flavor and desired consistency.	Lecithin, mono- and diglycerides, gum arabic, pectin, modified food starch, cellulose derivatives, alginates, propylene glycol.	Baked goods, cake mixes, salad dressings, frozen desserts, ice cream, chocolate milk, beverages, whipped toppings, sauces, gravies, fruit products, chewing gum.
To improve nutritive value. Medical and public health authorities endorse this use to aid in the reduction and prevention of certain diseases. For example, iodized salt to reduce the incidence of simple goiter, vitamin D in dairy products and infant foods to reduce the incidence of rickets, niacin in bread, and cornmeal and cereals to reduce the incidence of pellagra in the southern states.	Vitamin A, thiamin, niacin, riboflavin, ascorbic acid, vitamin D, iron, potassium iodide.	Wheat flour, bread and biscuits, breakfast cereals, corn meal, macaroni and noodle products, margarine, milk, iodized salt.
To enhance flavor. Many spices and natural and synthetic flavors give us a desired variety of flavorful foods such as spice cake, gingerbread, and sausage.	Spices, cloves, ginger, citrus oils, amyl acetate, carvone, benzaldehyde, vanilla (natural), vanillin (synthetic), MSG (monosodium glutamate).	Spice cake, gingerbread, ice cream, candy, soft drinks, fruit-flavored gelatins, fruit-flavored toppings, sausage, canned meats, soups, gravies, canned vegetables.
As leavening agents. Leavening agents are used in the baking industry in cakes, biscuits, waffles, muffins and other foods. These affect cooking results: texture, increase in volume.	Yeast, sodium bicarbonate, sodium aluminum sulfate, baking soda.	Cakes, cookies, quick breads, crackers.

Purpose	Additives	Foods
To control acidity or alkalinity. These can affect texture, taste, and wholesomeness.	Acetic acid, citric acid, lactic acid, tartaric acid, fumaric acid, adipic acid.	Candies, beverages, powdered soft drinks, butter, cheeses, condensed milk.
To maintain appearance, palatability, and wholesomeness by delaying deterioration of food due to microbial growth caused by mold, bacteria, and yeast is prevented or slowed by certain additives. Antioxidants keep fats from turning rancid and certain fresh fruits from darkening during processing when cut and exposed to air.	Propionic acid, sodium and calcium salts of propionic acid, ascorbic acid, butylated hydroxyanisole (BHA), butylated hydroxytoluene (BHT).	Bread, cheese, syrup, pie fillings, crackers, fruit juices, frozen and dried fruit, margarine, lard, shortening, potato chips, cake mixes.
To give desired and characteristic color to increase acceptability and attractiveness to the consumer. May not be used to cover up an unwholesome food or used in excessive amounts.	FDA approved colors such as: annatto, carotene, cochineal, caramel, beet powder, and synthetic approved colors	Confections, bakery goods, soft drinks, cheeses, ice cream, jams and jellies.
To mature, bleach flours, to modify gluten to improve baking, to improve the appearance of certain cheeses, and to meet the desire for white wheat flour by changing the natural yellow pigments.	Chlorine dioxide, chlorine, potassium bromate and iodate, sodium stearyl fumarate, various peroxides.	Cereal flour, certain cheeses, breads, instant potatoes, processed cereals, breads, and rolls.
Other functions, such as humectants, to retain moisture in some foods and to keep others, including salts and powders, free-flowing (anti-caking agents).	Glycerine, magnesium carbonate, calcium silicate, iron ammonium citrate.	Coconut, table salt, various powdered foods.

Sources: Food Additives—Who Needs Them? Booklet from Manufacturing Chemists Association, 1825 Connecticut Ave NW, Washington, DC. Lehman P: More Than You Ever Thought You Would About Food Additives . . . Part III. FDA Consumer, 13, June 1979

Questions: Food Additives

1. There are toxic substances in some foods which occur naturally in that food.
    a. True
    b. False

2. The interaction between some ingested substances can sometimes neutralize the otherwise toxic effect of one or more of the substances.
    a. True
    b. False

3. The Food Additive Amendment of 1958 to the Food, Drug, and Cosmetic Act established that testing the safety of food additives for human consumption must be completed when?

4. The Delaney Clause forbids the use of a food additive in what amount if it is found to induce cancer when ingested by experimental animals or humans?
    a. toxic amount
    b. large amount
    c. any amount

5. Which of the following are legal functions of the FDA?
    a. reviewing public opinion on proposed regulations or regulation changes involving food additives
    b. setting of tolerance levels to which chemicals may be added in foods
    c. judging whether a sweetener is needed for use in a certain food product
    d. regulating additives on the basis of safety only

6. An average American consumes about 100 pounds of sucrose (sugar), 15 pounds of salt, 8½ pounds of corn syrup, and four pounds of dextrose as food additives per year. In addition, ten pounds of various other additives are consumed, of which nine pounds are spices and chemicals naturally found in foods. Approximately one pound consists of chemicals (more than 1,800) intentionally added to foods and approximately one-half of these are each consumed in amounts less than one-half of a milligram per person per year.[26]
    a. Are chemical additives consumed in minor amounts?
    b. When some media source refers to the "huge" amounts of additives we consume in the average American diet, is it more accurate to associate "huge" with amounts of additives consumed or numbers of different manufactured chemical additives consumed?
    c. Which substance is used as a food additive in the greatest amount?

7. Can vitamins and minerals be food additives?

8. What factors beside the level (amount) of consumption operate to lessen the toxic effect of potentially harmful substances in foods?

9. Why do some persons challenge the animal feeding tests used for food additives using large amounts of the chemical additive?
    a. because the tests are costly
    b. because the tests are time-consuming
    c. because the amounts of chemicals used are unrealistic in terms of human consumption for that chemical

10. An individual has the opportunity to influence an FDA decision to enact or change a regulation regarding food additives.
    a. True
    b. False

11. GRAS list additives are "guaranteed regulated and safe."
    a. True
    b. False

12. GRAS list items cannot be banned from use.
    a. True
    b. False

13. Identify the numbered items as either intentional or incidental additives:

    _____ 1. paper fibers from packaging wrap   a. intentional
                                                   b. incidental

    _____ 2. enrichment with thiamin, riboflavin, niacin, and iron

    _____ 3. red food coloring in strawberry ice cream

    _____ 4. trace pesticides from food production use

    _____ 5. calcium proprionate in bread to delay food spoilage caused by mold

    _____ 6. chemicals in meat as a result of their addition to the feed of livestock

    _____ 7. sodium bicarbonate as a leavening agent for biscuits

    _____ 8. pectin to thicken fruit products

14. If you are concerned about the numbers and the safety of the amounts of chemical additives in foods you should:
    a. become informed on additives and then express your views to your legislative representative and the FDA
    b. not purchase foodstuffs containing additives unacceptable to you in an effort to encourage a food producer, through economic means, to curtail production of those foodstuffs
    c. eat a variety of foods daily in order to avoid consuming hazardous levels of toxic chemicals found in any one food, class of foods, or similar foods

15. Which of the four purposes for the use of intentional food additives is the most controversial? What are some of the additives in that class?

Answers: Food Additives

1. a
2. a
3. before commercial use and the marketing of food products
4. c
5. a, b, d
6. a. yes
   b. number of different manufactured chemical additives consumed
   c. sucrose (a sugar)

7. yes, in enriched, restored, or fortified foods
8. detoxification mechanisms of the body; interaction between chemicals consumed; the variety of total diet consumed.
9. c
10. a
11. b
12. b. (If a review of newer test data warrants removal from use, on the basis of questionable safety, the FDA can remove a substance from GRAS and even ban its use entirely as demonstrated by the case of cyclamate.)
13. 1. b
    2. a
    3. a
    4. b
    5. a
    6. b
    7. a
    8. a
14. a, b, c
15. to make foods more appealing; coloring agents, flavoring agents, flavor enhancers

REFERENCES

[1] Kautter DA and Lynt, Jr. RK: Botulism. FDA Papers, 5, November 1971. pp. 16-24
[2] Vail GE et al: Foods, 6th ed. Boston, Houghton Mifflin Company, 1973, p. 149
[3] Getoff MM: Unsafe food practices in the kitchen. Journal of Home Economics, 70, January 1978, pp. 45-47
[4] The following are the various references used to compile the list of safe food-handling procedures.
    Brown bag lunches: Questions and answers. USDA Publication No. 1975-679-275/198, Meat and Poultry Inspection Program, November 1973
    Food safety in the kitchen. USDA, DHEW (FDA), Publication No. 0-532-095, January 1974
    Heenan J: Can your kitchen pass the food storage test? Reprint from FDA Consumer, March 1974, DHEW Publication No. (FDA) 74-2052
    Heenan J: Please don't eat the mold. FDA Consumer, November 1974
    Morrison M: Don't let foodborne illness spoil your Christmas feast. Reprint from FDA Consumer, December 1973-January 1974, DHEW Publication No. (FDA) 74-2020
[5] Because an increasing number of processed meats and luncheon meats are being made without the addition of nitrite as a curing and preservative agent, the US Department of Agriculture recommends the following procedures when using no-nitrite meats:
    1. Prepare and freeze sandwiches the night before consumption as they will thaw in time for lunch.
    2. Pack such a sandwich in an insulated container.
    3. Double wrap such a sandwich and pack it with another cold food item.
    4. Put a cold-keeping device in the lunch container such as a frozen freezer gel, a plastic bag full of ice cubes, or a small plastic container of solid ice.
[6] Naturally occurring toxicants in foods. Food Technology, 29, March 1975, p. 68
[7] Strong FM: Toxicants occurring naturally in foods. Nutrition Reviews, 32, August 1974, p. 225
[8] Naturally occurring toxicants in foods. Food Technology, 29, March 1975, p. 69

[9] The summary of information on toxicants within foods was obtained from information in the following references:

Gross RL and Newberne PM: Naturally occurring toxic substances in foods. Clinical Pharmacology and Therapeutics. (Part 2) 22, November 1977

Hall RL: Safe at the plate. Nutrition Today, 10, November-December 1977

Newberne PM: Naturally occurring food-borne toxicants. In Goodhart RS and Shils ME (eds): Modern Nutrition in Health and Disease. Philadelphia, Lea and Febiger, 1980

Sapeika N: Pharmacodynamic action of natural food. World Review of Nutrition and Dietetics, 29 (Toxicology and Nutrition), New York, S. Karger, 1978

Strong FM: Toxicants occurring naturally in foods. In Present Knowledge in Nutrition, 4th ed. New York and Washington, D.C.; The Nutrition Foundation, Inc., 1976

Tannenbaum SR: Ins and outs of nitrites. The Sciences, 20, January 1980, pp. 7-9

Wilson BJ: Naturally occurring toxicants of foods. Nutrition Reviews, 37, October 1979, pp. 305-312

[10] **Alkaloids** are organic heterocyclic substances which are also nitrogen-containing bases. Some alkaloids have pharmacological properties and are important drugs such as quinine, morphine, and cocaine. Some alkaloids are extremely toxic compounds like strychnine, nicotine, and curare.

[11] **Laetril,** the controversial substance purported to be useful in treating cancer, is made from apricot pits and consequently contains cyanogens in concentrated form.

[12] Graham DM: Caffeine-Its identity, dietary sources, intake and biological effects. Nutrition Reviews, 36, April 1978, pp. 97-102

[13] Mayer J and Dwyer J: Limit your caffeine; It lurks everywhere. The Denver Post, July 27, 1980, p. 42

[14] "Workshop on caffeine—special report," Nutrition Reviews, 37, April 1979, pp. 124-26

[15] Weininger J and Briggs GM: Nutrition Update, 1979. Journal of Nutrition Education, 12, January-March, 1980, p. 4

[16] Weathersbee PS, Olsen LK and Lodge JR: Caffeine and pregnancy—A retrospective survey. Postgraduate Medicine, 62, 1977, pp. 64-69

[17] Hall RL: Food additives. Nutrition Today, 8, July-August, 1973, p. 20

[18] Coon JM: Natural food toxicants—A perspective. In Present Knowledge in Nutrition, 4th ed. New York and Washington, D.C.; The Nutrition Foundation, Inc., 1976, pp. 531-532

[19] Oser BL: Chemical additives in foods. In Goodhart RS and Shils ME (eds): Modern Nutrition in Health and Disease. Philadelphia, Lea and Febiger, 1980

[20] Schmidt AM: Food and Drug Law: A 200-year perspective. Nutrition Today, 10, April 1975, pp. 30-31

[21] Lehmann P: More than you ever thought you would know about food additives . . . part 1. FDA Consumer, 13, April 1979, p. 11

[22] A consumer guide to FDA. HEW Publication No. (FDA) 78-1013, pp. 4-5

[23] Pines WL: The cyclamate story. FDA Consumer, 8, December 1974-January 1975, pp. 19-27

[24] Lehmann P: More than you ever thought you would know about food additives . . . part I. FDA Consumer, 13, April 1979, pp. 10-11

[25] No-nitrite processed meats are now available due to consumer demand. However, since they lack the nitrite preservative they must be treated with as great a care as given fresh meat. They must be kept refrigerated and they should be used within four to seven days. They may be frozen but then should be used within three to four days after thawing (and kept in the refrigerator, of course). Source: No-nitrite meats: Handle safely. USDA, Food Safety and Quality Service, PA-1238, August 1979

[26] Hall RL: Food additives; Nutrition Today, 8, July-August 1973, pp. 21 and 26

16
THE LABELING OF FOOD

HISTORY
The history of food labeling laws and regulations are given here in outline form in order to condense the information and make this section an easy-to-use reference source. Current nutrition labeling regulations are examined more closely in the following subsection. An emphasis is given on how to use nutrition labeling to the advantage of the consumer.

I. Food and Drug Act of 1906
   A. First comprehensive pure food law encouraged and supported by Dr. Harvey W. Wiley, chief food chemist in the U.S. Department of Agriculture.
   B. First regulation providing definitions and differentiations of food and drugs.
   C. Prevented interstate commerce of misbranded or adulterated foods and drugs.
   D. In time this law became obsolete due to increased technology in food and sanitation and consequent inadequacies of the law.[1]

II. Federal Food, Drug, and Cosmetic Act of 1938
   A. This Act remains the basis for current food labeling regulation.
   B. Required certain information to be stated on labels.
      1. The common name of the product.
      2. The name and address of the manufacturer, packer, or distributor.
      3. The net contents in terms of weight, measure, or count (or appropriate combination of these).
      4. The ingredients listed in order of descending predominance (for foods not having an established standard of identity).[2]
   C. Contained three major amendments which shifted the burden for demonstrating proof of safety in ingredients and food products from the government to the manufacturer. The government accepted the responsibility for evaluating test evidence for safety. Thus, food ingredients had to be tested and proven safe for consumption before they could be marketed.
      1. The pesticide amendment of 1954.
      2. The food additive amendment of 1958.
         a. Includes intentional and incidental[3] food additives.
         b. Contains the Delaney Clause which forbids the use of any food additive, in any amount, if it is found to induce cancer when ingested by experimental animals or humans.[4]
         c. Excluded from the testing requirement established by the food additive amendment were numerous substances which had been used for a long time with no apparent ill effects. These were the "generally recognized as safe" (GRAS) substances.[5]
      3. The color additive amendment of 1960.

III. Fair Packaging and Labeling Act, passed 1966, adopted 1967.
   A. Contains five regulations regarding label information.
      1. *Statement of identity.* A statement of the food's identity must appear on the principal display panel in bold type. It shall be stated as the common or usual name of the food, such as "beets" or "peaches."
      2. *Identification of manufacturer, packer, or distributor.* A statement of the name and address of the manufacturer, packer, or distributor shall be conspicuously stated.
      3. *Standard measurement of contents.* The net contents must be given in standard measure without any qualifying term such as "Giant Quart" or "Jumbo Pound" and placed within the bottom 30 percent area of the principal display panel as a distinct item.
      4. *A statement of the net contents of a serving.* If the label of any food package represents the contents in terms of the number of servings, then this statement shall be accompanied by a description of the size of each serving.
      5. *A statement listing ingredients.* Ingredients must be listed on required food labels on a single panel of the label and shall be legible by virtue of type size, design, etc. It shall list the ingredients by their common name in decreasing order of predominance.[6]
IV. The Food and Drug Administration
   A. Is under the Department of Health and Human Services, U.S. Public Health Service.
   B. Enforces laws and regulations which require that food be safe and wholesome and properly labeled.[7]
   C. FDA enforces the laws by:
      1. Inspecting plants where food and drugs are processed to assure that they are safe for consumer use.
      2. Obtains samples of foods, drugs, and the other products it regulates and tests and analyzes them to make sure they are safe for consumer use and are properly labeled.
      3. Sets standards for certain foods that are required to be made according to a set recipe and tests such products to assure that they meet the standards.
      4. Establishes regulations for the labeling of products so consumers will know what they consist of and will be informed of any hazards associated with their use.
      5. Promotes the use of nutritional information on food labels to aid consumers in selecting a healthful diet.
      6. Investigates consumer complaints about the sanitation, safety, and labeling of the products it regulates.[8]
   D. Sets Standards of Identity.
      1. Originally established to benefit the consumer.
      2. Intended to produce a uniform product.[9]
      3. Federal law exempts foods with a Standard of Identity from listing ingredients on the label.
         a. The standards can be obtained by individuals from FDA.
         b. The FDA is presently encouraging full ingredient labeling of these foods though it cannot require such.
      4. Foods with a Standard of Identity must meet all defined standards in order to claim the commonly used name (such as mayonnaise or peanut butter).
   E. Sets Standards of Quality.
   F. Sets Standards for Fill (of containers).
   G. Sets Enrichment Standards.[10]

H. FDA undertook a comprehensive review of food labeling and the regulations controlling labeling:[11,12]
   1. Published new regulations in the Federal Register, January 19, 1973.
   2. Nutrition Labeling (to be discussed in depth later).
   3. Food label information panel. Standardized location, type size, and other technical details to make labeling more consistent and easier to understand.
   4. Cholesterol, Fat, and Fatty Acid Labeling. Allowed voluntary listing of cholesterol, fat, and fatty acid information.
      a. If listed must be according to set guidelines and must give the following statement: "Information on fat (and/or cholesterol where appropriate) content is provided for individuals who, on the advice of a physician, are modifying their total dietary intake of fat (and/or cholesterol, where appropriate)."
      b. If listed, then full nutritional labeling must be given.
   5. Special Dietary Use Label Statements. Established U.S. RDA as official measurement of nutritional intake. Set prohibition of certain nutritional claims. Identifies products intended for special dietary use.
   6. Proposed Nutrition Labeling for Certain Standardized Foods. Required standardized foods which have nutrients added to be labeled according to nutrition labeling regulations.
   7. Dietary Supplements of Vitamins and Minerals. Established a standard of identity for dietary supplements.
      a. *Ordinary foods* (require full nutrition labeling). Contain less than 50 percent of the U.S. RDA per serving for all added nutrients.
      b. *Dietary supplements.* Foods containing added vitamins or minerals from 50 to 150 percent of the U.S. RDA per serving.
   8. Regulates "Imitation" Foods.
      a. "Imitation" used only for foods nutritionally inferior to the traditional food product they are designed to replace.
      b. A new food product which is nutritionally equivalent according to FDA Standards to an established food can be marketed without the word "imitation" but must have its own descriptive and informative label. The word "imitation" was deemed to be uninformative.
   9. Established certain common or usual names for some nonstandardized foods.
   10. Set Nutritional Quality Guidelines.
      a. Established standards of nutrient and ingredient quality for certain classes of foods such as frozen "heat and serve" dinners.
      b. A product that meets the standards set forth in a nutritional quality guideline may include on its label a statement that it "provides nutrients in amounts appropriate for this class of food as determined by the U.S. Government."[13]

I. Other proposed and final FDA regulations.[14]
   1. Establishment of principles governing nutrient additions to foods by fortification, enrichment, or restoration.
   2. Establishment of nutritional quality guidelines for certain classes of fortified foods.
   3. Use of common names for certain formulated or fabricated food products such as meat extenders or replacements.
   4. Uniform procedure for listing ingredients on food labels.
      a. Includes ingredient disclosure for standardized *and* nonstandardized foods.

      b. Prohibit misleading vignettes (illustrations).
5. Declaration of colors and spices and flavors by specific name.
6. Source labeling for fats and oils by common or usual name such as beef fat instead of animal fat.
      a. Helps consumers to differentiate between polyunsaturated and saturated fats, make food choices according to religion preferences, and to make food choices according to personal food preferences.
      b. Required for all processed foods entering interstate commerce on or after January 1, 1978.[15]
7. Proposed standard "serving" sizes for certain classes of foods.
8. Uniform method of declaration of percentage of ingredients in foods.
9. Special exemption from nutritional labeling of smaller packaged food units within a larger externally labeled package.
10. Currently, there is legislation pending which would require nutrient and ingredient disclosure for all packaged foods, processed meat food products, and poultry products and also encourages such disclosures for fresh fruits, vegetables, meats, and restaurant foods.[16]
11. Declaration of total sugar in a food product.
12. Require sodium and potassium content as part of nutrition labeling.
13. Require greater disclosure of fatty acid and cholesterol content information disclosure as part of nutrition labeling.
14. Require open date labeling.
15. Individuals, agencies, and organizations do have opportunities to voice opinions and exert influence for change in labeling laws and regulations.
      a. FDA solicits comments from consumer groups, industry, and professional organizations for professional and consumer opinion on regulatory changes including labeling changes. For example, the Society of Nutrition Education recently submitted a position statement on food labeling with the hearing clerk of the FDA for entrance into the food labeling hearing records.[17]
      b. A period of time for comment from consumers and other interested parties is allowed by the FDA following new regulation proposals and changes before these become final.

NUTRITION LABELING

Nutrition labeling is voluntary for processed foods except when:

1. A nutrition claim is made for a food.
2. Any nutrient is added to a food.

For these two circumstances full nutrition labeling is mandatory. When nutrition labeling is given it must be presented in a standard form, either in the information or principal display panel. The following information must be given:[18, 19, 20]

Serving size
Servings per container
Calories per serving
Protein per serving
Carbohydrate per serving
Fat per serving
The percentage of the U.S. RDA per serving for certain essential nutrients:
Protein

Vitamin A
Vitamin C
Thiamin
Riboflavin
Niacin
Calcium
Iron

Another 12 vitamins and minerals must be listed if added to the food, and may be claimed if present, whether added or not: vitamins D, E, B$_6$, folacin, vitamin B$_{12}$, phosphorus, iodine, magnesium, zinc, copper, biotin, pantothenic acid. Optional listings are sodium and cholesterol.

Serving size. The serving size is that quantity "suitable for consumption as part of a meal" or suitable for an adult male who engages in light physical activity.

Servings per container. Obviously the larger the serving size, the smaller the number of servings per container. From this figure estimates can be made for the number of containers to purchase to provide adequate servings for the total number of individuals for whom the food is planned.

Calories per serving. Gives the number of kilocalories per serving as listed.

Protein per serving. Gives total protein in grams per serving. Protein is listed a second time as a percentage of U.S. RDA further down the information panel.

Carbohydrate per serving. Gives total carbohydrate in grams per serving as listed.

Fat per serving. Gives total fat in grams per serving as listed. A food processor may choose to show the type and amount of saturated and polyunsaturated fat in grams as well. If the additional fat information is given, full nutrition labeling must also be given and the following statement must be provided: "Information on fat content is provided for individuals who, on the advice of a physician, are modifying their total dietary intake of fat." The two subtotals of fat may not add up in grams to the total grams listed for fat in the particular food product labeled because a third category of fats termed monounsaturated are not always sublisted.[21]

Cholesterol may also be listed. If it is listed then full nutrition labeling must be given. When cholesterol content is stated it must be given in two ways:

1. milligrams per serving
2. milligrams per 100 grams of the food

The cholesterol content must be stated to the nearest 5 mg increment.

Sodium. If sodium content is listed it appears below the statement of fat content. However, listing of the sodium content on the label does not require full nutrition labeling. If sodium is listed it must be given in two ways:

1. milligrams of sodium per serving
2. milligrams of sodium per 100 grams

The sodium content must also be stated to the nearest 5 mg increment.

The next section of the nutrition information panel requires the listing of eight essential nutrients in terms of the percentage of the U.S. RDA each supplies per serving of the labeled food. The U.S. RDA table used most often for nutrition labeling is the one for adults and children over four years of age. Remember, there are four sets of U.S. RDA tables:

1. One for adults and children over four years of age (intended for general nutrition labeling needs)

2. One for children under four years of age (intended for labeling needs of junior foods)
3. One for infants under 13 months of age (intended for labeling needs of baby foods)
4. One for pregnant or lactating females (intended for the special dietary labeling needs of this group of women).

Refer to Chapter Two, the U.S. RDAs, for more detailed information on how the U.S. RDA values for the various nutrients were determined, as well as to review the U.S. RDAs themselves. Generally, the U.S. RDA values express the highest amount of each nutrient recommended for any age/sex group.

The eight essential nutrients which must have their individual amounts shown as percentages of U.S. RDA per serving are: protein (the second listing for protein on the nutrition label), vitamin A, vitamin C, thiamin, riboflavin, niacin, calcium, and iron. Twelve other nutrients may be listed if the food processor wishes to disclose their natural occurrence in a food, but they must be given if they are added to the food: vitamin D, vitamin E, vitamin B_6 (pyridoxine), folacin (folic acid), vitamin B_{12} (cobalamin), phosphorus, iodine, magnesium, zinc, copper, biotin, and pantothenic acid.

The percentages of U.S. RDA are listed in a specific manner. The percentage is shown to the nearest ten percent when a serving of food provides more than 50 percent of the U.S. RDA for a nutrient. The percentage is shown to the nearest five percent when a serving of food provides ten to 50 percent of the U.S. RDA for a nutrient. When a serving of food supplies ten percent or less for a nutrient the percentage of that nutrient must be given to the nearest two percent.

When a serving of food supplies less than two percent of a nutrient the percentage of U.S. RDA for that nutrient may be expressed in one of two ways:

1. A percentage of "O" is shown
2. An asterisk (*) is used along with the footnote: "Contains less than two percent of the U.S. RDA of this (or these) nutrients." If a food provides less than two percent of the U.S. RDA for five or more nutrients the nutrients do not have to be listed. However, the following footnote must be used: "Contains less than two percent of the U.S. RDA of . . . (list of the five or more nutrients)."

If a food is normally consumed in a combined form with another food, the food processor may choose to provide nutrition labeling information for the labeled food alone in one column and for the labeled food together with the accompanying food in a second column. This form gives the food processor the chance to provide the improved nutrient values for the labeled food product in the combined form in which it is normally eaten. Most breakfast cereals are shown in this manner: cereal alone and cereal with milk.

The percentage of U.S. RDA for protein is shown as a single value but is computed by different means for different foods. The method of determination depends upon the PER of the protein in the food. PER is the "protein efficiency ratio" and its value indicates the quality of a protein according to how it meets the tissue growth needs of an animal. Refer to Chapter Five, Measurements of Protein Quality, for a more detailed description of PER. High quality proteins have a PER equal to or better than the PER for casein, the protein of milk. These are generally proteins of animal source. A food protein with a PER equal to or greater than the PER of casein has its percentage of U.S. RDA based upon 45 grams (of protein).

Proteins of lesser quality are recognized as having a PER value between the PER of casein and 20 percent the PER of casein. These are generally proteins of plant origin. A food containing a protein of this class has its percentage of U.S. RDA based upon 65 grams (of protein) because more of this type of protein is needed to help meet the growth needs of humans.

A food containing a protein with a PER less than 20 percent the PER of casein (a poor quality protein) cannot have any value listed for its protein as a percentage of the U.S. RDA on the nutrition label. In this case, there may be a listing of protein content in grams but no listing in percentage of U.S. RDA which this protein provides.

Advantages of nutrition labeling to consumers. Nutrition labeling provides consumers with substantial nutrition information about packaged and processed foods. Nutrition labeling assists in educating consumers in the complex area of nutrition.[22] Nutrition labeling encourages food producers to maintain the nutritional quality of their food products.[23] Food producers are encouraged by nutrition labeling to develop ''new'' foods of similar nutritional quality to the traditional foods they wish to replace. These so-called new foods may be less expensive and have longer keeping qualities. *However, a reminder is necessary here about the need to eat a variety of common foods in order to obtain trace nutrients or nutrients not yet recognized as necessary for human consumption.*

Nutrition labeling affords the consumer the opportunity to compare nutrient quantity, nutrient quality, and the price of foods which are similar in order to make the most economical and nutritious food choices. Nutrition labeling enables the consumer to learn relative food energy values of different foods, relatively good food sources of particular nutrients and the general composition of various foods. However, the effective use of nutrition labeling is dependent upon the willingness of the consumer to take time to study labels as well as to learn the basic principles involved in good nutrition practices.

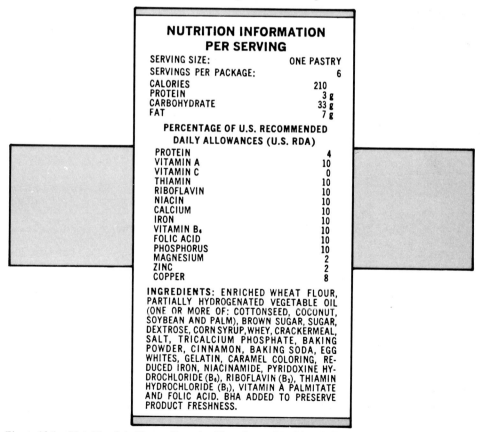

NUTRITION INFORMATION PER SERVING

SERVING SIZE:	ONE PASTRY
SERVINGS PER PACKAGE:	6
CALORIES	210
PROTEIN	3 g
CARBOHYDRATE	33 g
FAT	7 g

PERCENTAGE OF U.S. RECOMMENDED DAILY ALLOWANCES (U.S. RDA)

PROTEIN	4
VITAMIN A	10
VITAMIN C	0
THIAMIN	10
RIBOFLAVIN	10
NIACIN	10
CALCIUM	10
IRON	10
VITAMIN B$_6$	10
FOLIC ACID	10
PHOSPHORUS	10
MAGNESIUM	2
ZINC	2
COPPER	8

INGREDIENTS: ENRICHED WHEAT FLOUR, PARTIALLY HYDROGENATED VEGETABLE OIL (ONE OR MORE OF: COTTONSEED, COCONUT, SOYBEAN AND PALM), BROWN SUGAR, SUGAR, DEXTROSE, CORN SYRUP, WHEY, CRACKERMEAL, SALT, TRICALCIUM PHOSPHATE, BAKING POWDER, CINNAMON, BAKING SODA, EGG WHITES, GELATIN, CARAMEL COLORING, REDUCED IRON, NIACINAMIDE, PYRIDOXINE HYDROCHLORIDE (B$_6$), RIBOFLAVIN (B$_2$), THIAMIN HYDROCHLORIDE (B$_1$), VITAMIN A PALMITATE AND FOLIC ACID. BHA ADDED TO PRESERVE PRODUCT FRESHNESS.

Figure 16-1. Nutrition label from a ''new food'' product: a breakfast food pastry intended to replace a bread or cereal serving.

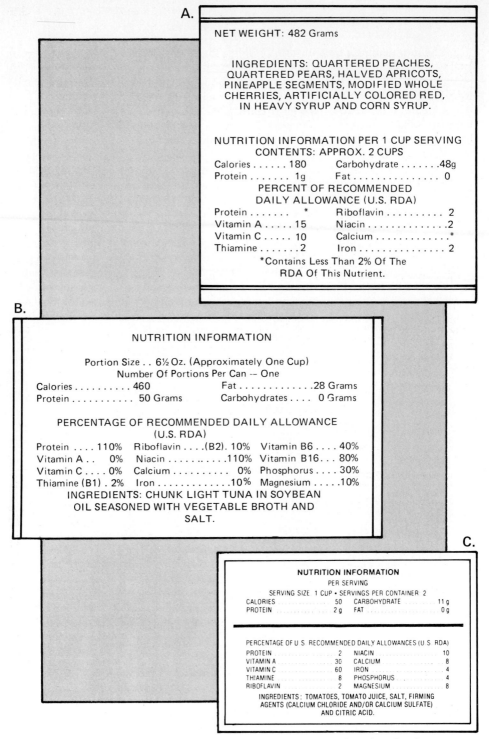

A.

NET WEIGHT: 482 Grams

INGREDIENTS: QUARTERED PEACHES,
QUARTERED PEARS, HALVED APRICOTS,
PINEAPPLE SEGMENTS, MODIFIED WHOLE
CHERRIES, ARTIFICIALLY COLORED RED,
IN HEAVY SYRUP AND CORN SYRUP.

NUTRITION INFORMATION PER 1 CUP SERVING
CONTENTS: APPROX. 2 CUPS

Calories 180	Carbohydrate 48g
Protein 1g	Fat 0

PERCENT OF RECOMMENDED
DAILY ALLOWANCE (U.S. RDA)

Protein . . . . *	Riboflavin 2
Vitamin A 15	Niacin 2
Vitamin C 10	Calcium . . . . *
Thiamine 2	Iron 2

*Contains Less Than 2% Of The
RDA Of This Nutrient.

B.

NUTRITION INFORMATION

Portion Size . . 6½ Oz. (Approximately One Cup)
Number Of Portions Per Can -- One

Calories 460	Fat . . . . 28 Grams
Protein . . . . 50 Grams	Carbohydrates . . . . 0 Grams

PERCENTAGE OF RECOMMENDED DAILY ALLOWANCE
(U.S. RDA)

Protein 110%	Riboflavin . . . . (B2). 10%	Vitamin B6 . . . . 40%
Vitamin A . . 0%	Niacin 110%	Vitamin B16 . . . 80%
Vitamin C 0%	Calcium 0%	Phosphorus 30%
Thiamine (B1) . 2%	Iron 10%	Magnesium 10%

INGREDIENTS: CHUNK LIGHT TUNA IN SOYBEAN
OIL SEASONED WITH VEGETABLE BROTH AND
SALT.

C.

NUTRITION INFORMATION
PER SERVING
SERVING SIZE 1 CUP • SERVINGS PER CONTAINER 2

CALORIES 50	CARBOHYDRATE . . . . 11 g
PROTEIN . . . . 2 g	FAT . . . . 0 g

PERCENTAGE OF U.S. RECOMMENDED DAILY ALLOWANCES (U.S. RDA)

PROTEIN	. . . 2	NIACIN 10
VITAMIN A	. . . 30	CALCIUM 8
VITAMIN C	. . . 60	IRON 4
THIAMINE	. . . 8	PHOSPHORUS 4
RIBOFLAVIN	. . . 2	MAGNESIUM 8

INGREDIENTS: TOMATOES, TOMATO JUICE, SALT, FIRMING
AGENTS (CALCIUM CHLORIDE AND/OR CALCIUM SULFATE)
AND CITRIC ACID.

Figure 16-2. Labels from three food products. A. Shows a nutrient supplying less than 2 percent U.S. RDA with an asterisk(*) and explanation (mixed fruit). B. Shows a nutrient supplying less than 2 percent U.S. RDA with 0% (chunk tuna). C. Shows a food supplying at least 2 percent U.S. RDA of all nutrients required to be listed on nutrition labeling (peeled tomatoes).

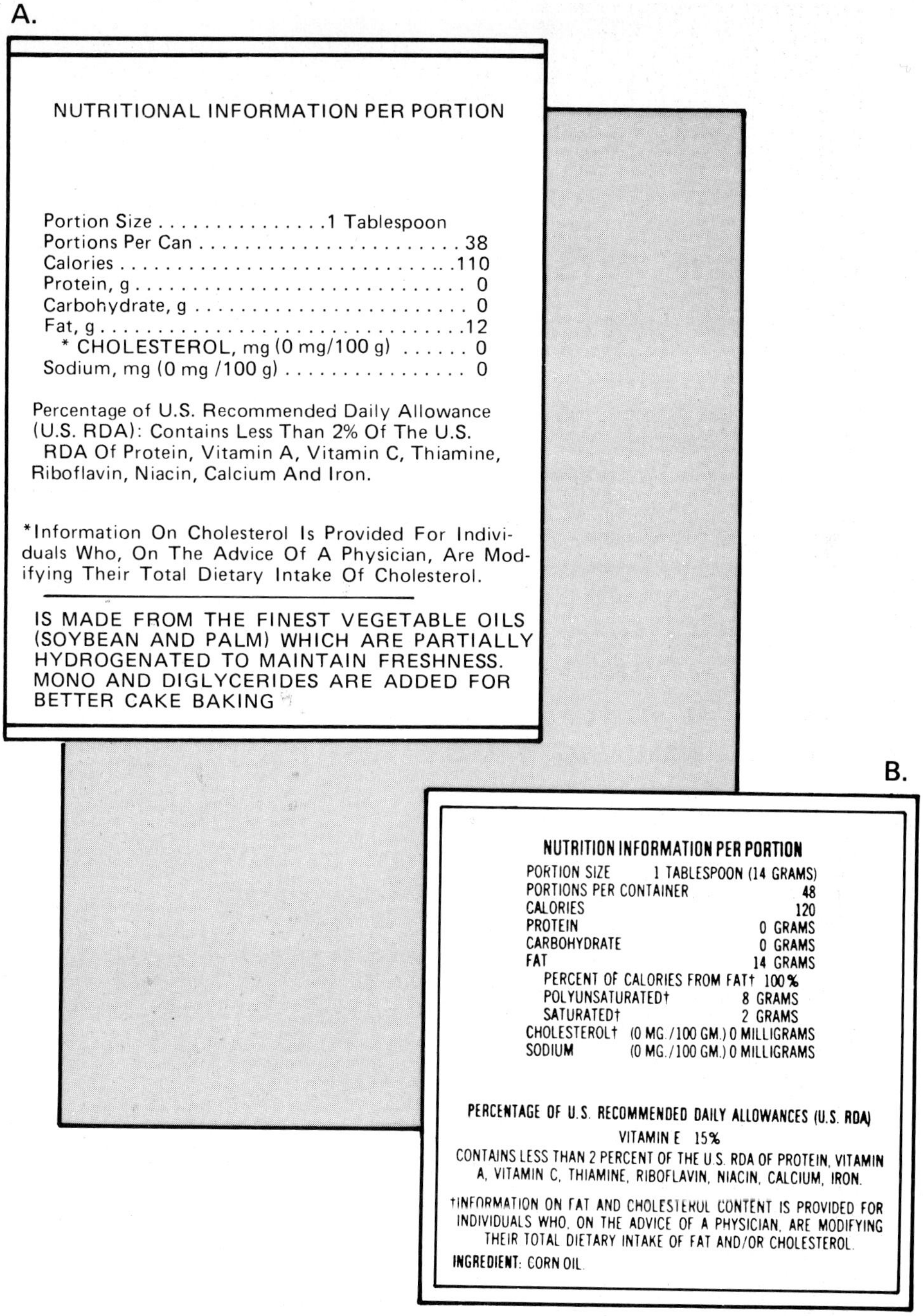

A.

NUTRITIONAL INFORMATION PER PORTION

Portion Size . . . . .1 Tablespoon
Portions Per Can 38
Calories 110
Protein, g 0
Carbohydrate, g 0
Fat, g 12
    * CHOLESTEROL, mg (0 mg/100 g) 0
Sodium, mg (0 mg /100 g) 0

Percentage of U.S. Recommended Daily Allowance
(U.S. RDA): Contains Less Than 2% Of The U.S.
  RDA Of Protein, Vitamin A, Vitamin C, Thiamine,
Riboflavin, Niacin, Calcium And Iron.

*Information On Cholesterol Is Provided For Indivi-
duals Who, On The Advice Of A Physician, Are Mod-
ifying Their Total Dietary Intake Of Cholesterol.
─────────────────────────────────
IS MADE FROM THE FINEST VEGETABLE OILS
(SOYBEAN AND PALM) WHICH ARE PARTIALLY
HYDROGENATED TO MAINTAIN FRESHNESS.
MONO AND DIGLYCERIDES ARE ADDED FOR
BETTER CAKE BAKING

B.

NUTRITION INFORMATION PER PORTION
PORTION SIZE   1 TABLESPOON (14 GRAMS)
PORTIONS PER CONTAINER   48
CALORIES   120
PROTEIN   0 GRAMS
CARBOHYDRATE   0 GRAMS
FAT   14 GRAMS
    PERCENT OF CALORIES FROM FAT† 100%
    POLYUNSATURATED†   8 GRAMS
    SATURATED†   2 GRAMS
CHOLESTEROL†   (0 MG./100 GM.) 0 MILLIGRAMS
SODIUM   (0 MG./100 GM.) 0 MILLIGRAMS

PERCENTAGE OF U.S. RECOMMENDED DAILY ALLOWANCES (U.S. RDA)
VITAMIN E   15%
CONTAINS LESS THAN 2 PERCENT OF THE U.S. RDA OF PROTEIN, VITAMIN
A, VITAMIN C, THIAMINE, RIBOFLAVIN, NIACIN, CALCIUM, IRON.

†INFORMATION ON FAT AND CHOLESTEROL CONTENT IS PROVIDED FOR
INDIVIDUALS WHO, ON THE ADVICE OF A PHYSICIAN, ARE MODIFYING
THEIR TOTAL DIETARY INTAKE OF FAT AND/OR CHOLESTEROL.
INGREDIENT: CORN OIL.

Figure 16-3.   *Labels from two fat products showing the different ways in which optional fat,*
cholesterol, and sodium information may be listed.

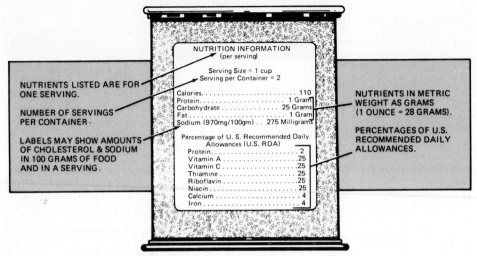

NUTRIENTS LISTED ARE FOR ONE SERVING.

NUMBER OF SERVINGS PER CONTAINER.

LABELS MAY SHOW AMOUNTS OF CHOLESTEROL & SODIUM IN 100 GRAMS OF FOOD AND IN A SERVING.

NUTRITION INFORMATION
(per serving)

Serving Size = 1 cup
Serving per Container = 2

Calories.......................... 110
Protein....................... 1 Gram
Carbohydrate .... 25 Grams
Fat .... 1 Gram
Sodium (970mg/100gm) .. 275 Milligrams

Percentage of U. S. Recommended Daily
Allowances (U.S. RDA)
Protein....................... 2
Vitamin A 25
Vitamin C 25
Thiamine 25
Riboflavin 25
Niacin 25
Calcium 4
Iron 4

NUTRIENTS IN METRIC WEIGHT AS GRAMS (1 OUNCE = 28 GRAMS).

PERCENTAGES OF U.S. RECOMMENDED DAILY ALLOWANCES.

Figure 16-4.   Nutrition labeling information. Any food to which a nutrient is added, or which makes a nutritious claim, must have a nutrition label. Adapted from: Read the Label, Set a Better Table. DHEW Publication No. (FDA) 75-4001.

A.

NUTRITION INFORMATION PER SERVING

Serving Size . . . . . . 20 oz. (57 g)
Servings Per Container. 5
Calories 35
Protein (Grams) 0
Carbohydrates (Grams) 4
Fat (Grams) 2

PERCENTAGE OF U.S. RECOMMENDED DAILY ALLOWANCES (U.S. RDA)

Contains Less Than 2% Of The U.S. RDA Of Protein, Vitamin A, Vitamin C, Thiamine, Riboflavin, Niacin, Calcium And Iron.

INGREDIENTS: Water, Mushrooms, Wheat Flour, Modified Food Starch, Partially Hydrogenated Vegetable Oil; (Soybean Oil; Palm Or Cottonseed Oil), Salt, Hydrolyzed Plant Protein, Caramel Color, Monosodium Glutamate, Natural Flavoring And Dehydrated Garlic.

B.

NUTRITION INFORMATION PER SERVING

Serving Size . . . . 2 oz. (57 g)
Servings Per Container. 5
Calories 30
Protein (Grams) 1
Carbohydrate (Grams) 3
Fat (Grams) 1

PERCENTAGE OF U.S. RECOMMENDED DAILY ALLOWANCES (U.S. RDA)
Niacin 2
Contains Less Than 2% Of The U.S. RDA Of Protein, Vitamin A, Vitamin C, Thiamine, Riboflavin, Calcium And Iron.

INGREDIENTS: Beef Stock, Wheat Flour, Water, Modified Food Starch, Beef Fat, Hydrolyzed Plant Protein, Salt, Caramel Color, Monosodium Glutamate, Natural Flavoring And Dehydrated Garlic.

Figure 16-5.   Two labels from different cans of prepared gravy: A. Mushroom gravy. B. Beef gravy.

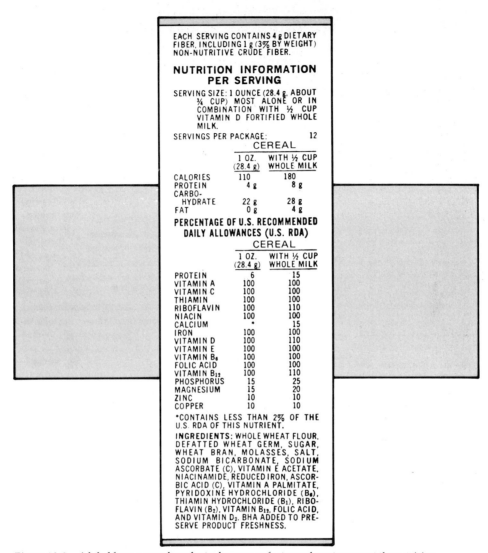

EACH SERVING CONTAINS 4 g DIETARY
FIBER, INCLUDING 1 g (3% BY WEIGHT)
NON-NUTRITIVE CRUDE FIBER.

NUTRITION INFORMATION
PER SERVING

SERVING SIZE: 1 OUNCE (28.4 g, ABOUT
¼ CUP) MOST ALONE OR IN
COMBINATION WITH ½ CUP
VITAMIN D FORTIFIED WHOLE
MILK.

SERVINGS PER PACKAGE: 12

CEREAL		
	1 OZ. (28.4 g)	WITH ½ CUP WHOLE MILK
CALORIES	110	180
PROTEIN	4 g	8 g
CARBO- HYDRATE	22 g	28 g
FAT	0 g	4 g

PERCENTAGE OF U.S. RECOMMENDED
DAILY ALLOWANCES (U.S. RDA)

CEREAL		
	1 OZ. (28.4 g)	WITH ½ CUP WHOLE MILK
PROTEIN	6	15
VITAMIN A	100	100
VITAMIN C	100	100
THIAMIN	100	100
RIBOFLAVIN	100	110
NIACIN	100	100
CALCIUM	*	15
IRON	100	100
VITAMIN D	100	110
VITAMIN E	100	100
VITAMIN B$_6$	100	100
FOLIC ACID	100	100
VITAMIN B$_{12}$	100	110
PHOSPHORUS	15	25
MAGNESIUM	15	20
ZINC	10	10
COPPER	10	10

*CONTAINS LESS THAN 2% OF THE
U.S. RDA OF THIS NUTRIENT.

INGREDIENTS: WHOLE WHEAT FLOUR,
DEFATTED WHEAT GERM, SUGAR,
WHEAT BRAN, MOLASSES, SALT,
SODIUM BICARBONATE, SODIUM
ASCORBATE (C), VITAMIN E ACETATE,
NIACINAMIDE, REDUCED IRON, ASCOR-
BIC ACID (C), VITAMIN A PALMITATE,
PYRIDOXINE HYDROCHLORIDE (B$_6$),
THIAMIN HYDROCHLORIDE (B$_1$), RIBO-
FLAVIN (B$_2$), VITAMIN B$_{12}$, FOLIC ACID,
AND VITAMIN D$_2$. BHA ADDED TO PRE-
SERVE PRODUCT FRESHNESS.

*Figure 16-6.   A label from a cereal product whose manufacturer chose to present the nutrition
information for his cereal product alone and in combination with the milk normally
served with this food product.*

MADE WITH NATURAL SESAME SEEDS
AND PURE CLOVER HONEY
CONTAINS NO SUGAR

Figure 16-7.   Descriptive information from the label of a candy bar.

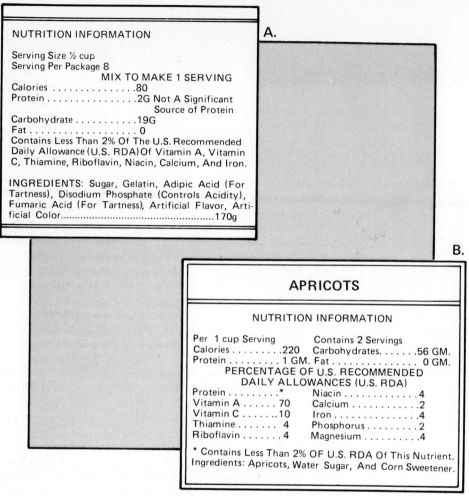

NUTRITION INFORMATION

Serving Size ½ cup
Serving Per Package 8
                 MIX TO MAKE 1 SERVING
Calories 80
Protein . . . . .2G Not A Significant
                          Source of Protein
Carbohydrate 19G
Fat 0
Contains Less Than 2% Of The U.S. Recommended
Daily Allowance (U.S. RDA) Of Vitamin A, Vitamin
C, Thiamine, Riboflavin, Niacin, Calcium, And Iron.

INGREDIENTS: Sugar, Gelatin, Adipic Acid (For
Tartness), Disodium Phosphate (Controls Acidity),
Fumaric Acid (For Tartness), Artificial Flavor, Arti-
ficial Color. 170g

A.

B.

APRICOTS

NUTRITION INFORMATION

Per 1 cup Serving   Contains 2 Servings
Calories 220   Carbohydrates. . . . . . .56 GM.
Protein . . . . 1 GM. Fat . . . . 0 GM.
            PERCENTAGE OF U.S. RECOMMENDED
                  DAILY ALLOWANCES (U.S. RDA)
Protein . . . .*   Niacin 4
Vitamin A 70   Calcium 2
Vitamin C 10   Iron 4
Thiamine 4   Phosphorus 2
Riboflavin 4   Magnesium 4

* Contains Less Than 2% OF U.S. RDA Of This Nutrient.
Ingredients: Apricots, Water Sugar, And Corn Sweetener.

Figure 16-8.   Two labels of food products supplying less than 2 percent U.S. RDA for protein. Each food manufacturer chose to present the information in a different manner.

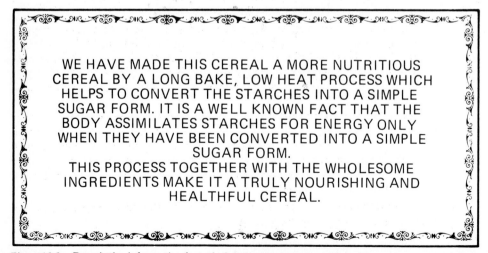

WE HAVE MADE THIS CEREAL A MORE NUTRITIOUS
CEREAL BY A LONG BAKE, LOW HEAT PROCESS WHICH
HELPS TO CONVERT THE STARCHES INTO A SIMPLE
SUGAR FORM. IT IS A WELL KNOWN FACT THAT THE
BODY ASSIMILATES STARCHES FOR ENERGY ONLY
WHEN THEY HAVE BEEN CONVERTED INTO A SIMPLE
SUGAR FORM.
THIS PROCESS TOGETHER WITH THE WHOLESOME
INGREDIENTS MAKE IT A TRULY NOURISHING AND
HEALTHFUL CEREAL.

Figure 16-9.   Descriptive information from the label on a prepared cereal product.

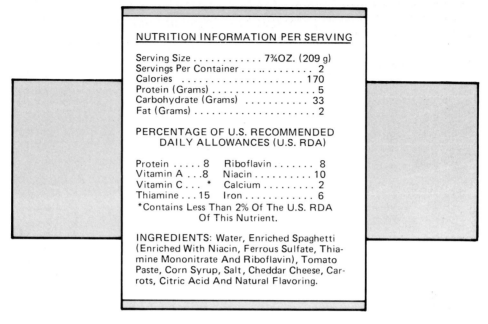

NUTRITION INFORMATION PER SERVING

Serving Size . . . . 7¾OZ. (209 g)
Servings Per Container 2
Calories 170
Protein (Grams) 5
Carbohydrate (Grams) 33
Fat (Grams) 2

PERCENTAGE OF U.S. RECOMMENDED
DAILY ALLOWANCES (U.S. RDA)

Protein 8   Riboflavin 8
Vitamin A . . .8   Niacin 10
Vitamin C . . . *   Calcium 2
Thiamine . . . 15   Iron 6
*Contains Less Than 2% Of The U.S. RDA
Of This Nutrient.

INGREDIENTS: Water, Enriched Spaghetti
(Enriched With Niacin, Ferrous Sulfate, Thiamine Mononitrate And Riboflavin), Tomato
Paste, Corn Syrup, Salt, Cheddar Cheese, Carrots, Citric Acid And Natural Flavoring.

Figure 16-10.   Label from a can of prepared spaghetti.

Key Points: The Labeling of Food

I. The Federal Food, Drug, and Cosmetic Act of 1938 remains the basis for current labeling regulations.

II. The Fair Packaging and Labeling Act set regulations for the appearance of information, format of information, and the content of labeling information. Specifically, it required disclosure of the common name of the food product, identification of manufacturer, packer, or distributor; standard measurement of contents, ingredients listed in decreasing order of predominance and, in some cases, serving information. It also required this information to be conspicuous and in legible type.

III. The Food and Drug Administration (FDA) enforces laws and regulations requiring food to be safe, wholesome, and properly labeled.

IV. Nutrition labeling regulations became effective after 1973.
    A. Nutrition labeling is voluntary for processed foods except when: (1) a nutrition claim is made for a food, (2) any nutrient is added to a food.
    B. Nutritional labeling uses the U.S. RDAs as standards for assessing the percentage of daily requirements which nutrients supply.
    C. Regulations provided a standardized format for presenting nutritional information.
    D. Advantages of nutritional labeling to consumers include: providing specific food product nutritional information, educating consumers about general nutrition principles, encouraging food producers to maintain a nutritionally high quality product, enabling a reasonable comparison of nutrient quality, quantity, and the price between food products, enabling identification of good sources for specific nutrients.

V. Consumer influence and expression of desires have effected labeling changes and inspired proposed labeling changes.

Questions: The Labeling of Food

1. Match the phrases on the right to the items on the left which they best describe:

    _____ 1. Food, Drug, and Cosmetic Act of 1938
    _____ 2. Fair Packaging and Labeling Act
    _____ 3. Food Additive Amendment of 1958
    _____ 4. GRAS
    _____ 5. Food and Drug Act of 1906
    _____ 6. Delaney Clause

    a. forbids the use of *any* food additive in *any* amount if it is found to induce cancer in experimental animals or humans
    b. first regulation defining food and drugs and preventing interstate commerce of misbranded or adulterated food and drugs
    c. the act which remains the basis for current food labeling regulation
    d. shifted burden for establishing proof of safety from government to manufacturer for food additives
    e. food additives excluded from the testing requirement because they were used for a long time without apparent ill effects at the time of the Food Additive Amendment adoption, 1958
    f. required clear and legible statement of identity, list of ingredients, and manufacturer information on food product packaging

2. The Fair Packaging and Labeling Act required that ingredients be listed legibly on a single panel on food labels with ingredients in:
    a. alphabetical order
    b. decreasing order of predominance
    c. increasing order of predominance

3. The Food, Drug, and Cosmetic Act of 1938 provided that the net contents be given in terms of:
    a. ounces and pounds
    b. grams and kilograms
    c. weight, measure, or count

4. The Food Additive Amendment of 1958 included what two broad categories of additives?

5. The Delaney Clause does *not* allow for scientific judgment in weighing the risk of cancer development against possible beneficial limited usage of certain food additives.
    a. True
    b. False

6. Identify the incorrectly written labeling item on the package in Figure 16-11 shown according to the regulations of the Fair Packaging and Labeling Act.

7. Which Agency enforces the laws and regulations requiring food to be safe, wholesome, and properly labeled?

8. The FDA will investigate an individual consumer's complaint made to that Agency about the sanitation, safety, or labeling of the products FDA regulates.
    a. True
    b. False

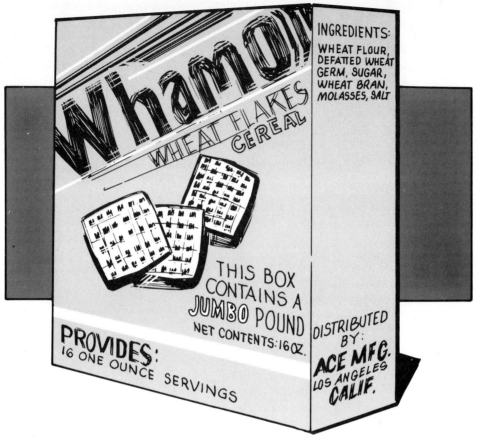

Figure 16-11. Cereal box illustrating package labeling.

9. Foods with a Standard of Identity and those which meet all the appropriate standards:
   a. do not have to list ingredients on the label.
   b. must have standards printed on the label.
   c. are uniform in quality and composition.

10. The FDA can inspect food processing plants, test samples of food products, set Standards of Identity, and establish regulations for food labeling.
   a. True
   b. False

11. Why was "imitation" dropped as a descriptive term for new food products *not* inferior to established foods according to FDA standards?

12. When "imitation" is on the label of a food product such as "imitation mayonnaise" that product is _____ to the established food it is meant to replace, such as mayonnaise.
   a. inferior
   b. equivalent
   c. superior

13. Standardized foods which contain added nutrients must comply with full nutrition labeling requirements.
    a. True
    b. False

14. Refer to Figure 16-6. Does this cereal product have to be listed as a dietary vitamin and mineral *supplement*?

15. Foods designated as "ordinary" contain less than what percentage of the U.S. RDA per serving for added nutrients (vitamins and minerals)?

16. Refer to Figure 16-3. The voluntary listing of cholesterol, percentage of calories from fat, polyunsaturated fat, and saturated fat content information does not *require* full nutrition labeling which just happens to be given.
    a. True
    b. False

17. Were the fat sources given in Figure 16-3 of corn, soybean, and palm oils voluntarily presented by the food processor?

18. If the package label on a heat and serve frozen dinner contains the statement "provides nutrients in amounts appropriate for this class of food as determined by the U.S. Government" you can be assured that:
    a. the dinner provides a high amount of calories.
    b. the dinner provides a high amount of fat.
    c. the dinner contributes a significant amount of nutrients for the total number of calories it provides.

19. Nutrition labeling is optional for use by food processors except under what two conditions?

20. What eight nutrients must be stated in terms of the percentage of U.S. RDA they provide per serving according to nutrition labeling regulations?

21. If sodium content is provided is full nutrition labeling required?

22. What serving information must be given in nutrition labeling?

23. Nutrient content in food per nutritional labeling must be given in the:
    a. English measurement system
    b. metric measurement system
    c. customary measurement system

24. Refer to Figure 16-3, item B. Why is the percentage for U.S. RDA of vitamin E given?

25. How many boxes of pastries in Figure 16-1 must be purchased to serve 12 persons one pastry for breakfast?

26. Compare the information below to the information in Figure 16-1.

Two slices whole wheat toast with one tablespoon butter.

		% U.S. RDA
kcal	212	
gm/protein	2.5	*
gm/carbohydrate	22.1	
gm/fiber	.8	
gm/fat	12.7	
mg/sodium	238	
mg/potassium	127	
mg/calcium	47	5%
mg/magnesium	36	9%
mg/phosphorus	106	*

mg/iron	.5	5%
mg/thiamin	.08	5%
mg/riboflavin	.04	2%
mg/niacin	1.2	5%
IU vitamin A	462	9%

*Contains less than 2% U.S. RDA for this nutrient.

a. Did the food processor of the pastries make a fair attempt to produce a new food product nutritionally equivalent to or better than the established food replaced (the toast with butter)?

b. The pastries were priced $1.89. The bread is 89 cents per loaf (twelve slices). The tablespoon butter is seven cents. Which food is cheaper, the pastries or toast?

c. Does the toast contain some nutrients not contained or identified in the pastries? Identify the ones shown.

d. Read the ingredients for the pastries. Do you think there is a significant amount of egg whites in the pastries?

27. Refer to Figure 16-3. Label (A) is from a solid shortening product. Label (B) is from a liquid oil.

 a. Why do you suppose the food processor for label (A) chose not to provide polyunsaturated/saturated fat information?

 b. Why in label (B) do the polyunsaturated/saturated fat quantities *not* add up to the total number of grams of fat given for that product?

28. Refer to Figure 16-8.

 a. Why was no figure allowed to be given for the percentage U.S. RDA for protein?

 b. Label (A) was from a gelatin dessert mix. What has the food processor done to help educate the consumer to correct the common misconception that gelatin is a good quality protein?

 c. Why is gelatin not a good quality protein? (Hint, refer to Chapter Five, Proteins "incomplete.")

29. Refer to Figure 16-3. In what two ways do amounts for cholesterol and sodium have to be stated?

30. Refer to Figure 16-6. Do the zinc and copper come from the cereal product or the milk?

31. Refer to Figure 16-2B and 16-10.

 a. The protein in the tuna is rounded off to what nearest unit percent?

 b. The protein in the spaghetti is rounded off to what nearest unit product?

 c. If a food product showed that it supplied 25 percent U.S. RDA for protein per serving that figure would actually have been rounded off to what nearest unit percent?

32. Inspect the labels and ingredients listed in Figure 16-2. Do you feel these foods would possibly supply some trace nutrients as well as other substances not yet identified as necessary nutrients?

33. Which of the nutrients listed with the percent U.S. RDA supplied per serving in Figure 16-8B were optionally given by the food processor?

34. a. Is the percent U.S. RDA per serving for protein in Figure 16-2B based on 45 or 65 g protein?

 b. Is the percent U.S. RDA per serving for protein in Figure 16-10 based on 45 or 65 g protein?

35. Refer to Figure 16-5A. A two once serving is approximately one-quarter of a cup. Therefore, one-quarter cup of this gravy contains 35 kcal.
     a. From what nutrients are these kcal derived?
     b. What ingredient is in the greatest quantity in this food product?
     c. Why are the percentages of U.S. RDA for the eight required nutrients not itemized?

36. Refer to Figure 16-10, the label from the canned spaghetti.
     a. What is the ingredient in greatest quantity in this product?
     b. Look down the list of ingredients. Where is cheddar cheese listed? Does this location for cheese lead you to conclude that there is a considerable amount, or a small amount, of cheese in this product?

37. Refer to Figures 16-2 and 16-8.
     a. Which foods are good sources of vitamin A?
     b. Which food is a very good source of vitamin B_{12} and niacin?
     c. Which food is a good source of vitamin C?
     d. Which food group supplies the smallest amount of protein: vegetables, fruit, or meats?

38. Refer to Figures 16-1, 16-2, 16-5, 16-6, 16-8, and 16-10.
     a. Which two foods supply the fewest nutrients per total calories per serving?
     b. What is the significant nutrient difference between the foods represented by labels (A) and (B) in Figure 16-5?
     c. Which food appears to have the greatest nutrient content per total kcal per serving?

39. Refer to Figure 16-9. This label was found on a granola type cereal product. This description appears to be intelligently informative, but in what way is this label information misleading? (If necessary, review Chapter Three, Digestion, Absorption, and Metabolism of Carbohydrates.)

40. Refer to Figure 16-7. This label was on a candy bar for sale in a university bookstore. In what way is this label misleading?

Answers: The Labeling of Food

1. 1. c
    2. f
    3. d
    4. e
    5. b
    6. a
2. b
3. c
4. intentional and incidental (unintentional) additives
5. a
6. illegal use of descriptor term "Jumbo Pound" associated with net contents information
7. Food and Drug Administration (FDA)
8. a
9. a, c
10. a
11. Imitation was deemed an uninformative term.
12. a
13. a

14.   Yes (and, in fact, it is on the main display panel of the package), because it supplies between 50 and 150 percent U.S. RDA of added nutrients (vitamins and minerals) per serving.

15.   50 percent

16.   b

17.   no; sources for fats and oils in processed foods are now required to be given by the common or usual name.

18.   c

19.   On any food to which a nutrient(s) is added or about which a nutritional claim is made.

20.   Protein, vitamin A, vitamin C, thiamin, riboflavin, niacin, calcium, and iron.

21.   no; use of nutritional labeling is voluntary when sodium information is given.

22.   serving size; servings per container

23.   b

24.   Vitamin E is an optional nutrient for which a food processor may elect to give percentage U.S. RDA per serving information.

25.   two

26.   a.   yes, it appears so
      b.   32 cents pastry ($1.98 ÷ 6)
           22 cents/2 slices toast with 1 tbsp. butter − 7½ cents per slice times two slices plus 7 cents butter; The toast and butter is cheaper.
      c.   yes: fiber, sodium, potassium, and probably others.
      d.   probably not; "Egg whites" is listed between the leavening agent (baking soda), gelatin, and a coloring agent (caramel), all of which are used in small quantities in bakery products.

27.   a.   There would be a relatively high proportion of saturated fat listed because the product is made by saturating vegetable oils with hydrogen to solidify the fat product. Refer to Chapter Three, Lipids "hydrogenation." Saturated fat is less desirable because most persons who modify their fat intake do so to increase the proportion of polyunsaturated fats they consume.
      b.   Because a third category, monounsaturated fats, is not subtotaled. In this case, monounsaturated fats would total 4 g.

28.   a.   Because whatever protein is present is either of quality below 20 percent the PER of casein (milk protein) or totals less than two percent U.S. RDA per serving.
      b.   The food processor noted on the label by the amount in grams of protein "not a significant source of protein."
      c.   Gelatin is an incomplete protein of low biological value because it is almost entirely deficient in the essential amino acid, tryptophan.

29.   milligrams per serving; milligrams per 100g of the food.

30.   It must be the cereal because the percent U.S. RDA is the same for zinc and copper in the cereal as in the cereal with milk.

31.   a.   10
      b.   2
      c.   5

32.   yes; These are fruits, a vegetable, and meat which have simply been canned to preserve the food. They are not "new" processed food products designed to replace an established food which has been fortified with only the nutrients required to be listed.

33.   phosphorus and magnesium

34.   a.   45g
      b.   65g

35. a. fat and carbohydrate
    b. water
    c. because five or more (actually all eight) are present in quantities less than amounts necessary to supply at least two percent U.S. RDA per serving
36. a. water
    b. Cheddar cheese is between salt and carrots (flavoring and coloring agents) and is probably in small quantity.
37. a. apricots and tomatoes
    b. tuna
    c. tomatoes
    d. fruit
38. a. Figure 16-8A, gelatin dessert; Figure 16-5A, mushroom gravy
    b. The mushroom gravy is water-based while the beef gravy base is actually from beef stock.
    c. tomatoes
39. This label states that its product is more nutritious because it has undergone a long-bake process which has broken down the starches into simpler sugars, the only form in which starch is "assimilated" by the body. In fact, our bodies normally contain enzymes and other substances necessary for the complete breakdown of dietary starch (digestion) to the monosaccharides (simple sugars) so they can be absorbed and metabolized by our bodies. No long-bake process is necessary in order to efficiently digest the starch in this cereal product. This label implies that the starch in other cereals not undergoing a long-bake process is not available to our bodies.
40. This label states that it contains honey but no sugar. In fact, honey is almost entirely of sugar composition: some sucrose, glucose, fructose, and water.

REFERENCES

[1] Schmidt AM: Food and drug law: A 200-year perspective. Nutrition Today, 10, April 1975, pp. 29-32

[2] Ross ML: What's happening to food labeling? Journal of the American Dietetic Association, 64, March 1974, p. 262

[3] An incidental food additive is one which is present in food in trace quantity as a result of some phase of production, processing, storage, or packaging. Finding trace amounts of a certain pesticide in a specific food is an example.

[4] Usually large amounts of a food additive are ingested by experimental animals which would far exceed the amounts normally expected to be ingested by humans. *However, if any food additive is found at any level to cause cancer in man or animal it cannot be used according to the Delaney Clause.*

[5] According to the FDA (Food ingredient review: Where it stands now. FDA Consumer, June 1974), the substances itemized on the GRAS list are currently being reevaluated. This is a painstaking and time-consuming process. This reevaluation resulted from President Nixon's order in 1969 to double-check the safety of food ingredients following the ban on the artificial sweetener cyclamate which had been on the GRAS list because newer scientific tests showed that it could cause cancer. After thorough retesting of individual GRAS list items, those substances found to comply with FDA criteria for acceptance as "generally recognized as safe" are intended to be added to a new FDA-affirmed GRAS list. The FDA released the first comprehensive review report in late 1980.

[6] Friedelson I: Fair packaging: Synopsis of food packaging and labeling regulations. FDA Papers, 1, October 1967, pp. 21-24

[7] The FDA also enforces laws requiring that drugs, medical devices, and cosmetics be safe, effective, and properly labeled.

[8] A consumer guide to FDA. HEW Publication No. (FDA) 78-1013

[9] Ross ML: What's happening to food labeling. Journal of the American Dietetic Association, 64, March 1974, p. 266

[10] Standards of identity. Nutrition Reviews, 32, January 1974, p. 29

[11] Food labeling regulations. Nutrition Today, 8, January-February 1973, pp. 14-15

[12] Food labeling. Dairy Council Digest, 45, March-April 1974

[13] The food labeling revolution. Reprint from FDA Consumer, April 1974, DHEW Publication No. (FDA) 74-2058

[14] Food Labeling: Phase IV. Journal of Nutrition Education, 6, July-September 1974, p. 86
Summary of food labeling notice. Department of HEW, Public Health Service, December 1979
Federal Register, Food labeling: tentative position of agencies. Friday, December 21, 1979

[15] Getting specific about fats and oils. FDA Consumer, 10, March 1976, p. 13

[16] Food labeling bills introduced. SNE Communicator (newsletter of the Society for Nutrition Education), Vol. 10 No. 3, September 1979, p. 4

[17] SNE board issues position statement on food labeling. SNE Communicator (newsletter of the Society for Nutrition Education), Vol. 9 No. 4, December 1978, p. 7
General information for nutrition labeling was obtained from the following sources numbered 18, 19, and 20.

[18] The food labeling revolution. Reprint from FDA Consumer, April 1974, DHEW Publication No. (FDA) 74-2058

[19] Food Labeling. Dairy Council Digest, 40, March-April 1974, pp. 7-12

[20] Nutrition Labeling—How It Can Work For You. National Nutrition Consortium, Inc. with Ronald M. Deutsch. Bethesda: The National Nutrition Consortium, Inc., 1975

[21] Monounsaturated fats are presently not deemed physiologically active in the development of circulatory or heart diseases. Monounsaturated fats contain fatty acids having only one double bond. Refer to Chapter Three for more information on fatty acid structure and the relationship of diet to heart and circulatory diseases.

[22] Nutrition Labeling. Nutrition Reviews, 32, August 1974, p. 251

[23] Johnson OC: The Food and Drug Administration and labeling. Journal of the American Dietetic Association, 64, May 1974, p. 473

17

SOME NUTRITIONAL CONSIDERATIONS FOR A FEW SPECIAL PHASES OF THE LIFE CYCLE

There are some periods in the life cycle which require special nutritional consideration. These considerations must be made in light of influencing factors unique to that special life cycle condition. This text will present some of the basic nutritional principles associated with good health and some nutritional problems associated with infancy, early childhood, adolescence, pregnancy and lactation, and old age.

This presentation is intended as an introduction to these life cycle periods with their special needs. It is hoped that you will become aware of the need for special nutritional considerations and diet modifications during these as well as other times, and be motivated to further your personal investigation into the needs and problems which affect most persons during such periods of increased physiological, emotional, and nutritional stress.

PREGNANCY AND LACTATION

Maternal weight gain and infant birth weight. It appears that infant birth weight is associated with maternal weight gain.[1] Low birth weight is associated with the increased incidence of infant mortality and impaired development. Low birth weight infants may be of average length, head circumference, and skeletal size, or may be below average in length and have a proportionately reduced head circumference and skeletal size. A head circumference measurement well below normal *suggests* hampered brain development.[2]

Research studies with animals suggest that inadequate food intake can cause a decrease in brain cell multiplication during the phase when brain cell growth is associated with permanent, irreversible limitation of functioning (brain damage or stunted brains).[3] Though the application of the results from these animal studies is limited when applied to humans, the possibility of damage to the growing fetus from maternal malnutrition does exist, especially when specific nutrient deficiencies occur to the fetus at associated critical stages of development.

Most researchers and doctors feel that total weight gain has been over-emphasized. *Of greater importance is the pattern of weight gain.*[4] The average total weight gain is approximately 11 kg (24 pounds) added at the rate of about two to three pounds the first three months (first trimester), 10 to 11 pounds the second three months (second trimester), and 11 pounds the last three months (third trimester). Excessive weight gain in the first trimester should not be compensated by curtailment of weight gain for the time remaining until pregnancy comes to term. Caloric needs are highest during the last trimester and are met, in part, by the normally decreased activity level of the pregnant woman at this time.

Increased risk occurs to infants of low birth weight whose mothers were underweight and undernourished before pregnancy and remain malnourished during pregnancy. Unfortunately, successive pregnancies of such poorly nourished mothers produce progressively more undernourished infants. It is also unfortunate that set patterns of inadequate nutrient intake frequently continue after birth for both mother and infant.

Weight gain during pregnancy is due to weight of the fetus, placenta, and amniotic fluid; increased uterus and breast tissue; and maternal blood volume and maternal interstitial fluid. It appears that with optimum nutrition these components of maternal weight gain can actually total about 26 pounds in a healthy woman.[5] Note that this total maternal weight gain with optimum nutrition throughout pregnancy is somewhat greater than recorded average total weight gain. Some researchers indicate that even a total weight gain of 26 to 30 pounds is justifiable due to optimal increase in maternal and fetal tissues as well as body fluids. The pregnant woman does add extra fat stores during pregnancy which probably are in physiological preparation of increased caloric needs during the last trimester and lactation. *Pregnancy is no time for a woman to try to lose weight.* Attempts to reduce maternal weight are best undertaken after the term of pregnancy, preferably two to three months following pregnancy in order to allow the body adequate time to return to normal nonpregnant functioning. At this time the woman is well advised to lose weight gained in order to avoid being overweight and obese as the result of cumulative weight gain from several pregnancies.

Nutrient needs of pregnancy. The Revised 1980 RDAs give an extra 300 kcal per day energy allowance for the pregnant woman to cover the energy cost of pregnancy, and allow for sufficient weight gain. An additional 500 kcal increase is allotted during lactation to cover the energy costs of this period. The RDA for protein in increased by 30g for the pregnant woman. This allowance is considered to be generous and covers the increased tissue growth needs of both mother and fetus. In malnourished women the provision of adequate energy food intake is especially important in order to spare whatever protein is available for tissue synthesis. The RDA protein during lactation is increased by 20g.

Almost a 30 percent increase in blood volume occurs during pregnancy which requires significantly increased iron for hemoglobin synthesis. The fetus and placenta also require additional iron. Even nonpregnant menstruating women find it difficult to meet their iron needs through dietary intake. The Ten-State Nutrition Survey found the most common nutritional deficiency was iron deficiency anemia. Therefore, the increased demand for iron probably is best met by supplementation during pregnancy.[6] The RDAs further recommend continued iron supplementation for two to three months following the term of pregnancy.

The RDA for folacin is doubled during pregnancy to 800 µg. If this amount is difficult to obtain from dietary sources a supplement is recommended. Some good sources for folacin are green leafy vegetables, asparagus, fruits, dairy products, non-leafy vegetables, beans, and cereals. A megaloblastic anemia[7] due to a deficiency of folacin can occur although it is not nearly as common as iron deficiency anemia.

The RDA for calcium is set at 1200 mg for the pregnant woman. Some researchers feel that the absorption of calcium is increased during pregnancy which helps to compensate for increased needs. This RDA level is maintained for the lactating woman. Milk fortified with vitamins and other high density calcium foods such as cottage cheese, cheese, yogurt, and dark green leafy vegetables are recommended sources for calcium.

Sodium restriction is no longer thought to be beneficial to health during pregnancy. It is now advised that women salt their food to taste during pregnancy. The RDAs for vitamins A and D are significantly increased during pregnancy and lactation, and other vitamins and minerals are increased slightly to correspond with increased caloric intake.

Toxemia of pregnancy. Toxemia of pregnancy is also termed preeclampsia or eclampsia. It is a complication of pregnancy involving hypertension (high blood pressure), proteinuria (protein components in the urine), and edema (tissue swelling). Though the exact cause of toxemia is not known it appears to be related to low income and poor nutritional status. Therefore, maintaining good nutritional status during pregnancy reduces the risk of toxemia. *The use of diuretics should be avoided in toxemia.*

Adolescent pregnancy. A girl younger than seventeen who is pregnant must meet the nutritional growth needs of her own body as well as that of the fetus. The adolescent girl is more likely to unduly restrict her caloric intake in an effort to control her weight. In addition, the likelihood of poor dietary habits is increased during adolescence.

Fetal death, low infant birth weight, anemia, toxemia, and infant and maternal death are increased risk factors for the pregnant teenager. For pregnant teenagers under 15 years of age, the death risk is 60 percent greater than for mothers 20 years and older.[8] If the pregnancy is out-of-wedlock the pregnant teenager may be under considerable emotional stress. Stress has been shown to cause a negative balance of some nutrients even in the face of adequate nutrient intake. Obviously, the pregnant teenager is in great need of psychological and emotional support as well as nutritional and medical care.

Key Points: Pregnancy and Lactation

   I. Maternal weight gain is associated with infant birth weight. Inadequate and prolonged maternal energy and nutrient intake can result in an infant of low birth weight. Low birth weight is associated with increased infant mortality and impaired development.

  II. Maternal weight gain averages about 24 pounds. Estimates of total gain from the components of maternal weight gain can average 26 pounds under optimal nutritional conditions for a healthy woman.
     A. The pattern of weight gain is more important than total weight gain.
     B. Weight gain during pregnancy, which is appropriate to allow for normal maternal and fetal tissue growth and increase in body fluids, is desirable even for a woman who is overweight at the beginning of pregnancy.
     C. Maternal weight loss is not recommended to be undertaken until several months following pregnancy.

 III. Nutritional supplements of iron and folacin are recommended if these nutrients are difficult to obtain from dietary sources.

 IV. Calcium requirements during pregnancy are increased but are somewhat compensated for by increased absorption during pregnancy.

  V. Sodium restriction, especially through restriction of salt intake, is no longer generally advised during pregnancy.

 VI. The incidence of toxemia of pregnancy is related to low income and poor nutritional status.

VII. Pregnancy during adolescence is especially stressful and increased nutrient needs of both the mother and the developing fetus must be met.

Questions: Pregnancy and Lactation

  1. Maternal weight gain during pregnancy is associated with infant birth weight.
    a. True
    b. False
  2. Low birth weight infants may be:
    a. average in length with average head circumference and skeletal size.
    b. below average in length, head circumference, and skeletal size.
    c. above average in head circumference measurement.
  3. Reduced infant head circumference *may*:
    a. be desirable for an easier delivery.

   b. indicate hampered brain development.
   c. be related to inadequate maternal food intake and inappropriately low weight gain during pregnancy.
4. Decreased brain cell growth in laboratory animals is associated with (reversible/irreversible) limitation of brain functioning.
5. The *pattern* of weight gain is more important than the total weight gain during pregnancy.
   a. True
   b. False
6. A recommended pattern of weight gain during pregnancy is:
   a. eight pounds (first trimester), eight pounds (second trimester), eight pounds (last trimester) = 24 pounds
   b. five pounds (first trimester), five pounds (second trimester), 14 pounds (last trimester) = 24 pounds
   c. three pounds (first trimester), 10 pounds (second trimester), 11 pounds (last trimester) = 24 pounds
7. When are calorie needs during pregnancy the highest?
   a. first trimester
   b. second trimester
   c. third trimester
8. If a pregnant woman gains 25 pounds in her first trimester she should avoid *any* further weight gain during the second and third trimesters.
   a. True
   b. False
9. The greatest risk to low birth weight infants occurs in infants whose mothers were (underweight/overweight) *before* pregnancy and were (malnourished/ adequately nourished) *during* pregnancy.
10. Development of extra fat stores is normal for the pregnant woman.
    a. True
    b. False
11. When should attempts to lose maternal weight gain begin?
12. What is the RDA energy allowance for the pregnant woman?
    a. 100 kcal above nonpregnant energy needs
    b. 300 kcal above nonpregnant energy needs
    c. 500 kcal above nonpregnant energy needs
13. What is the additional RDA allowance for the lactating woman above nonpregnant, nonlactating needs?
    a. 100 kcal
    b. 300 kcal
    c. 500 kcal
14. Why is adequate energy food intake especially important to the malnourished pregnant woman?
15. What was the most common nutritional deficiency found in the U.S. in the Ten-State Nutrition Survey?
16. In addition to dietary sources, what mineral is recommended to be supplemented during pregnancy?
17. What vitamin may need to be supplemented during pregnancy to prevent a type of megaloblastic anemia?
18. What factor is thought to assist the pregnant woman in meeting her calcium requirement?

19. What mineral intake is no longer thought beneficial to generally restrict during pregnancy?
    a. iron
    b. sodium
    c. calcium

20. Mary is in her sixth month of pregnancy. In the last few days she has gained seven pounds. Her face, hands, and ankles appear puffy. Her blood pressure has risen and a lab test shows Mary's urine contains significant amounts of protein components. Her husband has been out of work throughout most of her pregnancy and their finances have been tight.
    a. What condition might you *suspect* Mary has?
    b. What is Mary's probable nutritional status?
    c. Should Mary take a diuretic to help her lose the excess water she is retaining?

21. Why is pregnancy during adolescence especially stressful physiologically?

22. What are some of the increased risks for the pregnant teenager?

23. Stress can cause a negative nutrient balance in spite of an adequate intake of that nutrient.
    a. True
    b. False

Answers: Pregnancy and Lactation

1. a
2. a, b
3. b, c
4. irreversible
5. a
6. c
7. c
8. b
9. underweight; malnourished
10. a
11. several months after pregnancy has reached term
12. b
13. c
14. In the face of limited or below recommended intake of protein, adequate energy food intake can spare what protein is available for use in tissue growth and repair.
15. iron deficiency anemia
16. iron
17. folacin (folic acid)
18. increased absorption of calcium during pregnancy
19. b, sodium (especially through salt restriction)
20. a. toxemia of pregnancy (preeclampsia or eclampsia)
    b. probably poor
    c. No, unless specifically prescribed by her physician. A diuretic is not recommended in toxemia.
21. The adolescent girl must meet nutritional growth needs of both her body and that of the fetus.
22. fetal death, low infant birth weight, anemia, toxemia, and infant and maternal death
23. a

INFANCY

The infant's body is of higher water content than an adult's; skin surface area to body weight is proportionately higher than an adult's; and an individual's growth rate is higher in infancy than at any other time of life. *Consequently, nourishment for the infant must provide adequate fluids, adequate calories for increased metabolic rate, growth, and activity levels, and adequate protein for new tissue growth.* In addition, vitamins and minerals are necessary for hard tissue growth such as bones and teeth, energy production, and general tissue synthesis.

Breast milk confers some special advantages to the infant. *Colostrum,* the initial breast fluid secreted before mature breast milk contains antibodies which aid in protecting the infant from infection. Colostrum is a yellowish fluid and differs in composition from mature breast milk: it is somewhat lower in caloric value due to decreased amounts of carbohydrate and fat, and is higher in protein and vitamin A. Breast milk composition is more appropriate to the human infant's needs than cow's milk although suitable infant formulas can be prepared from cow's milk. Cow's milk is slightly lower in calories and carbohydrate than human milk but notably higher in protein, calcium, phosphorus, sodium, and potassium. The substantially increased amounts of these nutrients in cow's milk requires the dilution of cow's milk in infant formulas in order for it to be an appropriate food for the human infant. When cow's milk is appropriately diluted, additional carbohydrates must be added to bring the energy value of the formula to approximately 22 kcal per ounce. Table 3-2 compares the major nutrient composition of human and cow's milk.

When breast feeding is not or cannot be the method of infant feeding, bottle feeding is undertaken. Most researchers feel the importance of breast feeding in the U.S. lies equally in its naturally appropriate composition and in its promotion of a close mother-child bond. Breast feeding also supplies a product free of foodborne disease contaminants. However, bottle feeding can be accomplished in such a way as to be sterile and to develop warmth and closeness between the mother and child. In addition, other family members may feed the baby which helps to develop closer bonds between them and the baby.

For the infant in the United States, bottle feeding and breast feeding differences in terms of food quality and safety are probably minimal. Most doctors do feel that children with allergies[9] or certain gastrointestinal disorders receive greater benefits from breast feeding. Unfortunately, in many developing countries where the economic and health status of families is much lower than in the United States, breast feeding is frequently giving way to increased bottle feeding. Commercial formulas, though more costly, are seen as more prestigious than breast milk. Overdilution and contamination of formulas are problems which hinder the health and safety of infants receiving commercial formulas in developing countries.[10]

It appears that overfeeding with bottle formulas may occur because the mother can see the volume of milk consumed and encourages the baby to take all the milk in a bottle. Since breast feeding does not allow the mother to see the amount of milk taken, the mother is much more likely to accept the appearance of satiety in the infant and allow the infant to decide when he or she has had enough to eat. Bottle-propping is emphatically discouraged because of its association with infant aspiration (taking of fluid into the lungs), lack of physical human contact, and an increase in dental caries. (See Chapter three for more information about dental caries in infancy.)

Breast milk is relatively low in iron, ascorbic acid, and vitamin D. Commercial formulas are usually fortified with these nutrients. However, iron is more readily absorbed from breast milk, allowing greater utilization of this nutrient. Ascorbic acid levels in breast milk are associated with the lactating woman's ascorbic acid intake. A breast fed infant is usually given a vitamin D supplement, though a water-soluble form of vitamin D may be present in human milk, reducing need for such supplementation. Orange juice or a vitamin C supplement (to avoid allergic reactions associated with orange juice intake) may be recommended for the breast fed infant at about three months of age. Iron is recommended to be obtained first from supplementation at about three to four months of age and later from solid foods (enriched cereals, egg yolk, and meats) at about six months. Iron stores in the full-term infant generally provide adequate iron for the first few months of life. Because little fluoride crosses the placenta during pregnancy, fluoride supplementation is recommended for infants in areas where the fluoride content of water and foods is marginal.

The Committee on Nutrition of the American Academy of Pediatrics is currently encouraging breast feeding with appropriate vitamin D, iron, and fluoride supplementation; use of an iron fortified commercial formula as an alternative to breast feeding with appropriate fluoride supplementation; delaying the introduction of solid foods until the sixth month of life; and no cow's milk before the end of the first year of life.[11]

Key Points: Infancy

I. Principles to consider when planning nourishment for an infant.
   A. Adequate fluids
      1. Body water content is higher than an adult's.
      2. Skin surface area is proportionately higher than an adult's allowing for greater loss of water through evaporation.
   B. Adequate calories
      1. Metabolic rate is higher than an adult's.
      2. The greater skin surface area of an infant allows for greater heat loss.
      3. Growth and activity levels are high.
   C. Adequate protein
      1. Growth rate is highest in infancy.
      2. High quality protein is required for new tissue synthesis.
   D. Adequate vitamins and minerals for proper development of bones and teeth, energy production, proper enzyme action, and general tissue synthesis.

II. The initial breast fluid is colostrum
   A. Yellowish fluid lower in carbohydrate and fat but higher in protein and vitamin A than breast milk.
   B. Contains antibodies which help protect the infant against infection.

III. Breast feeding
   A. Breast milk is the most appropriate food in composition to meet human infant needs.
   B. Breast feeding promotes the development of a close mother-child bond.
   C. Breast feeding provides an uncontaminated food source of high quality.
   D. Breast feeding is especially beneficial for infants with allergies or certain gastrointestinal disorders.
   E. Breast milk is relatively low in iron, ascorbic acid, and vitamin D.

IV. Bottle feeding
   A. Cow's milk is lower in carbohydrate but higher in protein and mineral content than human milk, and must be diluted and then supplemented with carbohydrate to make appropriate infant feeding formulas.
   B. Bottle fed formulas can be made to be nourishing and sterile.
   C. Bottle feeding can be performed in such a way as to be a warm, loving experience for the infant with all family members.
   D. Bottle feeding may promote overfeeding of infant.
   E. Commercial formulas are supplemented with various nutrients to meet infant needs.

V. The Committee on Nutrition of the American Academy of Pediatrics currently recommends:
   A. Breast feeding with appropriate vitamin D, iron, and fluoride supplementation.

    B.   Iron-fortified commercial formula with appropriate fluoride supplementation as an alternative to breast feeding.

    C.   Delaying the introduction of solid foods until the sixth month of life.

    D.   No cow's milk before the end of the first year of life.

Questions: Infancy

1. The highest growth rate for an individual occurs during infancy.
   a. True
   b. False

2. The highest BMR for an individual occurs during infancy.
   a. True
   b. False

3. Why is fluid intake especially important for an infant?

4. The initial breast fluid is called _____ .

5. Colostrum is higher than breast milk in:
   a. carbohydrate
   b. fat
   c. protein and vitamin A

6. Why do infant formulas made from cow's milk require dilution before they can be appropriately used as infant foods?

7. In addition to supplying appropriate nutrient composition in breast milk, breast feeding promotes _____ .

8. A lack of adequate nutrition and sanitation knowledge, as well as proper cooking and refrigeration facilities, leads to what problems in using commercial formulas for infants in developing nations?

9. Children with allergies or certain gastrointestinal disorders are probably most benefited by (breast feeding/commercial formula feeding).

10. Overfeeding that leads to overweight and obesity in infancy may be promoted by (breast feeding/bottle feeding).

11. One good way a mother can gain some time to complete her increased workload is to prop a bottle up for a baby to drink while the infant lies in the crib.
    a. True
    b. False

12. An infant is breast fed to one year of age. This child appears pale and somewhat listless. This child may also be susceptible to infections. This child has been receiving a vitamin D and ascorbic acid supplement.
    a. What condition may the child have?
    b. The deficiency of what nutrient is the cause of this condition?
    c. What foods could the child have received to improve the intake of this nutrient (in b above)?

13. Supplementation of what mineral is advised in order to help protect the infant's teeth from caries, if it is not naturally found in the food and water source at adequate levels?

14. The American Academy of Pediatrics is currently recommending:
    a. preferred use of what first infant food?
    b. delaying the introduction of solid foods until when?
    c. delaying the introduction of cow's milk until when?

Answers: Infancy

1. a
2. a
3. Because the infant's body maintains a high proportion of water to body weight; the infant's body has a high proportion of skin surface area to body weight and, therefore, experiences relatively high body water loss.
4. colostrum
5. c
6. Because the amounts of calcium, phosphorus, protein, sodium, and potassium in cow's milk are inappropriately high for human infant consumption.
7. the formation of a close mother-child bond
8. overdilution and contamination of the formula
9. breast feeding
10. bottle feeding, if the mother always tries to feed the infant all the milk in a bottle, whether or not the child seems satisfied
11. b
12. a.   iron deficiency anemia
    b.   iron
    c.   enriched cereals and later enriched breads, egg yolk and meats (see Table 12-2) from about six months of age
13. fluoride
14. a.   breast milk
    b.   six month's of age
    c.   after one year of age

EARLY CHILDHOOD

The years from ages one to five are filled with curiosity, exploration, assertion of independence, and attempts to define oneself in terms of his or her environment. Food comes to awareness as something to touch, grasp, poke, examine, smell, and to put in the mouth. This can make for great messiness!

Parents need to develop a tolerance of the havoc created while a child enjoys a new food experience and learns to eat using hands and, later, eating utensils. Experimentation with food and independence in eating are encouraged by providing durable, appropriately-sized eating utensils, plates, and cups. Plastic sheeting under a high chair to facilitate clean-up from spills will ease frustration when these inevitable accidents occur.

It is important that mealtimes be pleasant times of shared conversation as well as food. Eating habits formed now will continue throughout later life. The environment should be attractive, but tablecloths and decorations should be able to withstand considerable wear. Avoid confrontations over disliked foods and table manners. Vary the eating environment to stimulate appetite and interest in eating. Try eating in the yard, picnicking in the park, eating by a window, and other pleasant sites.

Children find it easier to eat moist foods than dry foods. Try to serve a relatively dry food with moist food or drink to facilitate consumption of both foods by the child. Snacks are useful in meeting energy and nutrient needs of children while their stomachs are small and unable to hold large amounts of food served only during the customary three meals a day. Snacks should be nutritious, appropriate in quantity, and served at times which will interfere the least with meals. Avoid small, hard foods such as peanuts which a small child may easily choke on.

Each child develops food preferences which influence his or her food consumption.

Food preference is highly correlated with food consumption by the young child.[12] Introduce different foods slowly and with genuine interest and enthusiasm. Parental gestures and facial expressions convey as much, if not more, as words to the child concerning their own feelings about certain foods. One study found that parental attitudes condition the child's familiarity with a variety of foods and that this variable is the single most important one in determining the child's acceptance of new foods at school.[13]

Children need the same nutrients from the same food sources as adults but in proportionately smaller amounts. Energy nutrients are needed in amounts necessary to meet growth and individual activity levels. High quality proteins are needed to support new tissue growth. The intake of adequate amounts of carbohydrate and fat to meet energy needs spares dietary protein for tissue synthesis.

Fats contribute calories needed for the high energy needs of small children, and also makes food more moist and palatable. Fats are generally recommended to supply about 35 percent of the energy intake of children. Excess fat intake is discouraged in order to avoid development of overweight, obesity, and possibly some lipid-related health problems in adulthood.

Carbohydrates should supply approximately one-half of the total daily caloric intake of a child. Intake of complex carbohydrates and simple sugars in fruit is recommended. Excess consumption of simple sugars in concentrated sweets should be discouraged in order to avoid overweight, obesity, and to reduce the incidence of dental caries.

Three surveys have especially contributed information about food consumption of small children: the Ten-State Nutrition Survey, the Preschool Nutrition Survey, and the Health and Nutrition Examination Survey. It was found that nutritional status was strongly correlated to socioeconomic status, that inadequate consumption of nutrients was more reflective of decreased food intake by all family members due to inadequate money to purchase sufficient food than race, economic status, or geographic location. These surveys found most children to be adequately nourished. However, deficiencies of nutrients identified as intakes in amounts less than two-thirds RDA were: iron, ascorbic acid (vitamin C), calcium, and vitamin A. Iron intake was the most frequently identified as inadequate.[14] Protein intake was generally more than adequate. Obesity was also noted as a nutrition-related problem and was associated with higher family income.

Overconsumption of milk by children is strongly related to the development of iron deficiency leading to iron deficiency anemia. Milk is a poor source of iron and large amounts of milk displace solid foods which do contain iron in the diet of the small child. Intake of iron-rich solid foods may be increased by withholding fluids at the beginning of the meal, offering liver, enriched breads and cereals, legumes, and other meats. Calcium and iron intake can also be enhanced by offering milk products such as yogurt, ice cream, and cheese, as well as dried fruits at snack times.

The following table briefly summarizes the major correlations between age, developmental level, and the food intake of small children.

Table 17-1. Factors associated with food intake of toddler and preschool children.

1 year of age	Birth weight is tripled, length is increased about 50%, more than six teeth.	Introduce new foods singly to identify allergy or other food-associated health problems.	Child prefers finger foods; likes to feel, smell, and mouth foods.	Child is involved in exploring his or her environment.
2 years of age	Gains another 5 pounds, grows another 3 to 4 inches, 8 to 10 more teeth = 14 to 16 teeth.	Likes foods separate— do not mix. Child likes interestingly shaped foods, introduce new foods gradually, maybe first of meal while child is hungry.	Child is learning to feed self. Child has a decreased appetite because of a decreased growth rate.	Child is concerned with asserting his or her independence; child often expresses negativism.
2-5 years of age	Gains 4½ to 5 pounds per year, has 20 teeth by fifth year. Rule for height and weight assessment for ages 1 to 6 yrs.: wt in lbs = (age x 5) + 17, ht in ins = (age x 2½) + 30	Serve bite-size portions; soups in cups; difficult-to-pick-up foods like peas with easy-to-pick-up foods like mashed potatoes. Likes food that is: colorful, different in texture, mild-flavored, of moderate temperature.	Child learning to use eating utensils. Snacks are helpful in meeting total daily energy and nutrient needs.	Child is now self-regulating in eating, sleeping, toileting; motor skills are improving and becoming more finely tuned. Regularity of physiological functions aided by regular mealtimes.

Sources: Kreutler PA: Nutrition in Perspective. Englewood Cliffs, NJ: Prentice-Hall, Inc., 1980, pp. 520-539.
Hussy CG and Kanoff N: Toddler and Preschool Nutrition. *In* Slatery JS, Pearson GA, and Torre CT (eds): Nutrition: Assessment and Counseling. New York, Appleton-Century-Crofts, 1979, pp. 103-140.
McWilliams M: Nutrition for the Growing Years, 2nd ed. New York, John Wiley and Sons, Inc., 1973, pp. 187-257.

Key Points: Early Childhood

I.   Children not only satisfy their curiosity about food by eating it, but also by touching, manipulating, examining, smelling, and mouthing it.

II. Parents need to be tolerant of the messiness of a curious child who is experimenting with food and to provide sturdy, appropriately-sized eating utensils, plates, and cups which facilitate the learning of skills necessary to feed his or her self.

III. A pleasant atmosphere and attractive environment are conducive to food intake by most persons, including small children.

IV. Nutritious snacks can supply added energy and various nutrients to a small child's diet. The stomach capacity of a small child is limited. It is advantageous to offer smaller, more frequent meals and nutritious between-meal snacks which contain foods that help to meet the child's total daily required nutrient intake. Food needed to supply necessary nutrients is difficult for a small child to consume from substantial-sized, infrequent meals.

V.   Each child's food preferences should be respected although encouragement to try new foods should be given. Parental attitudes have a marked influence on the food preferences of their children.

VI. Carbohydrates and fats help to meet the increased energy needs of children and at the same time spare protein for tissue synthesis; protein should be of high quality to properly support new tissue growth.

VII. Young children in the U.S. are generally well nourished. When deficiencies are identified, iron deficiency is most often the one noted. Other nutrient intakes more often identified as somewhat deficient are calcium, ascorbic acid, and vitamin A.

Questions: Early Childhood

1. A dry food is made easier to eat by a young child if it is served with a
   _____ .
   a. spicy food
   b. moist food
   c. chewy food

2. Which snacks are the best sources of energy and nutrients for a three to five year-old child?
   a. strips of cheese
   b. fresh orange sections
   c. two pieces of chocolate fudge
   d. small sandwiches
   e. peanut butter on slices of raw apple
   f. carrot sticks
   g. a peppermint stick

3. Food preferences are highly correlated with food consumption by the young child.
   a. True
   b. False

4. The most important variable in determining a child's acceptance of new foods is:
   a. color and shape of food
   b. parental attitudes about familiarity with a variety of foods
   c. social interactions at mealtime

5. In general, foods which best supply nutrients for a small child are different foods than those which best supply nutrients for adults.
   a. True
   b. False

6. Why are high quality proteins found in animal source foods such as milk, cheese, meat, poultry, and fish especially recommended for consumption by young children?

7. Why are high fat diets discouraged for young children?

8. Though most young children were found through three extensive surveys to be generally healthy, what nutrient intake was most frequently found to be deficient?
   a. thiamin
   b. phosphorus
   c. iron

9. Excessive consumption of what food by small children is associated with the development of iron deficiency anemia?

10. Using the general rule for height and weight assessment for children ages one to six, what would be the average height and weight of a five year-old child?

11. In order to more easily identify a possible allergic reaction to the offending food, what is the best method of presenting new foods to a young child?

12. While a child's motor skills are developing and becoming more refined, what are several ways of serving foods which are difficult to eat with utensils?

13. Regularity of meal and snack times is important to a child's development of regularity in physiological functions.
   a. True
   b. False

14. At one year of age a child has some teeth with which to chew food.
   a. True
   b. False

15. At what age does a normal decrease in the appetite of a small child occur? Why?

16. Many of the vitamins and minerals most often noted as deficient in a young child's diet could be met by eating what foods?

Answers: Early Childhood

1. b
2. a, b, d, e, f
3. a
4. b
5. b
6. High quality proteins supply all essential amino acids as well as most nonessential amino acids in the proportions and amounts best suited for building body proteins and, therefore, enabling adequate growth of human tissues.
7. to avoid overweight and obesity and possibly some lipid-related health problems in adulthood.
8. c
9. milk
10. height= (5 x 2½) + 30 =42.5 inches
    weight= (5 x 5) + 17 = 42 pounds

11. singly, for several days; This gives time for possible allergy symptoms to appear and a clearer indication of the offending food.

12. Cut food into bite-size portions; serve soups in cups or mugs; serve difficult-to-pick-up foods such as peas with easy-to-pick-up foods like mashed potatoes—these foods can be mixed together if the child will accept them that way or pushed one into the other with a fork.

13. a

14. a

15. Sometime in the toddler years (one to three years) when the child's energy needs are decreased due to a slower rate of growth than experienced in infancy.

16. Milk and milk products, citrus fruits, meat (especially organ meats such as liver), enriched grain products, dark green and leafy vegetables, and dark yellow/orange fruits and vegetables.

ADOLESCENCE

Adolescence is a transition stage between childhood and adulthood. This is a period of time when physical stresses associated with growth and puberty occur simultaneously with the emotional and psychological stresses encountered in the struggle to assert themselves as adults, and in the awareness of their growing sexuality. They are learning to make their own decisions and are establishing their own identities. Food habits may be only one of a number of areas in which teens and their parents disagree.

Adolescence is also a time of greater social awareness when both boys and girls are concerned about their appearance. They are particularly concerned about their body weight, size, and complexion. Adolescents experience formidable peer pressures. Food choices may represent the values and opinions of their peer group. Desires to participate in athletics or other special activities may cause a teen to take drastic measures to alter weight or appearance. Under such pressures, adolescents are often likely to succumb to food fads and fad diets which promise quick and easily obtained desired results.

Boys want physically developed bodies which they feel appear more manly. They have increased energy needs for growth and activity. Boys undergo a growth spurt at puberty (somewhere between 12 to 15 years of age). During this spurt, height increases along with a substantial increase in lean tissue (muscle tissue). The need for iron is great during this period of increased growth. After this growth spurt the caloric needs of older adolescent boys and young men require a food intake which is generally sufficient in iron to meet body maintenance needs.

Girls, too, experience a growth spurt although it is not as long lasting as in adolescent boys. The female's growth spurt generally occurs earlier than for boys, before the onset of menstruation (somewhere between 10 to 12 years of age). With the advent of menses, girls have an increased need for iron. The Ten-State Nutrition Survey found adolescent girls to be generally deficient in iron. During adolescence hormonal changes influence the increased formation of fat pads in girls. In addition, girls often have decreased activity levels due to inactivity while in school or doing homework. As a group, girls participate less often in sports than boys. Consequently, girls are highly concerned about, and somewhat at risk, of becoming overweight.

The 1968 to 1970 Ten-State Nutrition Survey found some intakes of vitamin A, riboflavin, calcium, and iron to be below RDAs for adolescents in general.[15] Ascorbic acid intake was low for some adolescent groups. However, the 1977 to 1978 Nationwide Food Consumption Survey found that ascorbic acid intake increased considerably for all persons, including adolescents, over intakes in 1965.[16] One survey found that the teens with the greater sound nutrition knowledge were the teens who had nutrient intakes which met at least two-thirds of the RDA for all nutrients.[17]

Adolescents are young adults who have a great deal of control over what they eat, when they eat, where they eat, as well as their comings and goings from home. They frequently have access to various forms of transportation. It is important to try to coordinate family eating times with the busy schedule of the adolescent in order to plan at least one meal a day in which all family members are present. This time together is important for the sharing of each individual's experiences, thoughts and plans and, if the time is pleasant, it also enhances food intake.

Many times the teen resorts to fast foods which are hurriedly gulped on the way to some activity. These fast foods, typically hamburgers, hotdogs, tacos, pizzas, shakes, colas, and french fries, are high in calories, especially due to fat content, but are low in several essential nutrients. Though fast food meals often supply ample protein they are most often deficient in vitamin A. A meal of a hamburger, fries, and shake (often a nondairy product) provides about half of a day's recommended calories but less than one-third of the RDA for vitamin A.[18]

Other nutrients often supplied in inadequate amounts by fast foods are calcium, niacin, thiamin, riboflavin, ascorbic acid, vitamin D, and some trace minerals. The limited variety of foods available from a fast food menu is, in large part, responsible for the general inadequacy of nutrients fast foods provide. Fruits and vegetables are often lacking in fast foods which decreases the fiber content of these foods as well as the ascorbic acid and vitamin A content. The lack of dairy products contributes to the low availability of calcium, riboflavin, and vitamin D. Sodium content of fast foods, however, is unusually high.[19]

Adolescents need to develop independence and to accept greater responsibility for making their own choices and decisions. In order to keep open the lines of communication between parents and their teens, it is important to avoid unnecessary conflicts and stress. Consequently, some of the following suggestions may be helpful in dealing with adolescents and their food selections and diet: encourage them to take time to enjoy food and mealtimes and to sample new foods; encourage eating breakfast, even if foods other than typical breakfast foods are preferred; encourage their participation in food preparation as well as their presence at family gatherings for meals; praise the teen's selections of nutritious foods and refrain from criticizing poor food choices; present sound nutrition information without a judgmental attitude and try to relate these principles to appropriate food practices which offer some of the more immediate health benefit rewards.[20]

It seems more effective to provide a food environment that expresses principles of good nutrition than to lecture the adolescent about good food choices and nutrition. Leave nutritious snacks in the cupboards and refrigerator within easy reach, keep quickly prepared but nutritious foods available (especially for breakfast and snacks), keep fresh fruits and vegetables on hand and encourage their consumption for snacks, and provide congeniality and a welcome atmosphere for the adolescent and his or her friends (when possible) at mealtimes. The parental *practice* of good nutrition and food habits speaks most convincingly for the credibility of information and advice about nutrition given by parents.

Key Points: Adolescence

I. Adolescence is a transition period in development which is represented by increased emotional, psychological, social, as well as physical stresses.

II. Because of pressures from peers and desires to improve their appearance, adolescents may adopt food fads and fad diets which promise improvements and changes in a short time. These diets are often directly opposed to principles of good health and, probably, impossible to attain.

III. Males undergo a growth spurt at puberty which increases their height and substantially increases their lean body mass (muscle tissue). The need for iron is demanding during this period of increased growth.

IV. Females experience a growth spurt prior to the onset of menses. Menstruation increases the iron requirement of females which continues to be difficult to meet through diet alone until the end of the child-bearing years.

V. Involvement of the adolescent in meal preparation and shared meal experiences with other family members may encourage the adolescent to consume a more nutritionally adequate diet.

VI. Because of the demands on their time for school, sports, and other activities teens often resort to frequent consumption of fast foods. These foods are high in fat and calories while notably low in vitamin A, and are somewhat low in niacin, thiamin, riboflavin, ascorbic acid, vitamin D, trace minerals, and fiber.

VII. Nutrients often lacking in the diets of teens can be obtained from increased intakes of dairy products, fruits, vegetables, organ meats, and enriched grains.

VIII. In order to encourage the development of independence and a competence in decision-making, as well as to reduce the incidence of stress and conflict, it is recommended for the parent to provide the teen with objective nutrition information and a good nutrition environment, rather than personal opinions, lectures, and negative criticisms of food habits.

Questions: Adolescence

1. In an attempt to improve their personal appearance, physique, and shape, dissatisfied and impatient adolescents are likely to choose what kind of diets?

2. Adolescent boys have the (highest/lowest) energy intake recommendation of all sex and age categories. (Hint: refer to the Mean Heights and Weights and Recommended Energy Intake of the RDAs in Chapter Two.)

3. What nutrient intakes, in general, were found to be low for adolescents in the Ten-State Nutrition Survey?

4. The advent of menses (menstruation) increases the need for what nutrient by adolescent girls?

5. Why do adolescent boys have an increased need for iron?

6. Because of their decreased activity level, adolescent girls have difficulty in maintaining a nutrient dense calorie level which will not lead to overweight.
    a. True
    b. False

7. It is normal for an adolescent girl to increase the size of fat pads in breasts, hips, and thighs.
    a. True
    b. False

8. There is a trend toward increased ascorbic acid intake by all persons in the U.S., even adolescents.
    a. True
    b. False

9. Checking the activity schedule of the adolescent and then planning at least one meal a day when he or she can be present with all other family members, is effective both in increasing the teen's food intake and providing time for congenial family discussions.
    a. True
    b. False

10. A moderate intake of fast foods is of no real nutritional consequence. However, a constant diet of fast foods may result in a diet which provides inadequate intakes

of fiber, some minerals, and vitamins, especially, _____ .
   a.   vitamin E
   b.   vitamin K
   c.   vitamin A

11.   What are some immediate health benefits of good nutrition practices which a teen might appreciate and aspire to attain?

12.   Fast foods are generally high in caloric value, especially due to fat content, and often what mineral?

13.   Choose the method which is probably most helpful in assisting an adolescent in learning good nutritional principles and attaining good nutritional status.
   a.   Require the adolescent to read about nutrition and restrict his or her eating to supervised times.
   b.   Nag the adolescent until he or she changes a present, unacceptable diet pattern.
   c.   Provide accurate nutrition information, well-balanced meals, and nutritious foods in cupboards and the refrigerator for snacks and let the teenager make his or her own food choices.

Answers: Adolescence

1.   fad diets which promise quick results and maximum change
2.   highest
3.   vitamin A, riboflavin, calcium, and iron
4.   iron
5.   because adolescent boys experience a growth spurt which includes a large increase in muscle tissue; muscle tissue formation requires myoglobin, an iron-containing protein complex
6.   a
7.   a
8.   a
9.   a
10.   c
11.   increased energy, alertness, feeling of well-being, and physical endurance
12.   sodium
13.   c

OLD AGE

Individuals often face major changes in their physical, social, and economic status during old age. They generally have physiological changes due to aging which decrease functioning ability. It is difficult to find a population of aged persons free from disease. Psychological factors influence health as well. The elderly person may be unhappy with his or her living conditions. He or she may be desirous of increased security or family attentiveness. He or she may be despondent due to loneliness, lack of meaningful work or activity, or the restrictions of a sedentary life. Most elderly persons have limited economic resources.

   Physical changes due to old age greatly affect dietary habits, food intake, and nutrient utilization. Many older persons have missing teeth, painful caries, peridontal disease, loose teeth, or ill-fitting dentures. These persons have difficulty chewing and if they will not accept ground or pureed foods are likely to restrict their diet to repetitious, naturally soft textured food choices. The elderly experience a loss in the sense of taste and smell. Consequently, eating pleasure is diminished and a poor appetite is often the result. Neuromuscular coordination may decline or conditions such as arthritis may be so severe that difficulty is experienced in food preparation and the use of eating utensils. Loss of physical function may produce gastrointestinal problems such as maldigestion and malabsorption.

A reduced, limited income may prevent the purchase of nutritionally adequate foods. An elderly person may be able to afford housing that consists only of a rented room with no cooking or food storage facilities. Reduced finances may even limit means of transportation. Shopping may be restricted to markets near the elderly person's home and these may be higher-cost markets. If an elderly person lives alone his or her desire to cook or eat may be reduced. *Researchers have found that eating in the social company of other persons increases food intake of the elderly.*

Some elderly persons use food to manipulate family or friends. More attention is given to the elderly person who refuses to eat or expresses food complaints. Many elderly persons are enticed to purchase foods from a health food store at the urging of commercial advertising. They are often convinced that such foods impart special health benefits. In truth, these consumers often pay a higher price for food of equal nutritional quality to that found in grocery stores or supermarkets.

Elderly persons experience a reduced caloric need due to a reduced rate of metabolism and a reduced level of activity. The Revised 1980 RDAs Table Three, Mean Heights and Weights and Recommended Energy Intake, includes a category for persons over age 76. This population group has a caloric level reduced even from that of persons age 51 to 75.[21] See Chapter Three for this table.

Examination of the RDAs reveals that the nutrient requirements for the elderly are the same as for younger adults. Consequently, the diets of elderly persons need to be reduced in energy (calorie) value while still consisting of foods that are nutrient-dense.

Due to the reduced activity and calorie need, obesity is a common problem among the elderly.[22] Previous eating patterns which are not altered to conform to newer, reduced caloric needs lead to overweight and obesity. Obesity is likely to complicate existing and developing health problems as well as to interfere with movement and increase the risk of harmful falls.

A recent evaluation of nutrition programs has identified specific nutritional needs of the elderly including a need for the consumption of meat for protein and iron content, a need for iron-rich foods because of the high incidence of anemia in the elderly, the need for consumption of vitamin A and ascorbic acid-rich fruits and vegetables, and a need for increased intake of milk, cheese, and other calcium-rich foods.[23] There is also a need for further study of the interaction of diet with drugs commonly used by the elderly, especially because of the high incidence of drug use by this age group.[24]

Some of the nutrition programs provided by government and volunteer funds are Food Stamps, Meals-on-Wheels, and the Nutrition Program for the Elderly. Food Stamps increases food purchasing power, Meals-on-Wheels supplies meals to persons confined to their homes, and the Nutrition Program for the Elderly encourages social activity by providing congregate meals at various community meal sites and offers some nutrition education as well.

Table 17-2.   Tips for better nutrition, food preparation, and meal planning for the elderly.

---

1. Divide food consumption into more frequent meals if food is more easily tolerated and enjoyed this way.
2. Eat the heavier meal at noon rather than in the evening if this relieves discomfort or sleeping problems.

Table 17-2. **Tips for better nutrition, food preparation, and meal planning for the elderly (continued).**

3. Purchase foods in small container sizes if storage and/or refrigeration facilities are limited.

4. Use baby or junior foods in recipes that call for small amounts of a vegetable or fruit.

5. Use nonfat dry milk, reconstituted, to provide a less expensive but nutritious source of milk.

6. Use enriched bread products. Many specialty breads such as sweet rolls, french or sour dough are not made with enriched flour.

7. Use frozen dinners that meet nutrition quality guidelines and supplement these meals with fruit or juices, milk, and bread.

8. Season with lemon juice and tolerated herbs to spark the flavor of foods and to reduce excess caloric intake of fats such as butter or margarine. Exclude the use of spices, condiments, or food which causes distress.

9. Use casserole dishes, that can be used on the range and in the oven, as serving dishes and individual service dishes in order to reduce food preparation and service equipment.

10. Eat at a desirable and comfortable location, that is, by a window, outside, on a patio, or on a porch, where food is more likely to be eaten slowly and with enjoyment.

Adapted from: Food Guide for Older Folks. U.S. Department of Agriculture, Home and Garden Bulletin No. 17, revised 1973.

Key Points: Old Age

I. Elderly persons face major changes in their physical, social, and economic status from younger years; these changes have great impact on their dietary habits, food intake, and nutrient utilization.

II. Reduced health condition, presence of disease, increased dental problems, and loss of physical functions greatly alter food needs and nutrient utilization.

II'. Reduced income not only affects the type and nutritional quality of foods purchased, but place of purchase, cooking, and storage facilities.

IV. Eating in the presence of social company tends to increase the food and, therefore, nutrient consumption of the elderly.

V. Psychological factors have an impact on the elderly person's expectations of food, especially as a source of emotional rewards and often unrealistic health benefits.

VI. The elderly person has a need for nutrient dense foods in order to obtain required nutrients within a reduced calorie need.

VII. Obesity is often the result of a failure to reduce energy intake proportionately to reduced energy needs. Obesity complicates existing health problems, interferes with movement, and increases the risk of injurious falls.

VIII. Specific nutritional needs of the elderly are for consumption of meat for protein and iron, fruits and vegetables for ascorbic acid and vitamin A, and milk and milk products for calcium.

IX. High drug use by the elderly warrants further research into diet/drug interactions.

Questions: Old Age

1. The elderly person is likely to experience reduced body functioning due to physiological changes, disease, and/or psychological factors.
   a. True
   b. False
2. Why may some elderly persons need ground or pureed foods?
3. Taste and smell acuity decreases with advancing age.
   a. True
   b. False
4. A person with a decline in neuromuscular coordination or severe arthritis may find difficulty in _____ .
   a. food preparation
   b. use of eating utensils
   c. shopping for food
5. Why may an elderly person find it necessary to shop for food at markets which may be higher-cost but close to their home?
6. Isolation and loneliness will likely cause (decreased/increased) food intake.
7. Identify a possible disadvantage of shopping for food at a health food store?
8. A need for attentiveness and overt expression of caring may be expressed in what way by an elderly person in relation to food?
9. What are two contributing factors to the reduced calorie needs of elderly persons?
10. Nutrient needs remain the same for elderly persons but _____ needs decrease compared to younger adults.
11. Refer to the U.S. RDA Table. Why is the iron requirement for women over age 51 reduced to the requirement for men of that age category?
12. Obesity is an increased risk for many elderly persons, especially women. What are three problems experienced by obese elderly persons?
13. What might be one factor contributing to iron deficiency anemia in the elderly?
14. What three nutrients besides iron are often found deficient in the diets of elderly persons?
15. What are two unique benefits of food supplementation through the Nutrition Program for the Elderly?
16. Refer to Table 17-2 to answer the following questions:
    a. If food storage and refrigeration facilities are limited, in what size containers should food be purchased?
    b. If a person is uncomfortable or cannot sleep after eating a heavy evening meal, when should he or she try eating a heavier meal?
    c. Eating what foods will increase some B vitamins and iron intake?
    d. If eating alone, how can food eating enjoyment be increased?
    e. If food preparation is difficult, use of what processed foods might be advised?

Answers: Old Age

1. a
2. because of poor teeth or missing teeth
3. a

4. a, b, c
5. Though the elderly may have the time for shopping trips further away, they may not have transportation and/or the stamina for lengthy shopping trips.
6. decreased
7. The food is equal in nutritive value to food for sale in grocery stores or supermarkets, while at the same time the food is generally higher priced than food available in larger grocery stores or supermarkets.
8. complaints about food; refusal to eat
9. reduced BMR; reduced activity level
10. calorie
11. Because of the cessation of menses and reduced blood loss, most women over 51 retain more iron in their body and require less replenishment for iron than younger women.
12. a. complication of existing or developing health problems
    b. interference with movement
    c. increased risk of injurious falls
13. decreased consumption of meat (perhaps due to high cost or difficulty in eating) and other iron-rich foods
14. vitamin A, ascorbic acid (vitamin C), and calcium
15. food is provided in a group social setting; some nutrition education is provided
16. a. small
    b. at noon
    c. enriched bread products
    d. eating in pleasant surroundings such as by a window, on a patio, or on a porch
    e. heat and serve meals (TV dinners) with added fruits, milk, and bread

REFERENCES

[1] Worthington BS, Vermeersch J, and Williams SR: Nutrition in Pregnancy and Lactation. St. Louis, The C. V. Mosby Company, 1977, p. 26
[2] Scientists estimate one million children have stunted brains. CNI Weekly Report (Community Nutrition Institute), 5, November 6, 1975, p. 1
[3] Pitkin RM: What's new in maternal nutrition? Nutrition News, 42, April-May 1979, p. 5
[4] Nutrition in maternal health care. Chicago, The American College of Obstetricians and Gynecologists, 1974
[5] Scoloveno MA: Nutrition During Pregnancy. *In* Slatery JS, Pearson GA, and Torre CT (eds): Maternal and Child Nutrition: Assessment and Counseling. New York, Appleton-Century-Crofts, 1979, pp. 18-19
[6] Gibbs CE and Seitchik J: Nutrition in pregnancy. *In* Goodhart RS and Shils ME (eds): Modern Nutrition in Health and Disease. Philadelphia, Lea and Febiger, 1980, p. 749
[7] **Megaloblastic anemia** is characterized by unusually large and immature red blood cells.
[8] Teenage pregnancy. Public Health Currents, 18, June-July 1978, p. 10
[9] Incidence of allergy to milk proteins is higher for cow's milk than human milk.
[10] Worthington BS, Vermeersch J, and Williams SR: Nutrition in Pregnancy and Lactation. Saint Louis, The C. V. Mosby Company, 1977, p. 157
[11] Data obtained from Infant Nutrition—A Foundation for Lasting Health Symposium sponsored by Mead Johnson Nutritional Division, Mead Johnson and Company (US), Houston, Texas, September 26, 1979
[12] Birch LL: Preschool children's food preferences and consumption patterns. Journal of Nutrition Education, 11, October-December 1979 pp. 189-192
[13] Yperman AM and Vermeersch JA: Factors associated with children's food habits. Journal

of Nutrition Education, 11, April-June 1979, pp. 72-76

[14] Owen G and Lippman G: Nutritional status of infants and young children: USA. Pediatric Clinics of North America, 24, February 1977, p. 212

[15] Snyderman SE; Nutrition in infancy and adolescence. *In* Goodhart RS and Shils Me (eds): Modern Nutrition in Health and Disease. Philadelphia, Lea and Febiger, 1980, p. 774

[16] Pao EM: Nutrient consumption patterns of individuals, 1977 and 1965. Family Economics Review, Spring 1980, p. 19

[17] Axelson JM and DelCampo DS: Improving teenager's nutrition knowledge through the mass media. Journal of Nutrition Education, 10, January-March 1978, p. 30

[18] Perspectives on fast foods. Public Health Currents, 19, January-February 1979, p. 7

[19] Shannon BM and Parks SC: Fast foods: A perspective on their nutritional impact. Journal of the American Dietetic Association, 76, March 1980, p. 245

[20] Suitor CW and Hunter MF: Nutrition: Principles and Application in Health Promotion. Philadelphia, J. B. Lippincott Company, 1980, pp. 94-99

[21] Recommended energy intake for males age 51 to 75 is 2,400 kcal and for ages 76 and over is 2,050 kcal; recommended energy intake for females age 51 to 75 is 1,800 kcal, and for ages 76 and over is 1,600 kcal.

[22] Shannon B and Smiciklas-Wright H: Nutrition education in relation to the needs of the elderly. Journal of Nutrition Education, 11, April-June 1979, p. 85

[23] Kohrs MB: The nutrition program for older Americans. Journal of the American Dietetic Association, 75, November 1979, pp. 543-546

[24] Munro HN: Major gaps in nutrient allowances: The status of the elderly. Journal of the American Dietetic Association, 76, February 1980, p. 140

APPENDIX A

THE METRIC SYSTEM

Upon perusal of the RDA and U.S. RDA tables it becomes evident that the measurements of nutrients are given in metric terms. Although the metric system is an international system of measurements used by many countries since the 1800s, the Metric Conversion Act was not passed by the U.S. Congress until 1975.[1] Because of this delayed adoption, the metric system is still not readily familiar to much of the American public. It seems advantageous to present a review section of metric terms, equivalents, and conversion factors here.

The metric system is a more simplified system than the customary or English system which has been used in the U.S. The key to learning the system lies in memorizing the basic quantities and their symbols, and the prefixes which stand for the various factors of ten and their corresponding symbols. Table A-1 illustrates this key using units associated with the study of nutrition. Table A-2 lists conversions for measurements frequently used in nutrition study and food preparation.

The metric system is a decimal system based on the powers of ten. This means that a second unit will be ten times as large as the basic unit, a third will be ten times as large as the second, and so on. Therefore, the third unit is 10×10 or 10^2 times the basic unit, the fourth is $10 \times 10 \times 10$ or 10^3 times the basic unit. Each unit represents a multiple of the basic unit; the multiples are powers of ten. Other units are chosen so that the first is 0.1 (that is, one-tenth) the size of the basic unit, and each successive unit is 0.1 the size of the preceding. These smaller units are respectively 0.1×0.1, $0.1 \times 0.1 \times 0.1$, and so on, times the basic unit. In mathematical shorthand, 0.1 is represented by 10^{-1}, 0.1×0.1 by 10^{-2}, and so on, so the smaller units represent quantities which are respectively 10^{-1}, 10^{-2}, 10^{-3}, and so on, times the basic unit.[2] Therefore, you can change from one unit to another by multiplying or dividing by ten.

Conversions of home recipes to metric measurements are complicated slightly due to the fact that most solids are not measured in volume but rather by weight. For example, there is a need to think in terms of grams rather than cups when measuring such foodstuffs as solid shortening, flour, or sugar.[3] Table A-3 gives average or standardized equivalents which are helpful in making acceptable home recipe conversions from volume to weight measurements.

It is with practice and usage that the metric system will become easier to use. Many companies in converting to metrication on the job have found that training . . . is less of a problem than was once anticipated. Instead of giving all employees a course in metrics, these companies give instruction on a need-to-know basis, and only on aspects related to specific jobs.[4] Likewise, the emphasis in the following practice section will be on the metric measurements most often used in nutrition and food preparation study.

Table A-1.

Basic Quantity:	Length		Mass		Volume		Temperature		Energy	
	meter	Symbol	gram	Symbol	liter	Symbol	°Celsius	Symbol	joule	Symbol
		m		g		L		°C		J

Prefix:	Symbol:	Factor Multiplied by:	Means:	Which Equals:
tera	T	1,000,000,000,000	One trillion times	10^{12}
giga	G	1,000,000,000	One billion times	10^{9}
mega	M	1,000,000	One million times	10^{6}
kilo	k	1,000	One thousand times	10^{3}
hecto	h	100	One hundred times	10^{2}
deka	da	10	Ten times	10^{1}
deci	d	0.1	One tenth of	10^{-1}
centi	c	0.01	One hundredth of	10^{-2}
milli	m	0.001	One thousandth of	10^{-3}
micro	μ	0.000 001	One millionth of	10^{-6}
nano	n	0.000 000 001	One billionth of	10^{-9}
pico	p	0.000 000 000 001	One trillionth of	10^{-12}

Consequently, use of the numerical prefix symbol in front of the basic quantity symbol tells how many of what unit:

kg = kilogram (1,000 grams)   mL = milliliters (1/1000 liter)

Adapted from: Brief History of Measurement Systems with a Chart of the Modernized Metric System. United States Department of Commerce, National Bureau of Standards Special Publication 304A, (revised August 1976)

***

Table A-2.   Some frequently used approximately equivalents.

***

Length: 1 inch = 2.54 centimeters
            1 foot = 30.48 centimeters
            3.3 feet = 1 meter

Weight: 1 ounce = 28.35 grams
                     (round off to 30 for most calculations)
            2.2 pounds = 1 kilogram

Volume: 1.06 quarts = 1 liter
            1 cup = 236 milliliters
                     (round off to 240 for most calculations)
            1 teaspoon = 5 milliliters
            1 tablespoon = 15 milliliters
            1 gallon = 3.8 liters
            1 milliliter = 1 cc (cubic centimeter)

Temperature: 212°F = 100°C (boiling point of water)
              98.6°F = 37°C (body temperature)
              32°F = 0°C (freezing point of water)

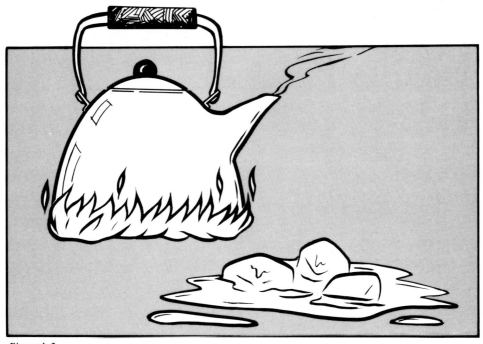

Figure A-2.

Temperature
Conversion
Equation: °C = 5/9 (°F-32)
            °F = 9/5° C + 32

Energy: 1 calorie = 4.2 joules
            (this calorie = the amount of heat energy necessary to raise 1 gram of
            water 1°C)

Table A-2.   Some frequently used approximately equivalents (cont'd.).

---

1 kilocalorie (kcal) = 4.2 kilojoules (kJ)
(kilocalorie = the amount of heat energy necessary to raise 1 kilogram of water 1°C)

Adapted from: Metrics Made Easy, © 1977, with permission of Barron's Educational Series, Inc., Woodbury, New York.

Table A-3.   Suggested volume to weight conversions for simple recipe adjustments.

Ingredient	English Measure	Metric Measure
Water	One cup	240 grams
Shortening	One cup	200 grams
Sugar	One cup	205 grams
Flour	One cup	112 grams
Milk	One cup	240 grams
Salt	Teaspoons	5 mL
Spices	or	
Baking powder	Tablespoons	15 mL

Questions: The Metric System

1. A metric conversion act has been passed by the U.S. Congress to facilitate the adoption of the metric system of measurement in the U.S.
   a. True
   b. False
2. How many grams would the following foods weigh?
   a. an 8 oz glass of milk
   b. a 10 oz steak
   c. a 4 oz serving of carrots
3. How many kilograms do the following weigh?
   a. a 120 lb woman
   b. a 160 lb man
4. Kilocalorie is the unit meant when calculating the caloric content of foods or energy requirement of an individual.
   a. What is the metric equivalent of kilocalorie?
   b. What is the conversion factor for kilocalorie to the metric equivalent?
5. Convert the following temperatures from Fahrenheit to Celsius:
   a. a moderate oven temperature of 350°F
   b. a simmering temperature of 200°F
6. Convert the following temperatures from Centigrade to Fahrenheit:

a. moderate oven temperature of 190°C
b. a simmering temperature of 90°C

7. Match each of the numerical values on the right to its proper prefix designator on the left.

_____ 1. kilo (k) a. 1/1,000 (10^{-3})
_____ 2. deci (d) b. 10 (10^1)
_____ 3. micro (μ) c. 1/100 (10^{-2})
_____ 4. hecto (h) d. 1/10 (10^{-1})
_____ 5. deka (da) e. 1,000,000 (10^6)
_____ 6. milli (m) f. 1,000 (10^3)
_____ 7. centi (c) g. 100 (10^2)
_____ 8. mega (M) h. 1/1,000,000 (10^{-6})

8. Name the metric unit and identify the corresponding abbreviation for the following quantities:
a. length
b. mass
c. volume
d. temperature
e. energy

9. Match each of the following terms on the right to its appropriate abbreviation on the left:

_____ 1. kg a. millimeter
_____ 2. mg b. kilojoule
_____ 3. cm c. dekaliter
_____ 4. mm d. milliliter
_____ 5. mL e. microgram
_____ 6. kJ f. centimeter
_____ 7. daL g. kilogram
_____ 8. μg h. milligram

10. Convert the following recipe into metric measurements using mass measurements for the solids instead of volume measurements (See Table A-3):
Homemade Biscuits
a. 2 cups sifted flour
b. 2½ teaspoons baking powder
c. 1 teaspoon salt
d. ⅓ cup shortening
e. ¾ cup milk

11. How many kilojoules do the following persons need daily?
a. a 44 inch tall 5 year-old girl weighing 44 pounds.
b. a 69 inch tall 15 year-old adolescent boy weighing 145 pounds.
c. a 62 inch tall 14 year-old adolescent girl weighing 101 pounds.
d. a 64 inch tall, pregnant 25 year-old woman normally weighing 120 pounds.
e. a 70 inch tall 80 year-old man weighing 154 pounds.

12. The following exercise helps to visualize the volume size of a liter. (Use the metric ruler given in Figure A-1.)
a. Cut a piece of paper 16 cm x 28 cm and tape the two 16 cm sides together.
b. You now have a cylinder exactly the size of a liter. What foods might one purchase that would come in this size of a container?

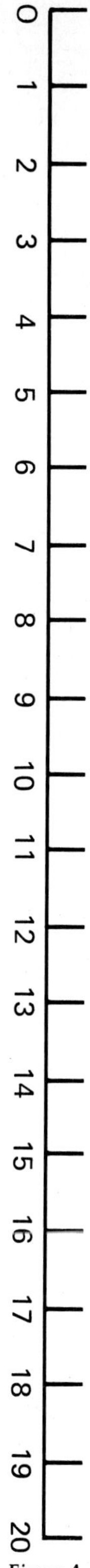

0 1 2 3 4 5 6 7 8 9 10 11 12 13 14 15 16 17 18 19 20

Figure A-1.

Answers: The Metric System

1. a
2. a. 30 x 8 = 240 grams
    b. 30 x 10 = 300 grams
    c. 30 x 4 = 120 grams
3. a. 120 ÷ 2.2 = 54.5 kg
    b. 160 ÷ 2.2 = 72.7 kg
4. a. kilojoule
    b. 4.2 x kcal = kJ (because 1 kcal = 4.2 kJ)
5. a. 176.7°C [C° 5/9 (350-32)]
    b. 93.3°C [C° 5/9 (200-32)]
6. a. 374°F [F° 9/5 (190) + 32]
    b. 194°F [F° 9/5 (90) + 32]
7. 1. f
    2. d
    3. h
    4. g
    5. b
    6. a
    7. c
    8. e
8. a. meter (m)
    b. gram (g)
    c. liter (L)
    d. Celsius (°C)
    e. joule (J)
9. 1. g
    2. h
    3. f
    4. a
    5. d
    6. b
    7. c
    8. e
10. a. 224g
    b. 12.5mL
    c. 5mL
    d. 67g
    e. 180g
11. a. 1,700 x 4.2 (1,300 x 4.2 − 2,300 x 4.2) = 7,140 (5,460 − 9,660)
    b. 2,800 x 4.2 (2,100 x 4.2 − 3,900 x 4.2) = 11,760 (8,820 − 16,380)
    c. 2,200 x 4.2 (1,500 x 4.2 − 3,000 x 4.2) = 9,240 (6,300 − 12,600)
    d. 2,300 x 4.2 (1,900 x 4.2 − 2,700 x 4.2) = 9,600 (7,980 − 11,340)
    e. 2,050 x 4.2 (1,650 x 4.2 − 2,450 x 4.2) = 8,610 (6,930 − 10,290)
12. b. some suggestions:
        1 quart (plus) milk
        juices
        soda drinks
        mineral waters

REFERENCES

[1] Brief history of measurement systems with a chart of the modernized metric system. United States Department of Commerce, National Bureau of Standards Special Publication 304A (Revised), August 1976

[2] Reprinted from Metrics Made Easy, ©1977, with permission of Barron's Educational Series, Inc., Woodbury, New York

[3] Miller BS and Trimbo HB: Use of metric measurements in food preparation. Journal of Home Economics, 64, ©February 1972, pp. 20-21

[4] Going metric: A lot easier and cheaper than expected. US News and World Report, 81, ©July 5, 1976; p. 114

APPENDIX B

The following are common methods for figuring the retinol equivalents of vitamin A from retinol, β-carotene, and other provitamin A sources. Exercises are provided to clarify the methods for determining retinol equivalents.

1 retinol equivalent = 1 μg retinol
= 6μg β-carotene
= 12μg other provitamin A
= 3.33 IU vitamin activity from retinol
= 10 IU vitamin A activity from β-carotene

For example:

1. If retinol and β-carotene are given in micrograms, then:

$$\mu g \text{ retinol} + \frac{\mu g \text{ } \beta\text{-carotene}}{6} = \text{retinol equivalents}$$

2. If both are given in IU, then:

$$\frac{\text{IU of retinol}}{3.33} + \frac{\text{IU of } \beta\text{-carotene}}{10} = \text{retinol equivalents}$$

3. If β-carotene and other provitamin A carotenoids are given in micrograms, then:

$$\frac{\mu g \text{ } \beta\text{-carotene}}{6} + \frac{\mu g \text{ other carotenoids}}{12} = \text{retinol equivalents}$$

Questions: Appendix B

1. Calculate the amount of retinol equivalents in a diet containing 500μg of retinol and 1800μg of β-carotene. For which adults does this amount meet the RDA?

2. Calculate the amount of retinol equivalents provided by 1,665 IU of retinol and 3,000 IU of β-carotene.

3. Calculate the amount of retinol equivalents provided by 1,800 μg β-carotene and 6,000 μg of other carotenoids.

Answers: Appendix B

1. $500 + \dfrac{1800}{6} = 800$ R.E.; the female

2. $\dfrac{1{,}665 \text{ IU of retinol}}{3.33} + \dfrac{3{,}000 \text{ IU of } \beta\text{-carotene}}{10} = 800$ R.E.

3. $\dfrac{1{,}800 \text{ } \mu g\beta\text{-carotene}}{6} + \dfrac{6000 \mu g \text{ other carotenoids}}{12} = 800$ R.E.

APPENDIX C

The Kidneys

The nephron is the functioning unit of the kidney. It consists of:

A. *Bowman's capsule*—surrounds the glomerulus, a tuft of capillaries.
B. *Proximal convoluted tubule* (nearest Bowman's capsule).
C. *Loop of Henle*—a straighter portion of tubule.
D. *Distal convoluted tubule* (farthest from Bowman's capsule).
E. *Collecting tubules.*

The blood supply to the nephron is accomplished by:

A. *Afferent arteriole*—enters Bowman's capsule carrying blood from a larger artery
B. *Glomerulus*—a tuft of capillaries.
C. *Efferent arteriole*—exits from Bowman's capsule.
D. *Network of capillaries surrounding proximal and distal tubules.*
E. *Renal vein*—capillaries unite into a larger vein and return blood to general circulation.

Through a complex series of filtration, absorption, and reabsorption, the kidneys assist in the maintenance of the relative constancy of blood composition and volume.

A. *The glomerulus*—filters the blood and removes water and small solutes (blood cells, proteins, and other large molecules are not removed).
B. *The proximal tubule*—reabsorption of water, electrolytes, and other nutrients takes place here.
C. *Loop of Henle*—continued reabsorption including water and sodium.
D. *The distal tubule*—area of fine control of volume of urine and solutes in urine, as well as the area of secretion of acid or base compounds to maintain pH control of blood.
E. *Ureter*—larger tube into which tubule filtrate accumulates and is carried to bladder.
F. *Bladder*—temporary storage place of urine before it is excreted.

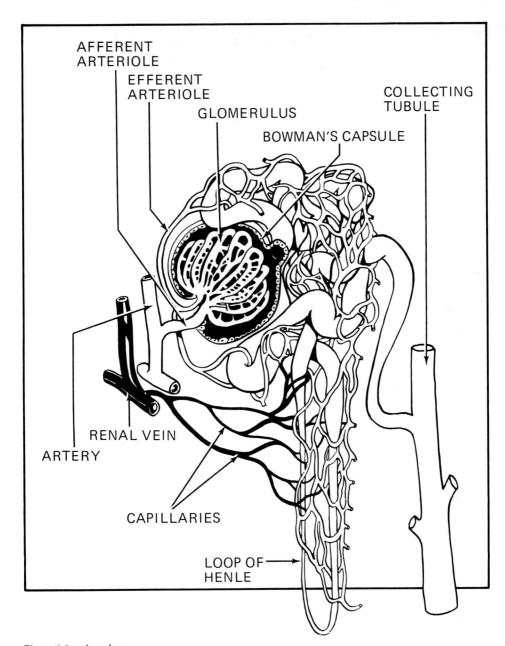

Figure C-1.   A nephron.

Although most of the glomerular filtrate is readily reabsorbed, the waste products are resistant to reabsorption. Reabsorption is accomplished by both diffusion and active transport systems. Concentration of filtrate increases as the filtrate proceeds through the tubules. Urine consists of about 95 percent water and five percent solids.[1] The kidneys filter the total blood supply many times in one day. In this way the kidneys effectively excrete waste products from the body while conserving needed water and nutrients.

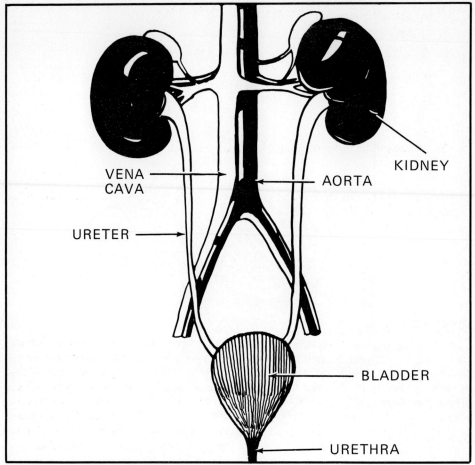

Figure C-2. Organs of urinary excretion.

Questions: Appendix C

1. Match the items on the right to the terms on the left which they best describe:

   _____ 1. distal tubule
   _____ 2. nephron
   _____ 3. proximal tubule
   _____ 4. efferent arteriole
   _____ 5. collecting tubules and ureters
   _____ 6. Bowman's capsule
   _____ 7. afferent arteriole
   _____ 8. glomerulus

   a. arteriole entering Bowman's capsule
   b. arteriole exiting Bowman's capsule
   c. surrounds the glomerulus
   d. tuft of capillaries where filtration of blood takes place
   e. secretion of acid or base compounds occurs here
   f. place of reabsorption of water, electrolytes, and other nutrients
   g. mechanisms by which urine filtrate is gathered and carried to bladder
   h. the functional unit of the kidney

2. Why are waste products not taken back into the blood system of the kidneys?

Answers: Appendix C

1. 1. e
    2. h
    3. f
    4. b
    5. g
    6. c
    7. a
    8. d
2. Waste products are resistant to reabsorption.

REFERENCES

[1] Robinson CH: Fundamentals of Normal Nutrition, 3rd ed. New York, The Macmillan Company, 1978, p. 134

APPENDIX D

DIETARY GOALS

The following are sets of dietary goals suggested by several different sources. Because there is not total agreement on the context of dietary goals for Americans in general, nor on the priorities of such goals, there is likely to be changes forthcoming in future revisions. Therefore, these goals are placed in this appendix section for your information with the advice that these goals represent efforts to interpret nutrition facts as they are known at present, into food practice recommendations for maximum health benefits. They are likely to be changed or modified (and should be) as additional nutrition knowledge is accumulated and analyzed, and its impact on food intake and dietary habits is understood.

DIETARY GOALS FOR THE UNITED STATES*

1. To avoid overweight, consume only as much energy (calories) as is expended; if overweight, decrease energy intake and increase energy expenditure.
2. Increase the consumption of complex carbohydrates and "naturally occurring" sugars from about 28 percent of energy intake to about 48 percent of energy intake.
3. Reduce the consumption of refined and processed sugars by about 45 percent to account for about 10 percent of total energy intake.
4. Reduce overall fat consumption from approximately 40 percent to about 30 percent of energy intake.
5. Reduce saturated fat consumption to account for about 10 percent of total energy intake; balance that with polyunsaturated and monounsaturated fats, which should account for about 10 percent of energy intake each.
6. Reduce cholesterol consumption to about 300 mg a day.
7. Limit the intake of sodium by reducing the intake of salt to about five grams a day.

In order to meet the Dietary Goals the following changes in food selection and preparation are suggested:

1. Increase consumption of fruits, vegetables, and whole grains.
2. Decrease the intake of sugars and foods containing large amounts of sugar (whether refined, corn sugar, syrups, molasses, or honey).
3. Decrease consumption of foods high in fat and substitute some saturated fat with polyunsaturated fat.
4. Increase consumption of poultry and fish while decreasing consumption of meats relatively high in saturated fat.
5. Except for young children, substitute nonfat milk and low-fat milk products for whole milk and whole milk products.
6. Decrease consumption of butterfat, eggs, and other high cholesterol sources. However, the egg is still recognized as a good source of protein for certain population groups.
7. Decrease consumption of salt and foods high in salt content.

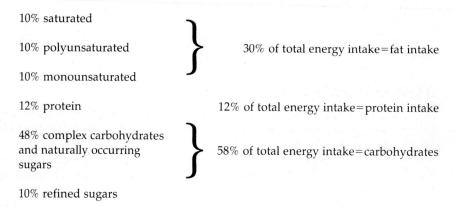

10% saturated

10% polyunsaturated

10% monounsaturated

} 30% of total energy intake=fat intake

12% protein

12% of total energy intake=protein intake

48% complex carbohydrates and naturally occurring sugars

} 58% of total energy intake=carbohydrates

10% refined sugars

Source: Senate Select Committee on Nutrition and Human Needs, Dietary Goals for the United States, 2nd ed. December, 1977.

NUTRITION AND YOUR HEALTH: DIETARY GUIDELINES FOR AMERICANS**

1. **Eat a variety of foods.** Include selections of: fruits; vegetables; whole grain and enriched breads, cereals, and grain products; milk, cheese, and yogurt; meats, poultry, fish and eggs; and legumes (dry peas and beans).
2. **Maintain ideal weight.** To improve eating habits: eat slowly, prepare smaller portions, and avoid "seconds." To lose weight: increase physical activity, eat less fat and fatty foods, eat less sugar and sweets, and avoid too much alcohol.
3. **Avoid too much fat, saturated fat, and cholesterol.** Choose lean meat, fish, poultry, dry beans, and peas as your protein sources. Moderate your use of eggs and organ meats (such as liver). Limit your intake of butter, cream, hydrogenated margarines, shortenings, coconut oil, and foods made from such products. Trim excess fat off meats. Broil, bake, or boil rather than fry. Read labels carefully to determine both amount and types of fat contained in food.
4. **Eat foods with adequate starch and fiber.** To eat more complex carbohydrates daily, substitute starches for fats and sugars and select foods which are good

sources of fiber and starch, such as whole grain breads and cereals, fruits and vegetables, beans, peas, and nuts.

5. **Avoid too much sugar.** Use less of all sugars, including white sugar, brown sugar, raw sugar, honey, and syrups. Eat less of foods containing these sugars such as candy, soft drinks, ice cream, cakes, and cookies. Select fresh fruits or fruits canned without sugar or light syrup rather than heavy syrup. Read food labels for clues on sugar content—if the names sucrose, glucose, maltose, dextrose, lactose, fructose, or syrups appear first, then there is a large amount of sugar. Remember, how often you eat sugar is as important as how much sugar you eat.

6. **Avoid too much sodium.** To avoid too much sodium, learn to enjoy the unsalted flavors of foods. Cook with only small amounts of added salt. Add little or no salt to food at the table. Limit your intake of salty foods such as potato chips, pretzels, salted nuts and popcorn, condiments (soy sauce, steak sauce, garlic salt), cheese, pickled foods, and cured meats. Read food labels carefully to determine the amounts of sodium in processed foods and snack items.

7. **If you drink alcohol, do so in moderation.**

**U.S. Department of Agriculture, U.S. Department of Health, Education, and Welfare, February 1980.

TOWARD HEALTHFUL DIETS***

1. Select a nutritionally adequate diet from the foods available by consuming each day appropriate servings of dairy products, meats or legumes, vegetables and fruits, and cereals and breads.

2. Select as wide a variety of foods in each of the major food groups as is practical in order to ensure a high probability of consuming adequate quantities of all essential nutrients.

3. Adjust dietary energy intake and energy expenditure so as to maintain appropriate weight for your height; if overweight, achieve appropriate weight reduction by decreasing total food and fat intake and by increasing physical activity.

4. If the requirement for energy is low (that is, reducing diet), reduce consumption of foods such as alcohol, sugars, fats, and oils, which provide calories but few other essential nutrients.

5. Use salt in moderation; adequate but safe intakes are considered to range between three and eight grams of sodium chloride daily.

***Source: Food and Nutrition Board, National Academy of Sciences-National Research Council, Washington, D.C., 1980.

APPENDIX E

SUGGESTED RESOURCES FOR ACCURATE NUTRITION INFORMATION

Books (*denotes those particularly helpful for the beginning student)

*Basic Nutrition and Diet Therapy, 4th ed., Robinson CH, 1980, Macmillan Publishing Co., Inc., NY

*Bogert's Nutrition and Physical Fitness, 10th ed. Briggs GM and Calloway, DH, 1979, W. B. Saunders, Philadelphia, PA

*Contemporary Nutrition Controversies. Labuza TP and Sloan AE (eds), 1979, West Publishing Co., St. Paul, MN

*Food and People, 3rd ed. Lowenberg ME, Todhunter EN, Wilson ED, Savage JR, and Lubawski JL, 1979, John Wiley & Sons, NY

 Food, Nutrition and Diet Therapy, 6th ed. Krause MV and Mahan LK, 1979, W. B. Saunders, Philadelphia, PA

*Fundamentals of Normal Nutrition, 3rd ed., Robinson CH, 1978, Macmillan Publishing Co., Inc., NY

*Introductory Nutrition, 4th ed. Guthrie HA, 1979, C. V. Mosby Co., Saint Louis, MO

 Nutrition, 9th ed., Chaney MS, Ross ML and Witschi, JC, 1979. Houghton Mifflin Co., Boston, MA

 Nutrition: An Applied Science. Reed PB, 1980, West Publishing Company, St. Paul, MN

 Nutrition and Diet Therapy, 3rd ed. Williams SR, 1977, C. V. Mosby Company, Saint Louis, MO

*Nutrition and Diet Therapy Reference Dictionary, 2nd ed. Lagua RT, Claudio VS, and Thiele VF, 1974, The C. V. Mosby Company, Saint Louis, MO

*Nutrition and Food Choices. McNutt KW and McNutt DR, 1978, Science Research Associates, Inc., Chicago, IL

*Nutrition: Concepts and Controversies. Hamilton EM and Whitney EN, 1979, West Publishing Co., St. Paul, MN

*Nutrition for the Growing Years, 3rd ed. McWilliams M, 1980, John Wiley & Sons, NY

 Nutrition in Health and Disease, 16th ed. Mitchell HS et al, 1976, J. B. Lippincott Company, Philadelphia, PA

*Nutrition in Perspective. Kreutler PA, 1980, Prentice-Hall, Inc., NJ

 Nutrition: Principles and Application in Health Promotion. Suitor CW and Hunter MF, 1980, J. B. Lippincott, Philadelphia, PA

*Programmed Nutrition, 2nd ed. Guthrie HA, and Braddock KS, 1978, C. V. Mosby Co., Saint Louis, MO

*Realities of Nutrition, Deutsch RM, 1976, Bull Publishing Company, Palo Alto, CA

*Understanding Nutrition, Whitney EN and Hamilton EMN, 1977, West Publishing Company, St. Paul, MN

Journals

(*denotes those particularly readable by the beginning nutrition student)

 American Journal of Clinical Nutrition
 American Journal of Public Health
*Diabetes Forecast
 Food Technology
 Journal of the American Dental Association

*Journal of the American Dietetic Association
*Journal of Home Economics
 Journal of the American Medical Association
 Journal of Nutrition
*Journal of Nutrition Education
*Nutrition Reviews
*Nutrition Today
*Science

Other periodicals
CNI Weekly Report
Contemporary Nutrition
Dairy Council Digest
Family Economics Review
Family Health
FDA Consumer
Food and Nutrition News
Nutrition Action
Nutrition News
Professional Nutritionist
Today's Health

Government Printed Materials:
Conserving the Nutritive Values in Food. USDA Home and Garden Bulletin #90, revised, November 1977

Family Fare: A Guide to Good Nutrition. USDA Home and Garden Bulletin #1 revised, June 1978

Family Food Budgeting . . . for good meals and good nutrition. USDA Home and Garden Bulletin #94 revised, July 1979

Food. USDA Home and Garden Bulletin #228

Food Guide for Older Folks. USDA Home and Garden Bulletin #17, revised August 1974

Food for the Family—A Cost-Saving Plan. USDA Home and Garden Bulletin #209, revised 1978

Food for Youth: Study Guide. USDA/Food and Nutrition Service, October 1975

Fruits in Family Meals: A Guide for Consumers. USDA, Home and Garden Bulletin #125, revised February 1975

Healthy People: The Surgeon General's Report on Health Promotion and Disease Prevention. US Dept. of Health, Education and Welfare, 1979

Keeping Food Safe to Eat: A Guide for Homemakers. USDA Home and Garden Bulletin #162, revised, October 1978

Nutrition: Better Eating for A Head Start. DHEW Publication No. (OHDS) 76-31009

Nutrition Education for Young Children. DHEW Publication No. (OHDS) 76-31015

Nutrition Labeling: Tools for Its Use. USDA Agriculture Information Bulletin #382, April 1975

Storing Perishable Foods in the Home. USDA Home and Garden Bulletin #78, revised April 1976

Storing Vegetables and Fruits. USDA Home and Garden Bulletin #119, revised January 1978

Soybeans in Family Meals. USDA Home and Garden Bulletin #208, June 1974

Vegetables in Family Meals: A Guide for Consumers. USDA Home and Garden Bulletin #105, revised 1975

What's to Eat? And Other Questions Kids Ask About Food. The US Department of Agriculture Yearbook, 1979

INDEX